D1698916

Edited by
Felix Kratz, Peter Senter,
and Henning Steinhagen

Drug Delivery in Oncology

Related Titles

Fialho, A., Chakrabarty, A. (eds.)

Emerging Cancer Therapy

Microbial Approaches and
Biotechnological Tools

2010
ISBN: 978-0-470-44467-2

Jorgenson, L., Nielson, H. M. (eds.)

Delivery Technologies for Biopharmaceuticals

Peptides, Proteins, Nucleic Acids and Vaccines

2009
ISBN: 978-0-470-72338-8

Airley, R.

Cancer Chemotherapy

Basic Science to the Clinic

2009
ISBN: 978-0-470-09254-5

Missailidis, S.

Anticancer Therapeutics

2009
ISBN: 978-0-470-72303-6

Dübel, S. (ed.)

Handbook of Therapeutic Antibodies

2007
ISBN: 978-3-527-31453-9

Knäblein, J. (ed.)

Modern Biopharmaceuticals

Design, Development and Optimization

2005
ISBN: 978-3-527-31184-2

Edited by Felix Kratz, Peter Senter, and Henning Steinhagen

Drug Delivery in Oncology

From Basic Research to Cancer Therapy

Volume 1

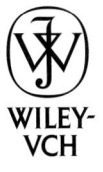

WILEY-VCH

WILEY-VCH Verlag GmbH & Co. KGaA

The Editors

Dr. Felix Kratz
Head of the Division of
Macromolecular Prodrugs
Tumor Biology Center
Breisacherstrasse 117
D-79106 Freiburg
Germany

Dr. Peter Senter
Vice President Chemistry
Seattle Genetics, Inc.
218, Drive S.E. Bothell
Seattle, WA 98021
USA

Dr. Henning Steinhagen
Vice President
Head of Global Drug Discovery
Grünenthal GmbH
Zieglerstr. 6
52078 Aachen
Germany

All books published by **Wiley-VCH** are carefully produced. Nevertheless, authors, editors, and publisher do not warrant the information contained in these books, including this book, to be free of errors. Readers are advised to keep in mind that statements, data, illustrations, procedural details or other items may inadvertently be inaccurate.

Library of Congress Card No.: applied for

British Library Cataloguing-in-Publication Data
A catalogue record for this book is available from the British Library.

Bibliographic information published by the Deutsche Nationalbibliothek
The Deutsche Nationalbibliothek
lists this publication in the Deutsche
Nationalbibliografie; detailed bibliographic
data are available on the Internet at
<http://dnb.d-nb.de>.

© 2012 Wiley-VCH Verlag & Co. KGaA,
Boschstr. 12, 69469 Weinheim,
Germany

All rights reserved (including those of translation into other languages). No part of this book may be reproduced in any form – by photoprinting, microfilm, or any other means – nor transmitted or translated into a machine language without written permission from the publishers. Registered names, trademarks, etc. used in this book, even when not specifically marked as such, are not to be considered unprotected by law.

Composition Laserwords Private Ltd., Chennai
Printing and Binding betz-druck GmbH, Darmstadt
Cover Design Schulz Grafik-Design, Fußgönheim

Printed in the Federal Republic of Germany
Printed on acid-free paper

ISBN: 978-3-527-32823-9
oBook ISBN: 978-3-527-63405-7

Foreword

It is highly likely that the reason our therapies so often fail our patients with cancer is that either (i) those therapies actually never get to their intended targets or (ii) those therapies are "intercepted" by similar targets on normal cells. If we want to understand why many of our therapies fail our patients, and what we can do to possibly remedy those failures, this book *Drug Delivery in Oncology* can help all of us achieve that understanding – and with this book it will be a state-of-the-art understanding.

Drs. Kratz, Senter, and Steinhagen have assembled a respectable breadth of both seasoned and precocious investigators to put together this very special treatise (49 chapters in all). The chapters are well written with basic science, preclinical, and clinical perspectives.

The book begins with a history and the limitations of conventional chemotherapy. Expert discussions of the vascular physiology of tumors that affect drug delivery (and how to defeat those issues) then follow. There are excellent discussions of the neonatal Fc receptor, development of cancer targeted ligands, and antibody-directed enzyme prodrug therapy (ADEPT).

A very special part of this book is the emphasis on tumor imaging. Again, the authors are major experts in this field, which undoubtedly will continue to mature to enable us to document whether or not our therapeutics actually make it to their intended target(s) – and if not, why not.

There are impressive chapters on macromolecular drug delivery systems, including biospecific antibodies, antibody–drug conjugates, and antibody–radionuclide conjugates. Up-to-date discussions of polymer-based drug delivery systems including PEGylation, thermoresponsive polysaccharide-based and even low-density lipoprotein–drug complexes are also presented.

Those with an interest in learning about nano- and microparticulate drug delivery systems can study liposomes to immunoliposomes, to hydrogels, micelles, albumin–drug nanoparticles, and even carbon nanotubes, which are all covered in this book.

Other special delivery systems covered include peptides–drug conjugates, vitamin–drug conjugates, and growth factor–drug conjugates, conjugates of drugs with fatty acids, RNA and RNA interference delivery, and specific targeted organ drug delivery.

As investigators who want to more effectively treat and indeed cure cancer we have many worries. The first of these is that many of our therapeutics just do not make it into the targets in the tumors. This book gives the reader a comprehensive insight into multiple ways to address this problem. A second major worry is that we are losing our pharmacologists who can solve those drug delivery issues. The editors and the authors of this incredible treatise give us comfort that these pharmacologists are alive and well, and thinking as to how they can contribute to getting control of this awful disease.

Daniel D. Von Hoff, MD, FACP
Physician in Chief and Distinguished Professor,
Translational Genomics Research Institute (TGen)
Professor of Medicine, Mayo Clinic
Chief Scientific Officer, Scottsdale Healthcare and US Oncology

Contents to Volume 1

Foreword V
Preface XVII
List of Contributors XIX
Drug Delivery in Oncology – Challenge and Perspectives LIX

Part I   Principles of Tumor Targeting 1

1   **Limits of Conventional Cancer Chemotherapy** 3
          Klaus Mross and Felix Kratz
1.1   Introduction: The Era of Cancer Chemotherapy 3
1.2   Dilemma and Challenge of Treating Malignant Diseases 14
1.3   Adverse Effects 16
1.3.1   Common Side-Effects 18
1.3.1.1   Depression of the Immune System 18
1.3.1.2   Fatigue 19
1.3.1.3   Tendency to Bleed Easily 19
1.3.1.4   Gastrointestinal Distress 19
1.3.1.5   Hair Loss 20
1.3.2   Damage to Specific Organs 20
1.3.2.1   Cardiotoxicity 20
1.3.2.2   Hepatotoxicity 21
1.3.2.3   Nephrotoxicity 22
1.3.2.4   Pulmonary Side-Effects 22
1.3.2.5   Vascular Adverse Effects 23
1.3.2.6   Tissue Damage (Extravasation) 23
1.3.2.7   Neurological Side-Effects 24
1.3.2.8   Secondary Neoplasms 25
1.3.2.9   Infertility 25
1.3.2.10 Other Side-Effects 25
1.4   Supportive Care 25
1.5   New Approaches Complementing Current Cancer Chemotherapy 26
1.6   Conclusions and Perspectives 28
          References 29

2	**Pathophysiological and Vascular Characteristics of Solid Tumors in Relation to Drug Delivery** 33
	Peter Vaupel
2.1	Introduction 33
2.2	Basic Principles of Blood Vessel Formation in Solid Tumors 34
2.2.1	Angiogenesis 34
2.2.2	Vascular Co-option 36
2.2.3	Vasculogenesis 36
2.2.4	Intussusception 36
2.2.5	Vascular Mimicry 36
2.2.6	Microvessel Formation by Myeloid Cells 36
2.3	Tumor Lymphangiogenesis 37
2.4	Tumor Vascularity and Blood Flow 37
2.5	Arteriovenous Shunt Perfusion in Tumors 38
2.6	Volume and Characteristics of the Tumor Interstitial Space 40
2.7	Interstitial Fluid Pressure in Tumors 42
2.8	Role of the Disorganized, Compromised Microcirculation as an Obstacle in Drug Delivery 43
2.8.1	Blood-Borne Delivery 43
2.8.2	Extravasation of Anticancer Agents 45
2.9	Interstitial Barriers to Drug Delivery 46
2.10	Pathophysiological Tumor Microenvironment as an Obstacle in Tumor Therapy 47
2.10.1	Hypoxia as an Obstacle in Drug Therapy 48
2.10.1.1	Direct Effects 48
2.10.1.2	Indirect Effects Based on Changes in the Transcriptome, in Differential Regulation of Gene Expression, and in Alterations of the Proteome 49
2.10.1.3	Indirect Effects Based on Enhanced Mutagenesis, Genomic Instability, and Clonal Selection 51
2.10.1.4	Tumor Hypoxia: An Adverse Parameter in Chemotherapy 51
2.10.2	Tumor Acidosis and Drug Resistance 53
2.11	Conclusions 56
	Acknowledgments 56
	References 56
3	**Enhanced Permeability and Retention Effect in Relation to Tumor Targeting** 65
	Hiroshi Maeda
3.1	Background and Status Quo 65
3.2	What is the EPR Effect: Mechanism, Uniqueness, and Factors Involved 66
3.3	Heterogeneity of the EPR Effect: A Problem in Drug Delivery 72
3.4	Overcoming the Heterogeneity of the EPR Effect for Drug Delivery and How to Enhance the EPR Effect 75
3.4.1	Angiotensin II-Induced High Blood Pressure 75

3.4.2	Use of NO-Releasing Agents	78
3.4.3	Use of Other Vascular Modulators	79
3.5	PEG Dilemma: Stealth Effect and Anti-PEG IgM Antibody	79
3.6	Concluding Remarks	80
	Acknowledgments	81
	References	81

4 Pharmacokinetics of Immunoglobulin G and Serum Albumin: Impact of the Neonatal Fc Receptor on Drug Design 85

Jan Terje Andersen and Inger Sandlie

4.1	Introduction	85
4.2	Discovery of FcRn	87
4.3	FcRn Structure	88
4.4	FcRn–Ligand Interactions	89
4.5	FcRn as a Multiplayer with Therapeutic Utilities	90
4.5.1	Directional Placental Transport	90
4.5.2	FcRn at Mucosal Surfaces	91
4.5.3	Systemic FcRn-Mediated Recycling	92
4.5.4	Role of FcRn in Antigen Presentation	93
4.5.5	FcRn at Immune-Privileged Sites	94
4.5.6	FcRn in the Kidneys	94
4.5.7	FcRn Expressed by the Liver	95
4.6	Engineering IgG for Altered FcRn Binding and Pharmacokinetics	95
4.6.1	IgG Fc Fusions	95
4.6.2	Engineered IgG Variants	96
4.6.3	Blocking FcRn Recycling	102
4.7	Targeting FcRn by SA	102
4.7.1	SA Fusions	102
4.7.2	Targeting SA	105
4.8	Considering Cross-Species Binding	111
4.9	Concluding Remarks	113
	Acknowledgment	113
	References	113

5 Development of Cancer-Targeting Ligands and Ligand–Drug Conjugates 121

Ruiwu Liu, Kai Xiao, Juntao Luo, and Kit S. Lam

5.1	Introduction	121
5.2	Overview of Cancer-Targeting Ligand–Drug Conjugates	122
5.3	Cancer-Targeting Ligands	125
5.3.1	Introduction	125
5.3.2	Phage-Display Library Approach	125
5.3.2.1	Phage-Display Library Screening and Decoding	127
5.3.2.2	Examples	127

5.3.3	OBOC Combinatorial Library Approach	*131*
5.3.3.1	OBOC Library Design	*132*
5.3.3.2	OBOC Library Construction	*135*
5.3.3.3	OBOC Library Screening	*137*
5.3.3.4	OBOC Library Decoding	*138*
5.3.3.5	Ligand Optimization	*139*
5.3.3.6	Examples	*140*
5.4	Linkers	*143*
5.4.1	Acid-Sensitive Linkers	*143*
5.4.2	Enzymatic Cleavage	*143*
5.4.3	Self-Immolative Spacers	*145*
5.4.4	Reductive Cleavage	*146*
5.4.5	On-Demand Cleavable Linker	*146*
5.5	Examples of Cancer-Targeting Ligand–Drug Conjugates	*147*
5.5.1	Folic Acid–Drug Conjugates	*147*
5.5.2	Peptide Ligand–Drug Conjugates	*148*
5.5.3	Peptide Hormone–Drug Conjugates	*150*
5.5.4	Antibody–Drug Conjugates	*151*
5.5.5	ADEPT	*154*
5.5.6	Polymer–Drug Conjugates	*156*
5.5.7	Targeting Liposomes and Nanoparticles	*158*
5.6	Conclusions and Perspectives	*159*
	Acknowledgments	*160*
	References	*160*

6 Antibody-Directed Enzyme Prodrug Therapy (ADEPT) – Basic Principles and its Practice So Far *169*
Kenneth D. Bagshawe

6.1	Introduction	*169*
6.2	Principles and the Components of ADEPT	*170*
6.2.1	Target	*170*
6.2.2	Antibody	*171*
6.2.3	Enzyme	*172*
6.2.4	Prodrug and Drug	*173*
6.3	Third Essential	*173*
6.4	ADEPT Studies Elsewhere	*175*
6.5	Reagents for First Clinical Trials in London (1990–1995)	*176*
6.5.1	First ADEPT Clinical Trial	*177*
6.5.2	Subsequent ADEPT Clinical Studies in London	*178*
6.5.3	Two-Phase ADEPT Clinical Studies in London	*179*
6.6	Technology Advances	*179*
6.7	ADEPT Future	*181*
	References	*181*

Part II Tumor Imaging 187

7 Imaging Techniques in Drug Development and Clinical Practice 189
John C. Chang, Sanjiv S. Gambhir, and Jürgen K. Willmann
7.1 Introduction 189
7.2 Cancer Biology 191
7.2.1 Tumor Genetic Heterogeneity 191
7.2.2 Altered Tumor Metabolism 191
7.2.3 Tumor Angiogenesis 192
7.2.4 Receptor Pathologies 194
7.3 Cancer Biomarkers 194
7.3.1 Histological Biomarkers 194
7.3.2 Hematological Biomarkers 196
7.3.3 Imaging Biomarkers 196
7.4 Imaging Techniques 197
7.4.1 SPECT 197
7.4.2 PET/PET-CT 198
7.4.3 MRI 198
7.4.4 CT 199
7.4.5 Ultrasound 199
7.4.6 Fluorescence/Bioluminescence 200
7.5 Examples of Imaging Assessment of Tumor Response 200
7.5.1 SPECT 200
7.5.2 PET/PET-CT 201
7.5.2.1 Microdosing 201
7.5.2.2 Cancer Metabolism and Proliferation 202
7.5.2.3 Hypoxia 204
7.5.2.4 Biomarker Imaging 205
7.5.2.5 Angiogenesis 207
7.5.2.6 Apoptosis 207
7.5.3 MRI 207
7.5.3.1 Cellular Structure 209
7.5.3.2 Metabolic Response 209
7.5.3.3 Tumor Perfusion 210
7.5.4 CT Imaging 211
7.5.5 Ultrasound 212
7.5.6 Fluorescence/Bioluminescence 213
7.6 Challenges of Imaging in Drug Development and Validation 214
7.7 Conclusions and Future Perspectives 215
References 217

8 Magnetic Nanoparticles in Magnetic Resonance Imaging and Drug Delivery 225
Patrick D. Sutphin, Efrén J. Flores, and Mukesh Harisinghani
8.1 Introduction 225

8.2	Passive Targeting of Nanoparticles	227
8.2.1	Mechanism of Action	229
8.2.2	Lymphotropic Nanoparticle MRI	229
8.3	Active SPIO Nanoparticle Targeting	232
8.3.1	Creating the Targeted Imaging Agents	233
8.3.1.1	Transferrin–USPIO Nanoparticles	233
8.3.1.2	Folate Receptor	235
8.3.1.3	Integrins	235
8.4	Nanoparticles in Targeted Therapy	236
8.4.1	Nanoparticles in Gene Therapy	237
8.4.2	Nanoparticles in Molecularly Targeted Drug Delivery	238
8.4.3	Conversion of Therapeutic Agent to Imaging Agent	239
8.4.4	Toxic Payload	240
8.5	Conclusions	240
	References	242

9 Preclinical and Clinical Tumor Imaging with SPECT/CT and PET/CT 247

Andreas K. Buck, Florian Gärtner, Ambros Beer, Ken Herrmann, Sibylle Ziegler, and Markus Schwaiger

9.1	Introduction	247
9.2	Technical Aspects of Functional and Molecular Imaging with SPECT and PET	249
9.2.1	Principles of Clinical PET and Hybrid PET/CT Imaging	249
9.2.2	Biomarkers for PET and PET/CT Imaging	250
9.2.3	Principles of Clinical SPECT and Hybrid SPECT CT Imaging	252
9.2.4	Biomarkers for SPECT and SPECT/CT Imaging	258
9.2.5	Principles of Preclinical Imaging with SPECT and PET	258
9.3	Preclinical and Clinical Developments	260
9.3.1	Imaging Neoangiogenesis	260
9.3.1.1	VEGF/VEGFR Imaging	261
9.3.1.2	Radiolabeled Integrin Antagonists (RGD Peptides)	262
9.3.1.3	Monomeric Tracer Labeling Strategies	262
9.3.2	Imaging the Proliferative Activity of Tumors	264
9.3.3	Imaging the Hypoxic Cell Fraction of Tumors	267
9.3.4	Imaging Receptor Expression	269
9.4	Clinical Applications of SPECT/CT and PET	272
9.4.1	Differentiation of Benign from Malignant Tumors and Cancer Detection	272
9.4.2	Staging of Cancer: Prognostic Potential of Imaging Biomarkers	273
9.4.3	Assessment of Response to Therapy	274
9.4.4	Restaging of Cancer and Detection of Recurrence	274
9.4.5	PET for Radiation Treatment Planning	275
9.4.6	PET for Cancer Drug Development	275
9.4.7	SPECT/CT for Mapping of SLNs	276

9.4.8	SPECT/CT for Detection of Bone Metastases *277*	
9.4.9	SPECT/CT in Thyroid Cancer *278*	
9.4.10	SPECT/CT for Imaging of Adrenocortical Tumors *279*	
9.4.11	SPECT/CT in Neuroendocrine Tumors *281*	
9.5	Conclusions and Perspectives *281*	
	References *282*	

Contents to Volume 2

Part III   Macromolecular Drug Delivery Systems   *289*

Antibody-Based Systems   *289*

10	**Empowered Antibodies for Cancer Therapy** *291* *Stephen C. Alley, Simone Jeger, Robert P. Lyon, Django Sussman, and Peter D. Senter*	
11	**Mapping Accessible Vascular Targets to Penetrate Organs and Solid Tumors** *325* *Kerri A. Massey and Jan E. Schnitzer*	
12	**Considerations of Linker Technologies** *355* *Laurent Ducry*	
13	**Antibody–Maytansinoid Conjugates: From the Bench to the Clinic** *375* *Hans Erickson*	
14	**Calicheamicin Antibody–Drug Conjugates and Beyond** *395* *Puja Sapra, John DiJoseph, and Hans-Peter Gerber*	
15	**Antibodies for the Delivery of Radionuclides** *411* *Anna M. Wu*	
16	**Bispecific Antibodies and Immune Therapy Targeting** *441* *Sergej M. Kiprijanov*	
	Polymer-Based Systems *483*	
17	**Design of Polymer–Drug Conjugates** *485* *Jindřich Kopeček and Pavla Kopečková*	
18	**Dendritic Polymers in Oncology: Facts, Features, and Applications** *513* *Mohiuddin Abdul Quadir, Marcelo Calderón, and Rainer Haag*	

19	**Site-Specific Prodrug Activation and the Concept of Self-Immolation** 553	

André Warnecke

20	**Ligand-Assisted Vascular Targeting of Polymer Therapeutics** 591	

Anat Eldar-Boock, Dina Polyak, and Ronit Satchi-Fainaro

21	**Drug Conjugates with Poly(Ethylene Glycol)** 627	

Hong Zhao, Lee M. Greenberger, and Ivan D. Horak

22	**Thermo-Responsive Polymers** 667	

Drazen Raucher and Shama Moktan

23	**Polysaccharide-Based Drug Conjugates for Tumor Targeting** 701	

Gurusamy Saravanakumar, Jae Hyung Park, Kwangmeyung Kim, and Ick Chan Kwon

24	**Serum Proteins as Drug Carriers of Anticancer Agents** 747	

Felix Kratz, Andreas Wunder, and Bakheet Elsadek

25	**Future Trends, Challenges, and Opportunities with Polymer-Based Combination Therapy in Cancer** 805	

Coralie Deladriere, Rut Lucas, and María J. Vicent

26	**Clinical Experience with Drug–Polymer Conjugates** 839	

Khalid Abu Ajaj and Felix Kratz

Part IV Nano- and Microparticulate Drug Delivery Systems 885

Lipid-Based Systems 885

27	**Overview on Nanocarriers as Delivery Systems** 887	

Haifa Shen, Elvin Blanco, Biana Godin, Rita E. Serda, Agathe K. Streiff, and Mauro Ferrari

28	**Development of PEGylated Liposomes** 907	

I. Craig Henderson

29	**Immunoliposomes** 951	

Vladimir P. Torchilin

30	**Responsive Liposomes (for Solid Tumor Therapy)** 989	

Stavroula Sofou

31	**Nanoscale Delivery Systems for Combination Chemotherapy** *1013* Barry D. Liboiron, Paul G. Tardi, Troy O. Harasym, and Lawrence, D. Mayer	

Polymer-Based Systems *1051*

32	**Micellar Structures as Drug Delivery Systems** *1053* Nobuhiro Nishiyama, Horacio Cabral, and Kazunori Kataoka
33	**Tailor-Made Hydrogels for Tumor Delivery** *1071* Sungwon Kim and Kinam Park
34	**pH-Triggered Micelles for Tumor Delivery** *1099* Haiqing Yin and You Han Bae
35	**Albumin–Drug Nanoparticles** *1133* Neil Desai
36	**Carbon Nanotubes** *1163* David A. Scheinberg, Carlos H. Villa, Freddy Escorcia, and Michael R. McDevitt

Contents to Volume 3

Part V Ligand-Based Drug Delivery Systems *1187*

37	**Cell-Penetrating Peptides in Cancer Targeting** *1189* Kaido Kurrikoff, Julia Suhorutšenko, and Ülo Langel
38	**Targeting to Peptide Receptors** *1219* Andrew V. Schally and Gabor Halmos
39	**Aptamer Conjugates: Emerging Delivery Platforms for Targeted Cancer Therapy** *1263* Zeyu Xiao, Jillian Frieder, Benjamin A. Teply, and Omid C. Farokhzad
40	**Design and Synthesis of Drug Conjugates of Vitamins and Growth Factors** *1283* Iontcho R. Vlahov, Paul J. Kleindl, and Fei You
41	**Drug Conjugates with Polyunsaturated Fatty Acids** *1323* Joshua Seitz and Iwao Ojima

Part VI Special Topics 1359

42 **RNA Drug Delivery Approaches** 1361
Yuan Zhang and Leaf Huang

43 **Local Gene Delivery for Therapy of Solid Tumors** 1391
Wolfgang Walther, Peter M. Schlag, and Ulrike Stein

44 **Viral Vectors for RNA Interference Applications in Cancer Research and Therapy** 1415
Henry Fechner and Jens Kurreck

45 **Design of Targeted Protein Toxins** 1443
Hendrik Fuchs and Christopher Bachran

46 **Drug Targeting to the Central Nervous System** 1489
Gert Fricker, Anne Mahringer, Melanie Ott, and Valeska Reichel

47 **Liver Tumor Targeting** 1519
Katrin Hochdörffer, Giuseppina Di Stefano, Hiroshi Maeda, and Felix Kratz

48 **Photodynamic Therapy: Photosensitizer Targeting and Delivery** 1569
Pawel Mroz, Sulbha K. Sharma, Timur Zhiyentayev, Ying-Ying Huang, and Michael R. Hamblin

49 **Tumor-Targeting Strategies with Anticancer Platinum Complexes** 1605
Markus Galanski and Bernhard K. Keppler

Index 1631

Preface

Modern oncology research is highly multidisciplinary, involving scientists from a wide array of specialties focused on both basic and applied areas of research. While significant therapeutic advancements have been made, there remains a great need for further progress in treating almost all of the most prevalent forms of cancer. Unlike many other diseases, cancer is commonly characterized by barriers to penetration, heterogeneity, genetic instability, and drug resistance. Coupled with the fact that successful treatment requires elimination of malignant cells that are very closely related to normal cells within the body, cancer therapy remains one of the greatest challenges in modern medicine.

Early on, chemotherapeutic drugs were renowned for their systemic toxicities, since they poorly distinguished tumor cells from normal cells. It became apparent to scientists within the field that further advancements in cancer medicine would require new-generation drugs that ideally targeted critical pathways, unique markers, and distinguishing physiological traits that were selectively found within the malignant cells and solid tumor masses. Several new areas of research evolved from this realization, including macromolecular-based therapies that exploit impaired lymphatic drainage often associated with solid tumors, antiangiogenesis research to cut the blood supply off from growing tumors, antibody-based strategies that allow for selective targeting to tumor-associated antigens, and new drug classes that attack uniquely critical pathways that promote and sustain tumor growth. A large proportion of both recently approved and clinically advanced anticancer drugs fall within these categories.

Beyond the generation of such drug classes, it has also been recognized that approved cancer drugs could be made more effective and less toxic through delivery and transport technologies that maximize tumor exposure while sparing normal tissues from chemotherapeutic damage. By doing so, existing or highly potent cytotoxic drugs may display improved therapeutic indices. This has attracted considerable attention and has spawned the area of macromolecular-based delivery strategies.

There are few places where those actively engaged in drug delivery or who may wish to enter the field can find the major advancements consolidated in one place. This prompted us to organize the series of books entitled *Drug Delivery in Oncology* comprised of 49 chapters written by 121 internationally recognized leaders in the field. The work within the book series overviews many of the major breakthroughs in cancer medicine made in the last 10–15 years and features many of the chemotherapeutics of the future. Included among them are recombinant antibodies, antibody fragments, and antibody fusion proteins as well as tumor-seeking ligands for selective drug delivery and tumor imaging, and passive targeting strategies using macromolecules and nano- and microparticulate systems.

One of the special distinguishing features of this series is that the chapters are written for novices and experts alike. Each chapter is written in a style that allows interested readers to not only to find out about the most recent advancements within the field being discussed, but to actually see the data in numerous illustrations, photos, graphs, and tables that accompany each chapter.

None of this would have been possible without the devoted efforts of the contributing authors, all of whom shared the common goal of creating a new series of books that would provide an important cornerstone in the modern chemotherapeutic treatment of cancer. We are all very thankful for their efforts.

We also wish to thank the publishing team at Wiley-VCH in Weinheim, Germany. In particular, we want to give our wholehearted thanks and kind acknowledgments to Frank Weinreich, Gudrun Walter, Bernadette Gmeiner, Claudia Nußbeck, Hans-Jochen Schmitt, and Ina Wiedemann, who were always helpful and supportive during the 2 years it took to put all this together. It is our hope that this series will provide readers with inspired ideas and new directions for research in drug delivery in oncology.

July 2011

Felix Kratz
Peter Senter
Henning Steinhagen

List of Contributors

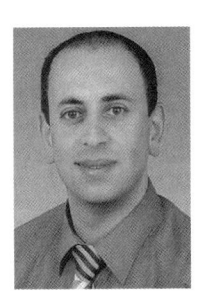

Khalid Abu Ajaj received his BSc from Yarmouk University (Jordan, 1991), his MSc from the University of Jordan (Jordan, 1995), and his PhD in Chemistry from the University of Leipzig (Germany, 2002). He then carried out a Postdoctoral Fellowship in the research groups of Professor Dr. A. Zychlinsky (Max Planck Institute for Infection Biology, Berlin) and Professor Dr. M. Bienert (Institute of Molecular Pharmacology, Berlin), developing bacterial lipopeptides to investigate the mechanisms of activation of Toll-like receptors. He joined the Macromolecular Prodrug Research Group of Dr. Felix Kratz at the Tumor Biology Center in Freiburg in 2006. His research in the group is focused on developing dual-acting prodrugs for circumventing multidrug resistance.

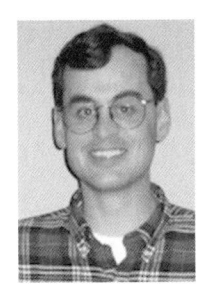

Stephen C. Alley received his PhD in Organic Chemistry from the University of Washington and completed a Postdoctoral Fellowship in Chemistry at Pennsylvania State University. He joined the Research Biology Department at Pathogenesis Corp. and then came to Seattle Genetics in 2003. His research has surrounded conjugation technologies and determination of the mechanisms by which antibody–drug conjugates work.

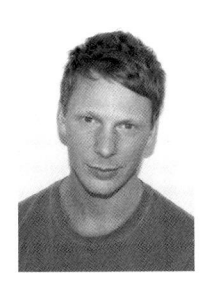

Jan Terje Andersen graduated in Molecular Immunology at the Department of Molecular Biosciences, University of Oslo, Norway in 2008. He has a postdoctoral position at the Department of Molecular Biosciences, University of Oslo, and the Center for Immune Regulation at the Institute for Immunology, Norway. His research areas are molecular biology and immunology, with a current focus on receptor interactions and receptor targeting. Specifically, the interactions of antibodies of the IgG class with the Fcγ receptors as well as the interactions of IgG and albumin with the neonatal Fc receptor. He has authored approximately 15 scientific publications, including book chapters and patent applications.

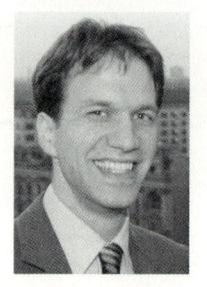

Christopher Bachran studied Biochemistry at the Freie Universität Berlin, Germany. He joined the laboratory of Hendrik Fuchs at the Charité–Universitätsmedizin Berlin as a PhD student to study targeted protein toxins for targeted tumor therapy in 2002 and obtained his PhD from the Freie Universität Berlin in 2006. He stayed in Hendrik Fuchs' group as postdoc to investigate the efficacy of saporin-based targeted toxins in mouse models and to analyze the impact of saponins for drastically improved drug delivery in tumor mouse models. During this time he co-organized with Hendrik Fuchs the 2nd and 4th Fabisch-Symposium for Cancer Research and Molecular Cell Biology on the topic of targeted tumor therapies in 2006 and 2009. In 2009, he joined the laboratory of Stephen Leppla at the National Institute of Allergy and Infectious Diseases, National Institutes of Health, in order to develop sophisticated anthrax toxin-based targeted tumor therapy approaches.

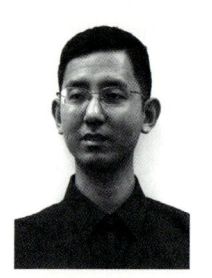

You Han Bae received his PhD degree in Pharmaceutics from the University of Utah in 1988, and has held a Full Professorship at the Department of Pharmaceutics and Pharmaceutical Chemistry of University of Utah since 2002. His research interests include self-assembled superintelligent nanoparticulates for multidrug-resistant tumors, acidic solid tumor targeting, protein drug stabilization and controlled release, polymeric vector design for genetic materials, and polymeric systems for rechargeable cell delivery. He has authored over 210 peer-reviewed scientific publications, book chapters, and US patents.

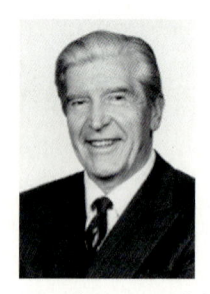

Kenneth D. Bagshawe is Emeritus Professor of Medical Oncology at Imperial College London. After service in the Royal Navy, he studied medicine at St. Mary's Hospital Medical School in London. He was a Research Fellow at Johns Hopkins Hospital Baltimore. He reported first use of combination chemotherapy resulting in cure of metastatic cancer. He established the first radioimmunoassay for human chorionic gonadotropin. He set up a national-scale registration scheme for patients with hydatidiform mole in 1973. He was Chairman of the Scientific Committee of the Cancer Research Campaign. He proposed ADEPT in 1987 and 1990, carried out the first clinical trial of ADEPT. He is a Fellow of the Royal Society.

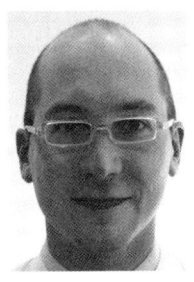

Ambros Beer studied Medicine at the Ludwig-Maximilians-Universiät in Munich, Germany. After his final exam in 1999, he performed his training in Radiology at the Department of Radiology at the Klinikum rechts der Isar of the Technical University in Munich (Professor Dr. E.J. Rummeny). Afterwards he performed his training in Nuclear Medicine at the Department of Nuclear Medicine at the Klinikum rechts der Isar of the Technical University in Munich (Professor Dr. M. Schwaiger). Currently he is working as Attending and Assistant professor at the Department of Nuclear Medicine at the Klinikum rechts der Isar of the Technical University in Munich. His main research interest is translational molecular imaging, with a focus on assessment of angiogenesis using targeted tracers, like $\alpha_v\beta_3$-specific tracers. Moreover, he is interested in multimodality molecular imaging, combining, for example, magnetic resonance imaging and positron emission tomography.

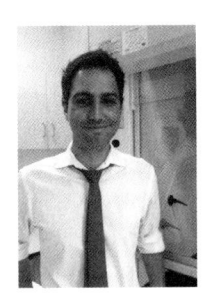

Elvin Blanco received his BS in Biomedical Engineering from Case Western Reserve University in Cleveland, OH. He received his PhD in Biomedical Engineering under the mentorship of Dr. Jinming Gao at the University of Texas Southwestern Medical Center at Dallas in 2008. In 2009, he began his postdoctoral training under the mentorship of Dr. Mauro Ferrari at the University of Texas Health Science Center at Houston. He is currently a Research Associate at the Methodist Hospital Research Institute in Houston under the mentorship of Dr. Mauro Ferrari.

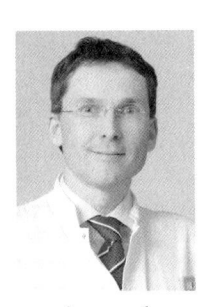

Andreas K. Buck graduated in Medicine at the University of Ulm, Germany in 1996. From 1997 to 2003 he worked as a Resident and from 2003 to 2006 as a Senior Physician at the Department of Nuclear Medicine at the University of Ulm. From 2006 to 2010 he worked as Associate Professor at the Department of Nuclear Medicine at the Technical University in Munich, Germany. Since 2011 he has been Director of the Department of Nuclear Medicine at the University of Wuerzburg, Germany. His research is focused on hemato-oncology and cancer treatment with radiopharmaceuticals.

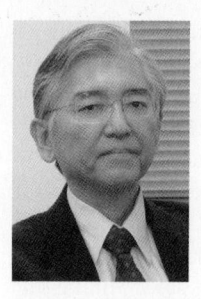

Horacio Cabral received his PhD under the supervision of Professor K. Kataoka in Materials Engineering from the University of Tokyo in 2007. He worked as an Assistant Professor at the Division of Clinical Biotechnology, Graduate School of Medicine, University of Tokyo until 2009. From 2010, he has been a Lecturer at the Bioengineering Department, University of Tokyo. His main research interests relate to smart nanodevices for the diagnosis and therapy of cancer.

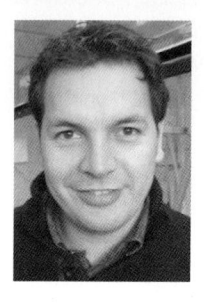

Marcelo Calderón received his PhD in Organic Chemistry in 2007 from the National University of Córdoba, Argentina, under the supervision of Professor Miriam Strumia. In the following years, he joined the Research Group of Professor Rainer Haag at the Free University of Berlin as a Postdoctoral Fellow. He is currently working as an Associate Researcher at the same University, with a research interest in the development of nanotransporters based on dendritic polyglycerol for intelligent delivery of drugs, gene, and imaging probes.

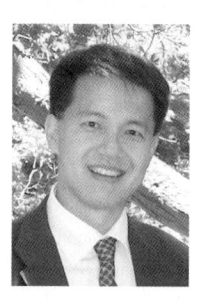

John C. Chang MD, PhD graduated from the University of Illinois at Urbana-Champaign with an MD and an Electrical Engineering PhD degree in 2004. During his graduate training, he has authored and coauthored five refereed articles focused on neural engineering. During his radiology residency at Stanford University, he pursued research in nanoparticle application in optical and magnetic resonance imaging with ultimate application in understanding cancer biology and novel therapy. He currently serves as a Clinical Instructor in Radiology at Stanford University.

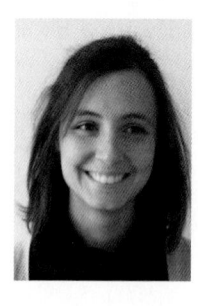

Coralie Deladriere studied Chemistry at the University Paris Sud (France) and obtained her Master's degree in Analytical Chemistry in 2006. She then joined the Polymer Therapeutics Laboratory headed by Dr. Vicent at the Centro de Investigación Príncipe Felipe, Valencia (Spain) as a PhD Student. Her PhD work is focused on the development of polymer–drug conjugates as a platform for combination therapy in the treatment of hormone-dependent breast cancer.

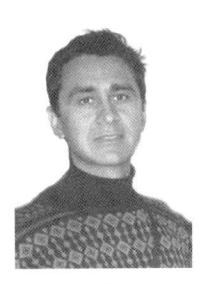

Neil Desai is currently Senior Vice President of Global Research and Development at Abraxis BioScience in Los Angeles, CA, where he is responsible for the development of the company's growing product pipeline and the development of the company's intellectual property portfolio. He is an inventor of ABI's nanotechnology and nanoparticle-albumin bound (*nab*™) drug delivery platform, and was primarily responsible for the development of its nanotechnology drug *nab*-paclitaxel and the discovery of the novel targeted biological pathway utilized by *nab*-drugs. Prior to joining ABI, he was Senior Director of Biopolymer Research at VivoRx Inc., where he developed novel encapsulation systems for living cells and was part of the team that performed the world's first successful encapsulated islet cell transplant in a diabetic patient. With more than 20 years of experience in the research and development of novel drug delivery systems and biocompatible polymers, he holds over 100 issued patents and peer-reviewed publications, has made over 150 presentations at scientific meetings, and has organized and chaired symposia in the areas of biocompatible polymers and nanotechnology-based delivery systems. He is a reviewer for several scientific journals, and an active participant in the US Food and Drug Administration (FDA) Nanotechnology Task Force and FDA-Alliance for Nanohealth initiatives. He holds a MS and PhD in Chemical Engineering from the University of Texas at Austin, USA, and a BS in Chemical Engineering from the University Institute of Chemical Technology in Mumbai, India.

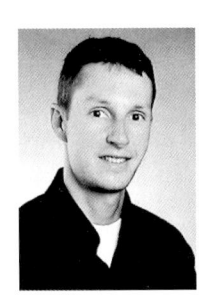

Laurent Ducry studied Chemistry at the University of Lausanne (Switzerland) and did his Diploma thesis with Professor T. Gallagher at the University of Bristol (UK). He obtained his PhD from the ETH Zürich (Switzerland) with Professor F. Diederich in 1998. During his graduate studies, he worked for 6 months with Dr. G. Olson at Hoffmann-La Roche in Nutley (New Jersey). He then held a Swiss National Science Foundation Postdoctoral Fellowship at the University of Pennsylvania in Philadelphia with Professor A.B. Smith III and Professor R. Hirschmann. He began his industrial carrier in process R&D at Lonza in Visp (Switzerland) in 2000 and became Project Leader the following year. His activities focused on the development and scale-up of chemical processes, as well as the production of pharmaceutical intermediates and active pharmaceutical ingredients under current Good Manufacturing Practices. In the second half of 2006 he trained the Lonza R&D team in Nansha (China) and was promoted to Senior Research Associate in 2007. Since 2008, he has been leading the antibody–drug conjugates R&D group of Lonza.

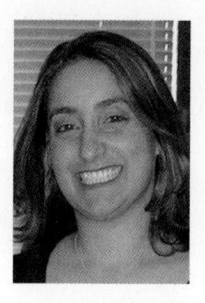

Anat Eldar-Boock is currently undertaking her PhD studies at Tel Aviv University under the supervision of Dr Ronit Satchi-Fainaro. Her thesis goal is to synthesize and characterize antiangiogenic and anticancer polymer therapeutics bearing paclitaxel and RGD peptidomimetics for the treatment of breast cancer. She graduated her MS studies from Tel Aviv University at the Department of Developmental Biology investigating the involvement of sphingolipid metabolism in aging and apoptosis of rat oocytes.

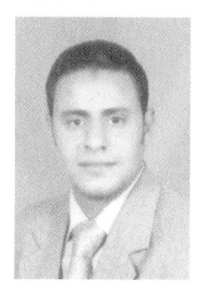

Bakheet Elsadek graduated in Pharmaceutical Sciences from Al-Azhar University, Egypt in 2001. He was then awarded the Master's degree in Biochemistry from the Faculty of Pharmacy, Assiut University, Egypt. In 2010 he received his PhD from the Faculty of Pharmacy, Assiut University, supervised by Dr. Felix Kratz, Head of the Division of Macromolecular Prodrugs, Clinical Research, Tumor Biology Center, Freiburg, Germany and Professor Dr. Tahia Saleem, Professor of Biochemistry and Molecular Biology, Faculty of Medicine, Assiut University. His PhD thesis was funded through the Egyptian Scientific Channel System and focused on the development of prodrugs for treating prostate cancer. His current research areas are angiogenesis, drug targeting, and drug delivery systems in oncology and prodrugs.

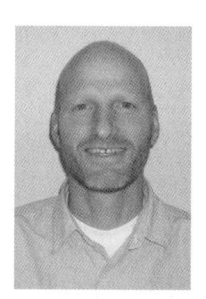

Hans Erickson received his PhD in Biochemistry from the University of California, San Diego. After a Postdoctoral Fellowship at the University of Utah, he joined ImmunoGen, Inc., where his efforts have focused on understanding the mechanisms associated with the efficacy and toxicity of antibody–drug conjugates.

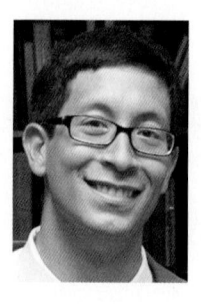

Freddie Escorcia is a MD PhD candidate at the Weill Cornell/Rockefeller/Sloan-Kettering Tri-Institutional Program. He has a BS in Chemistry and Bioengineering from the University of Illinois. His research interests are in understanding the mechanisms of action and therapeutic applications for targeting of tumor vasculature and tumor angiogenesis.

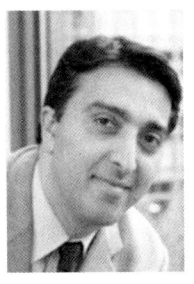

Omid C. Farokhzad received his MD and MA from Boston University School of Medicine. He completed his postdoctoral clinical and research training at Brigham and Women's Hospital/Harvard Medical School (HMS) and MIT in the laboratory of Professor Robert Langer. He is an Associate Professor at HMS, and directs the Laboratory of Nanomedicine and Biomaterials at Brigham and Women's Hospital. He pioneered the development of aptamer–nanoparticle conjugates for cancer therapy. His laboratory is currently focused on the high-throughput screening of targeting ligands and the development of multifunctional targeted nanoparticle platforms for medical applications.

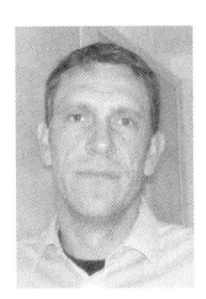

Henry Fechner studied Veterinary Medicine at the Humboldt University of Berlin and received his DVM in 1995 at the Free University of Berlin in the Institute of Virology. He then worked as an assistant in the Institute of Veterinary Pathology in the Free University of Berlin and as a postdoc in the "Lipidlabor" of the Charité Berlin from 1996 to 1998. From 1998 to 2010 he was postdoc and group leader in the Department of Cardiology and Pneumology of the Charité Berlin. In 2010 he received a senior group leader position at the University of Berlin in the Institute of Biotechnology. His research interests focus on the development of gene therapeutic strategies for the treatment of cardiovascular and tumor diseases.

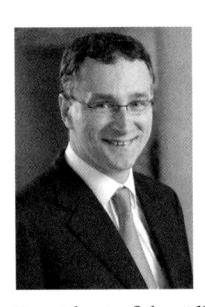

Mauro Ferrari obtained his Dottore in Mathematics from Università di Padova in Italy and received his PhD in Mechanical Engineering from the University of California at Berkeley. From 2003 to 2005, he served as an Expert on Nanotechnology at the National Cancer Institute (NCI), providing leadership into the formulation, refinement, and approval of the NCI's Alliance for Nanotechnology in Cancer. Currently, he is the President, CEO, and Director of the Methodist Research Institute, Ernest Cockrell Jr. Endowed Chair, and President of the Alliance for NanoHealth in Houston, TX.

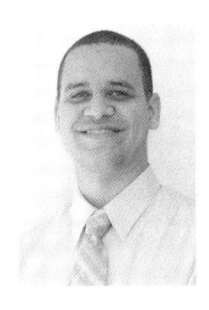

Efrén J. Flores MD received his medical degree at the University of Puerto Rico School of Medicine in 2005 and completed his Residency in Diagnostic Radiology at Massachusetts General Hospital in 2010. His relationship with Dr. Mukesh Harisinghani as a mentor has allowed him to developed a new interest in the future impact of magnetic nanoparticles in cancer treatment.

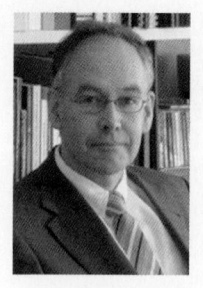

Gert Fricker graduated in Chemistry from the University of Freiburg, Germany in 1986. He then did postdoctoral research at the Department of Clinical Pharmacology, University Hospital Zurich, Switzerland. From 1888 to 1995, he worked as a Research Scientist at Sandoz, Basle, Switzerland. In 1995, he was appointed Professor of Pharmaceutical Technology and Biopharmacy at the University of Heidelberg, Germany. Since 2002 he has been Director of the Institute of Pharmacy and Molecular Biotechnology at the University of Heidelberg and the Steinbeis Technology Transfer Center Biopharmacy and Analytics. His research interests include drug delivery, membrane transport proteins, and the blood–brain barrier.

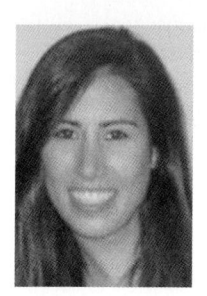

Jillian H. Frieder earned her Bachelor in Physiology from the University of Arizona in 2010. In July 2010 she joined Professor Omid Farokhzad's group at Brigham and Women's Hospital. Her current work involves aptamer–nanoparticle targeting for *in vivo* applications.

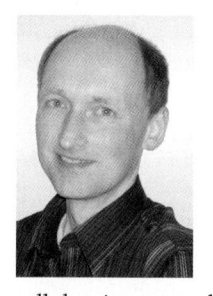

Hendrik Fuchs studied Biochemistry at the Freie Universität Berlin, Germany, and finished his PhD work on the human transferrin receptor in 1996 in the laboratory of Reinhard Geßner. After a short postdoc at the Rudolf Virchow University Hospital in Berlin, he became a group leader in 1997 at the Department for Clinical Chemistry and Pathobiochemistry, headed by Rudolf Tauber, at the Benjamin Franklin University Hospital in the same city. Since that time his research focus is on the investigation of systemic and cellular iron metabolism and on the development of protein-based targeted antitumor drugs. After his habilitation in 2002 he continued his research as a German Privatdozent and was appointed as Professor at the Department of Laboratory Medicine, Clinical Chemistry and Pathobiochemistry at the Charitè–Universitätsmedizin Berlin in 2010. He organized together with Christopher Bachran the 2nd and 4th Fabisch-Symposium for Cancer Research and Molecular Cell Biology on the topic of targeted tumor therapies in 2006 and 2009.

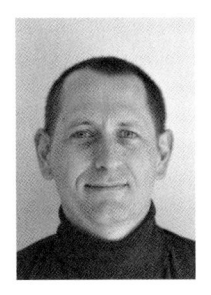

Markus Galanski graduated in 1994 and obtained his PhD degree in 1996, both from the University of Heidelberg. In 1996, he moved to the University of Vienna together with Bernhard Keppler and was promoted to the rank of Associate Professor in 2007. He is Deputy Head of the Institute of Inorganic Chemistry and working on the development of anticancer platinum complexes.

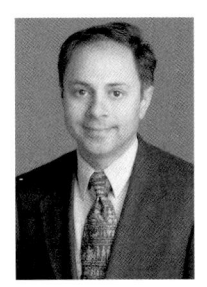

Sanjiv Sam Gambhir MD, PhD is Professor of Radiology, Bioengineering, and Materials Science and Engineering at Stanford University. He is Director of the Molecular Imaging Program at Stanford and Head of Nuclear Medicine. He has published over 375 articles in the field of molecular Imaging, edited three books, has over 30 patents granted or filed, and is a member of the Institute of Medicine of the US National Academies.

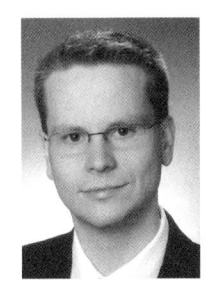

Florian Gärtner studied Medicine at the Technical University in Munich, Germany and received his Approbation in 2005. During his Doctorate thesis he worked on tumor targeting with radiolabeled compounds. Currently, he is working as a Resident in the Department of Nuclear Medicine at the Technical University in Munich. His current research subjects are neuroendocrine tumors, peptide receptor radionuclide therapy, and tumor hypoxia.

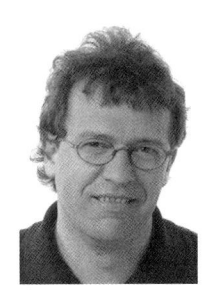

Hans-Peter Gerber received an MS in Biochemistry and a PhD in Molecular Biology from the University of Zurich, Switzerland. He joined Genentech in 1995 as a Visiting Scientist, where he spent 11 years in research studying the mechanisms involved in regulating blood vessel formation and developing therapeutic antibodies interfering with tumor angiogenesis. He was a member of several teams reviewing preclinical and clinical data from trials conducted with Avastin® (bevacizumab), a therapeutic antibody blocking the angiogenic factor VEGF-A. In March 2006, he joined Seattle Genetics as Head of the Translational Biology Department, where he contributed to the development of therapeutic antibodies and antibody–drug conjugates (ADCs) including

SGN-35, SGN-40, SGN-75, and SGN-19A targeting hematopoietic malignancies and solid tumors. In April 2009, he joined Wyeth Discovery Research Oncology in Pearl River, NY. After the acquisition by Pfizer in late 2009, he now leads the Vascular Biology/BioConjugate Development group at the Center of Integrative Biology and Biotherapeutics, where he is building a program to develop novel ADCs to target tumor and stromal cells.

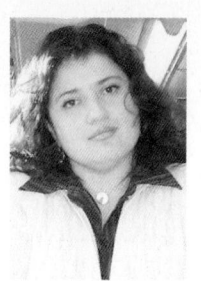

Biana Godin studied Pharmaceutical Sciences at the Hebrew University of Jerusalem (Israel) under the supervision of Professor Touitou. She conducted her research toward the PhD degree designing novel lipid nanovesicular carriers for treatment of challenging infectious diseases. After her graduation, she joined the group of Professor Ferrari at the University of Texas Health Science Center at Houston, focusing on the delivery of drugs and imaging agents from injectable porous silicon multistage nanovectors. She is currently an Assistant Member at the Methodist Hospital Research Institute in Houston, TX.

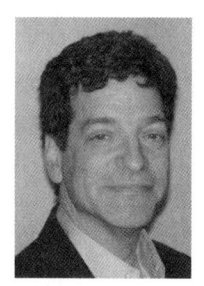

Lee M. Greenberger received his PhD from Emory University (Atlanta, GA) in 1984. He did Postdoctoral training at Albert Einstein College of Medicine (with Dr. Susan Horwitz) where he studied ABC transporters associated with resistance to cancer therapy. Since 1991 he has worked at various pharmaceutical companies identifying novel cancer therapeutics, including antimicrotubule agents, antiestrogens, erbB inhibitors, and transport inhibitors. As Vice President of Research at Enzon Pharmaceuticals since 2006, he oversees the preclinical development of RNA antagonists and novel drug conjugates to treat cancer.

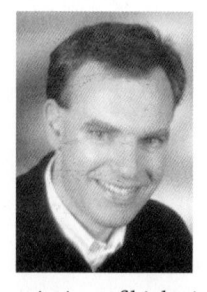

Rainer Haag obtained his PhD with A. de Meijere at the University of Göttingen in 1995. After postdoctoral work with S.V. Ley, University of Cambridge (UK), and G.M. Whitesides, Harvard University, Cambridge (USA), he completed his habilitation at the University of Freiburg in 2002. He then became Associate Professor at the University of Dortmund, and in 2004 was appointed Full Professor of organic and macromolecular chemistry at the Freie Universität at Berlin. His main research interests are in the mimicry of biological systems by functional dendritic polymers. Polyglycerol-based materials feature heavily in the diverse range of projects within the Haag group, with particular focus on applications in nanomedicine, such as drug, dye, and gene delivery, as well as regenerative medicine, such as nonfouling surfaces and matrix materials.

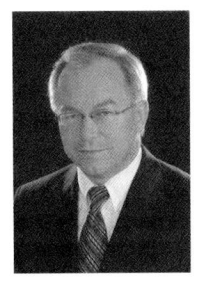

Gabor Halmos PharmD, PhD graduated in Pharmacy in 1986, and then received his pharmaceutical, biomedical, and biochemical training as well as his PharmD and PhD degrees from the University of Szeged and University of Debrecen (Hungary). In 1991 he was invited by Dr. Andrew V. Schally to work at the Endocrine, Polypeptide and Cancer Institute at the Veterans Affairs Medical Center and Tulane University, Department of Medicine, New Orleans, LA. He was the Head of the Receptor Section of the Institute (1991–2005), and his research work was focused on peptide hormone receptors and the development of new drugs targeting various human cancers. In 2005, he became Professor and Chair, Department of Biopharmacy at the University of Debrecen, Medical and Health Science Center (Hungary), retaining his research ties with Dr. Schally. In 2006, he also became a Visiting Professor at the University of Miami, Miller School of Medicine, Miami, FL, where he conducts cancer research for 2–4 months a year. His research areas are the expression and pathophysiological function of peptide hormone receptors and development of peptide hormone analogs for targeted cancer therapy. He has nearly 200 publications.

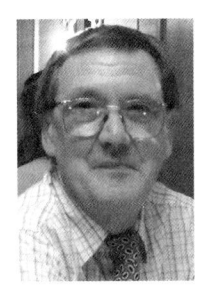

Michael R. Hamblin is a Principal Investigator at the Wellman Center for Photomedicine at Massachusetts General Hospital and an Associate Professor of Dermatology at Harvard Medical School. He was trained as a synthetic organic chemist and received his PhD from Trent University in the UK. His research interests lie in the areas of photodynamic therapy (PDT) for infections, cancer, and heart disease. In particular, he has worked on covalent photosensitizer conjugates, induction of antitumor immunity by PDT, PDT for vulnerable atherosclerotic plaque, and antimicrobial photoinactivation *in vitro* and *in vivo*. He is also interested in basic mechanistic studies in low-level laser (light) therapy, and its application to wound healing, traumatic brain injury, and hair regrowth. He has published over 120 peer-reviewed articles, over 150 conference proceedings, book chapters, and international abstracts, and holds eight patents.

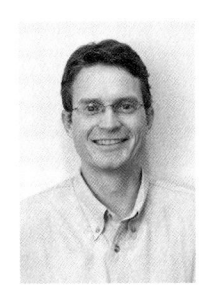

Troy O. Harasym is Director (Biological Evaluation) at Celator Pharmaceuticals. He received his BS and PhD degrees from the Department of Biochemistry at the University of British Columbia. He has 15 years experience in the biotechnology industry, and has held previous positions at The Canadian Liposome Company assessing liposomal drug carriers and Inex Pharmaceuticals developing liposomal antisense therapeutics. He joined Celator Pharmaceuticals in December 2000 as Director of Pharmacodynamics where he focused on developing external research collaborations and preclinical guidance in xenograft evaluations. He has since held key Director positions at Celator, including the Director of Drug Screening, where he developed Celator's automated process for the identification of synergistic drug ratios and, currently, as the Director of Biological Evaluation where he leads the team in pharmacokinetics/pharmacodynamics and efficacy evaluations.

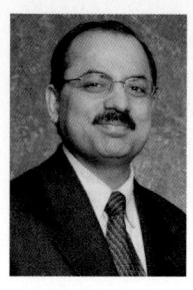

Mukesh Harisinghani MD completed his Diagnostic Radiology Residency at the Massachusetts General Hospital and Harvard Medical School in 2000. He then pursued an Abdominal Imaging and Intervention Fellowship at the Massachusetts General Hospital till 2001 and has been on Faculty in the same Division since then. He is an Associate Professor of Radiology at the Harvard Medical School and Director of Abdominal Magnetic Resonance Imaging at the Massachusetts General Hospital. He also leads the Translational Imaging Group, Clinical Discovery Program, at the Center for Molecular Imaging and Research. Since his radiology residency, he has been involved with clinical bench to bedside applications of magnetic nanoparticles, carrying out clinical trials using nanoparticle-enhanced magnetic resonance imaging for staging genitourinary malignancies.

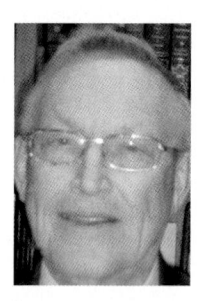

I. Craig Henderson is currently an Adjunct Professor of Medicine at UCSF and serves as a consultant to various biotechnology companies. In 1992, he founded the Bay Area Breast Cancer Translational Research Program and served as the principle investigator on the SPORE grant that funded that program. One of the key projects in that program was the creation of immunoliposomes using PEGylated liposomes and monoclonal antibodies directed toward HER2/*neu*. (This project within the SPORE was initially led by Dr. Demtri Papahadjopoulos and later by Dr. John Park). In 1993, he joined the Board of SEQUUS Pharmaceuticals, and in 1995, he became CEO and Chairman of the company. At SEQUUS he played a leadership role in shepherding Doxil®/Caelyx® through the regulatory process and in developing strategies that eventually demonstrated its value in ovarian and breast cancers and multiple myeloma. As CEO of SEQUUS he had oversight on both preclinical and clinical studies of SPI-77, a PEGylated liposomal platinum. He initiated the program to encapsulate topoisomerase I inhibitors. From 1975 to 1992, he was on the staff of the Dana-Farber Cancer Institute, where he founded the Breast Evaluation Center, and was a member of the Harvard Medical School Faculty. From 1992 to 1995, he was Chief of Medical Oncology and Deputy Director of the Cancer Center at UCSF. More recently he has been CEO of Access Oncology and President of Keryx Biopharmaceuticals where he developed an oral AKT inhibitor, perifosine. He has designed and conducted numerous phases I–III trials, and he has published nearly 300 books and papers.

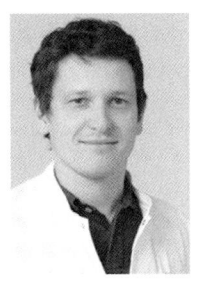

Ken Herrmann studied Medicine at the Universities of Berlin and Lausanne. In 2004 he graduated and started working under the supervision of Professor M. Schwaiger in Munich. After finishing his medical thesis in the Research Group of Cellular Neurosciences at Max Delbrück Centrum Berlin he joined Dr. Buck's team investigating molecular imaging of proliferation in a variety of different tumors, including lymphomas, sarcomas, gastric, and pancreatic cancer. Currently, he is finishing the Postdoctoral Lecture qualification.

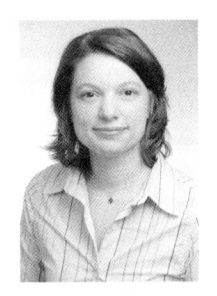

Katrin Hochdörffer studied Chemistry at the Technische Universität Kaiserslautern and received her Diploma at Boehringer Ingelheim Pharma (Ingelheim) in 2005. Under the supervision of Professor T. Schrader, she carried out her PhD thesis research on trimeric aminopyrazoles against the pathological aggregation of the Alzheimer peptide Aβ. After finishing her PhD thesis in 2009 she joined the research group of Dr. Felix Kratz at the Tumor Biology Center in Freiburg. She is currently working on the development of prodrugs for targeted cancer therapy.

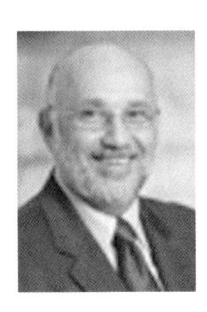

Ivan D. Horak received his MD from the University of Medicine, Bratislava, Czechoslovakia. He is Board-Certified in Internal Medicine and Medical Oncology. From 1999 to 2002, he acted as Clinical Vice President of Oncology in Research & Development at Pharmacia Corp. From 2002 to 2005, he was Chief Scientific Officer at Immunomedics where he led the development of monoclonal antibody therapy for cancer and autoimmune diseases including radiolabeled antibody for patients with solid tumors and hematologic malignancies. He joined Enzon in September 2005 as Executive Vice President and Chief Scientific Officer, and currently he is President of Research and Development. He has published extensively in the field of oncology and has served on the editorial boards of several scientific journals. He also has lectured extensively at scientific symposia and conferences.

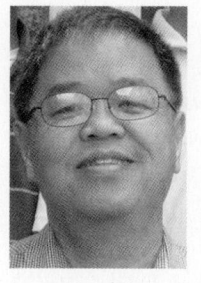

Leaf Huang PhD is the Fred N. Eshelman Distinguished Professor and Chair, Division of Molecular Pharmaceutics in the Eshelman School of Pharmacy, University of North Carolina at Chapel Hill. His research has been in the area of gene therapy and targeted drug delivery. He pioneered the liposome nonviral vector and produced the vector for the first nonviral clinical trial in 1992. His current work centers on further improvement of liposome vectors for gene transfer in tumor, liver, and lung. He also continues research in establishing a ligand targeted delivery system for siRNA and peptides for tumor growth inhibition, and for peptide vaccines in treating cervical cancer. He has authored or coauthored more than 300 peer-reviewed papers, and more than 120 reviews and book chapters. The *h*-index of his publications is 74. He is also the inventor or coinventor of 16 US and foreign patents. In 2004, he received the Alec D. Bangham MD FRS Achievement Award, which is the highest honor in the field of liposome research. He has also cofounded five biotech start-ups in the past.

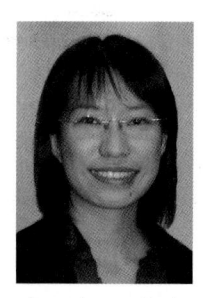

Yingying Huang received her MD degree of Clinical Medicine from Xiangya Medical College of Central South University (China) in 2004. In 2007 she received a Masters degree in Dermatology from Sun Yat-Sen University (China) and in April 2008 she joined the research group of Dr. Michael R. Hamblin at the Wellman Center for Photomedicine, Massachusetts General Hospital. She is currently investigating the mechanism of quantitative structure–activity relationships of photosensitizers for photodynamic therapy purposes.

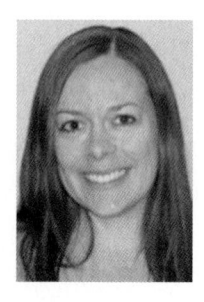

Simone Jeger obtained her MS degree in Pharmaceutical Sciences from the University of Basel, Switzerland, in 2005. In 2009, she received a PhD from the Swiss Federal Institute of Technology, Zurich for research in the area of novel conjugation methods to produce tumor-selective radioimmunoconjugates for diagnostics and therapy. In 2010, she started postdoctoral studies on antibody engineering and immunoconjugation technologies at Seattle Genetics.

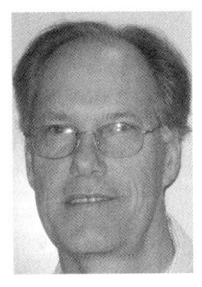

John DiJoseph is a Principal Research Scientist of Oncology at Pfizer Research in Pearl River, NY. He received his postgraduate training at Rutgers University and joined Ayerst Research in 1981. He has received many awards for his contributions, including the 1998 MMP13/TACE Discovery Teamwork Award, the Discovery Achievement Award (humanized anti-CD20 SMIP), and the 2007 Discovery Achievement Award (Anti-5T4 P2 Team). He has been instrumental in the development of CMC-544 (Inotuzumab ozogamicin). He has been an Invited Lecturer at oncology and hematology workshops and symposia. He holds four patents for his work, and has authored or co-authored numerous articles in national and international journals, including *Blood*, *International Journal of Oncology*, and *Journal of Pharmacology and Therapeutics*.

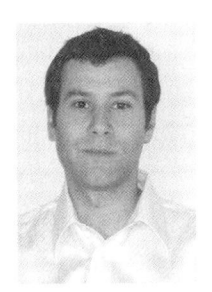

Kazunori Kataoka received his PhD from the University of Tokyo in 1979. He has been a Professor of Biomaterials at the Graduate School of Engineering, University of Tokyo, Japan since 1998. He has also been appointed in a joint position as a Professor of Clinical Biotechnology since 2004 at the Graduate School of Medicine, University of Tokyo. He is the author of more than 380 scientific papers in international journals and a recipient of many awards. His current major research interests include the development of new polymeric carrier systems, especially block copolymer micelles, for drug and gene targeting.

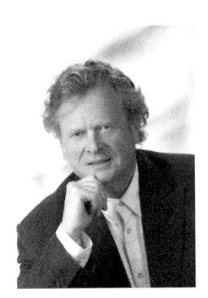

Bernhard K. Keppler received his Diploma and PhD in Chemistry from the University of Heidelberg in 1979 and 1981, respectively, and a PhD in Medicine from the German Cancer Research Center at Heidelberg in 1986 as well as the license to practice medicine (Approbation). He habilitated and gained the qualification of a University Lecturer in Inorganic Chemistry at the University of Heidelberg in 1990. In 1995, he joined the Institute of Inorganic Chemistry at the University of Vienna as a Full Professor. He is Head of the Institute of Inorganic Chemistry and Dean of the Faculty of Chemistry at the University of Vienna.

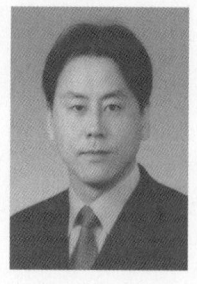

Kwangmeyung Kim graduated in Chemical Engineering from Sung Kyun Kwan University. He obtained his PhD under the supervision of Professor Youngro Byun at Gwangju Institute of Science and Technology in 2003. He then joined Dr. Ick Chan Kwon's group, and carried out postdoctoral research at the Korea Institute of Science and Technology (KIST) and developed cancer-specific optical imaging systems. Since 2004 he has been a Senior Research Scientist at KIST where he is now in charge of organizing and managing translational research from the laboratory to the clinic. His research interests are noninvasive and diagnostic imaging for various human diseases, molecular and cellular imaging for biological processes, and inorganic/organic nanoparticulate imaging probes. He has published over 80 peer-reviewed papers and four review articles.

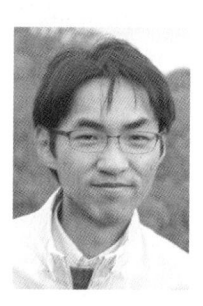

Sungwon Kim received his PhD in Materials Science and Engineering from Gwangju Institute of Science and Technology (Korea) in 2004. After postdoctoral research on drug delivery and molecular imaging at Korea Institute of Science and Technology (Korea), he joined Professor Kinam Park's group at Purdue University (USA), and has worked on polymer micelles and microfabrication since 2006. His research interests are nanomedicine, medical imaging, and tissue engineering.

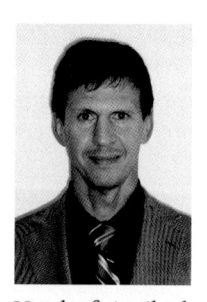

Sergej Kiprijanov graduated in Biochemistry and Molecular Biology from Novosibirsk State University (Novosibirsk, Russia) and received his PhD degree from the Institute of Genetics and Selection of Industrial Microorganisms (Moscow, Russia). He then carried out his postdoctoral research at the German Cancer Research Center (DKFZ) in Heidelberg (Germany), where he played a key role in the design and generation of the novel bispecific antibody formats useful for tumor therapy. During 2000–2006, he was Head of Antibody Engineering and then Head of Research and Development at Affimed Therapeutics AG (Heidelberg, Germany) focusing on engineering bispecific antibodies for cancer indications. He then served as Chief Scientific Officer at Novoplant GmbH (Gatersleben, Germany), a German plant biotech company developing antibodies for oral applications. In 2008, he joined Affitech AS (Oslo, Norway) as Vice President of Discovery, Research, and Preclinical Development, dealing with the generation of fully human therapeutic antibodies. He has authored more than 70 research articles, reviews, and book chapters, and is named as an inventor on 20 patents and patent applications.

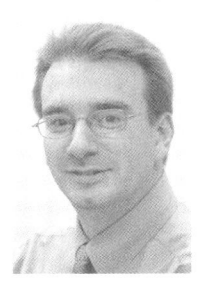

Paul J. Kleindl graduated from Marquette University in 1995 with a BS degree in Chemistry. Under the direction of Professor David R. Williams, he received a MS degree in Organic Chemistry in 1997 from Indiana University-Bloomington. Upon graduation, he was employed first at Great Lakes Chemical Co. and then Custom Synthesis Services (Madison, WI), as a Synthetic Organic Chemist. His work included the synthesis of flame retardants, polymer additives, stable-isotope mass standards, and the scale-up of processes to produce material for preclinical evaluation. In 2003, he joined Endocyte and is currently employed in the Discovery Chemistry Department as a Synthetic Scientist working on the synthesis of folate conjugates for the treatment of inflammation and cancer.

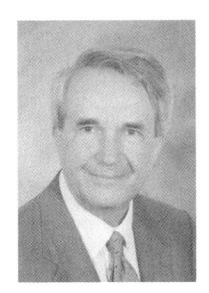

Jindřich Kopeček received his PhD in Macromolecular Chemistry and DSc in Chemistry from the Czechoslovak Academy of Sciences. He is currently Distinguished Professor of Pharmaceutical Chemistry and Distinguished Professor of Bioengineering at the University of Utah. His research focuses on biorecognition of macromolecules, bioconjugate chemistry, targetable macromolecular therapeutics, and self-assembly of block and graft copolymers into hybrid hydrogels.

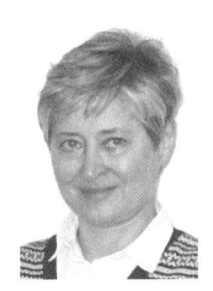

Pavla Kopečková received her PhD in Macromolecular Chemistry from the Institute of Macromolecular Chemistry, Czechoslovak Academy of Sciences in Prague. She is currently Research Professor of Pharmaceutics and Pharmaceutical Chemistry at the University of Utah. Her research centers on bioorganic polymer chemistry, biodegradability of polymers, and drug delivery systems.

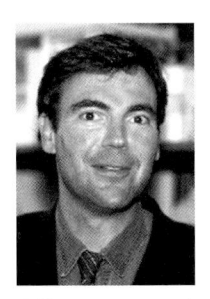

Felix Kratz graduated in Chemistry from the University of Heidelberg in 1991. He then carried out postdoctoral research at the Bioinorganic Institute of the University of Florence and developed tumor-specific carrier systems with Ru(III) complexes. Since 1994, he has been Head of Macromolecular Prodrugs at the Tumor Biology Center in Freiburg, Germany, where he is now in charge of organizing and managing translational research from the laboratory to the clinic. His research areas are drug targeting, drug delivery systems in oncology, prodrugs, receptor targeting, bioconjugate chemistry, and nanocarriers.

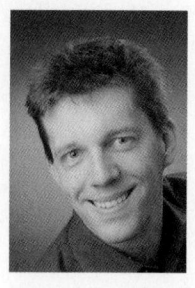

Jens Kurreck studied Biochemistry and Philosophy at the Free University of Berlin, and received his Doctorate in 1998 at the University of Technology Berlin. After a stay at Arizona State University he went to the Free University of Berlin, where he completed his Habilitation in 2006. From 2007 to 2009 he was Professor for Nucleic Acid Technology at the University of Stuttgart and since 2009 he has been Professor for Applied Biochemistry at the University of Technology Berlin. His work involves the application of RNAi for medically relevant topics, in particular virology and pain research.

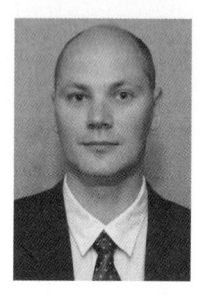

Kaido Kurrikoff is currently a Research Fellow at the Institute of Technology, University of Tartu, Estonia. He acquired his PhD degree (Neurosciences) at the University of Tartu in 2009. His main research areas have been molecular pain mechanisms and peptide-based drug delivery carriers. He has also worked as an Assistant Teacher in the Department of Medicine, University of Tartu. He is a coauthor of about 10 scientific publications.

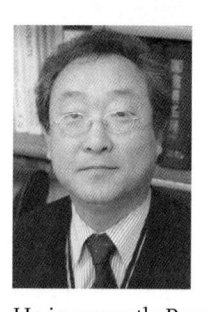

Ick Chan Kwon is currently Head of Biomedical Research Center at the Korea Institute of Science and Technology (KIST). He received his BS and MS degrees from the Department of Textile Engineering at Seoul National University in 1982 and 1984, and his PhD in Pharmaceutics and Pharmaceutical Chemistry from the University of Utah under the guidance of Professor Sung Wan Kim in 1993. After postdoctoral training in the Center for Controlled Chemical Delivery at the University of Utah, he joined KIST in 1994. He is currently President of the Korean Society of Molecular Imaging (2008–2010). He also serves as an Editor Asia of the *Journal of Controlled Release* (Elsevier), Asian Editor of the *Journal of Biomedical Nanotechnology* (American Scientific Publisher), and as a member of the Editorial Boards of *Journal of Biomedical Engineering Research* and *Journal of Biomaterials Science, Polymer Edition*. His main research interest is targeted drug delivery with polymeric nanoparticles and is now expanding to the development of smart nanoprobes for theranostic imaging. He is a project leader of "Real-time molecular imaging" supported by the Ministry of Science and Technology of Korea. He has published 140 peer-reviewed articles, 11 book chapters, and eight review articles.

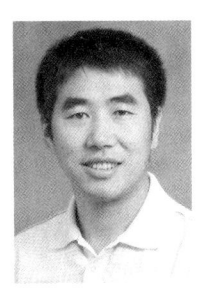

Kit S. Lam obtained his PhD in Oncology from McArdle Laboratory for Cancer Research, University of Wisconsin, and his MD from Stanford University School of Medicine. He completed his Internal Medicine residency training and Medical Oncology Fellowship training at the University of Arizona. He is board certified in both Internal Medicine and Medical Oncology. He was the Division Chief of Hematology/Oncology at UC Davis for over 10 years until recently when he became s the Chair of the Department of Biochemistry and Molecular Medicine. He is both a practicing medical oncologist and a laboratory investigator. He invented the "one-bead/one-compound" combinatorial library method. He has published over 258 scientific publications and is an inventor on 14 patents. He received the Cathay Award in 1998 and the Combinatorial Science Award in 2007. His research encompasses the development and applications of combinatorial chemistry to basic research and drug development.

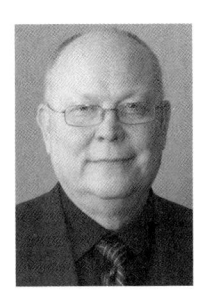

Ülo Langel is a Professor and Chairman at the Department of Neurochemistry, Stockholm University, Sweden. He graduated from Tartu University, Tartu, Estonia, as a Bioorganic Chemist in 1974; he has received his PhD degree twice: in 1980 from Tartu University (Bioorganic Chemistry) and in 1993 from Tartu University/Stockholm University (Biochemistry/Neurochemistry). His professional experience includes a career at Tartu University (from Junior Research Fellow to Associate Professor, Visiting Professor, and Adjunct Professor; 1974 till now); The Scripps Research Institute, La Jolla, CA, USA (Associate Professor and Adjunct Professor; 2000 till now); and Stockholm University (from Research Fellow to Associate Professor, Professor, and Chairman; 1987 till now). He is an Honorary Professor at Ljubljana University, Slovenia. He has been awarded a White Star Order, fourth class, by the Estonian Republic. He is a coauthor of more than 290 scientific articles and 15 approved patents or patent applications.

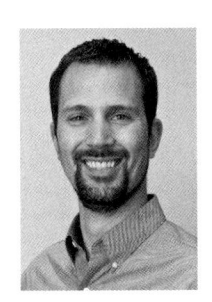

Barry D. Liboiron is Associate Director (Biophysical Characterization) at Celator Pharmaceuticals. He received his PhD from the University of British Columbia in 2002. Following a Postdoctoral Fellowship at Stanford University, he joined Celator Pharmaceuticals in 2006, as a Research Scientist in biophysics, and was promoted to his current position in 2008. Through the elucidation of key physicochemical properties of Celator's drug products and proprietary technologies, his work has furthered the development of the company's liposomal and nanoparticle drug platforms. His research interests include drug delivery, *in vivo* spectroscopy, and inorganic biochemistry. He is the author of 15 publications, including an invited review on the use of electron paramagnetic resonance as a tool to aid drug development for diabetes mellitus.

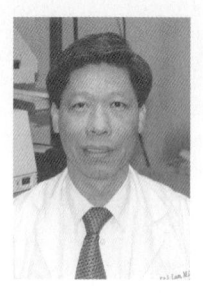

Ruiwu Liu is a Research Associate Professor of Chemistry at the Department of Biochemistry and Molecular Medicine, UC Davis School of Medicine. In 1990, he received his BA degree in Medicinal Chemistry from West China University of Medical Sciences, China. He obtained his PhD degree in Medicinal Chemistry in 1995 from the Institute of Materia Medica, Chinese Academy of Medical Sciences, China. He then joined the faculty of the Institute and spent a year at the Research Center of Taisho Pharmaceutical Co. Ltd., Japan as a Visiting Researcher. In 1998, he was promoted to Associate Professor at the Institute of Materia Medica where he worked on developing new antitumor taxoids. He received training on combinatorial chemistry in Dr. Kit Lam's laboratory at UC Davis in 1999. He and Dr. Lam have codeveloped several new methods for combinatory chemistry. He was appointed as a Research Assistant Professor, an independent investigator, at UC Davis in 2004 and promoted to Research Associate Professor in 2010. His primary research focus has been in methods development for combinatory chemistry and applying combinatory chemistry (e.g., the "one-bead/one-compound" library approach) for drug discovery. His current research projects include developing cancer-targeting imaging and therapeutic agents for lymphoma, glioblastoma, and prostate cancer, and developing novel amyloid imaging agents for Alzheimer's disease.

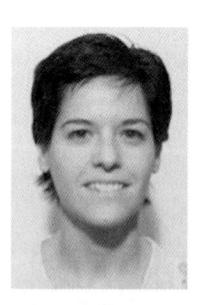

Rut Lucas studied Pharmacy at the Universitat de Valencia (Spain) and obtained her Doctoral degree in Pharmacy in 2002 under the guidance of M. Paya, working on the pharmacological study of new molecules from natural and synthetic origin controlling the inflammatory process. She then joined the group of J.A. Mitchell for postdoctoral research in the area of inflammation in the cardiovascular field. Her main expertise is based on the effect of hypoxia in human adult stem cells mimicking the cardiovascular system microenvironment At present she is a Senior Researcher funded by the Health Ministry of Spain in the Polymer Therapeutics Laboratory at the Centro de Investigación Príncipe Felipe.

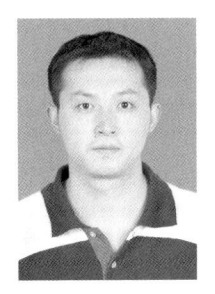

Juntao Luo is a Research Assistant Professor in the Department of Biochemistry and Molecular Medicine, UC Davis School of Medicine. In 2003, he received his PhD degree in Polymer Chemistry and Physics from Nankai University, Tianjin, China. Then, he pursued his first postdoctoral research in polymer and bioorganic chemistry, comentored by Dr. Julian Zhu and William D. Lubell at the University of Montreal, Montreal, Canada. In 2006, he moved to UC Davis Medical Center for his second postdoctoral training with Dr. Kit S. Lam in combinatorial chemistry and cancer treatment. In 2008, he became an independent researcher at UC Davis Medical Center. His research interest is nanomedicine and drug delivery in cancer treatment and cancer imaging. He is also interested in bioconjugation chemistry, combinatorial chemistry in drug discovery, and the development of biomaterials for biomedical applications.

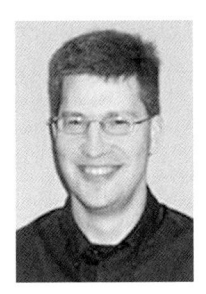

Robert P. Lyon received his PhD in Medicinal Chemistry from the University of Washington in 2002, where he studied the enzymology of drug-metabolizing enzymes. His postdoctoral work at Syntrix Biosystems involved the preparation and biophysical characterization of synthetic oligonucleotides designed for sequence-specific probe applications. He has been working in the antibody–drug conjugate field in the Chemistry Department at Seattle Genetics since 2005.

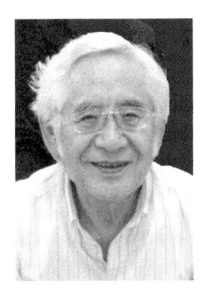

Hiroshi Maeda received his BS from Tohoku University, Sendai, Japan in 1962, and his MS from the University of California, Davis, USA in 1964 where he studied protein chemistry. Then, he worked on the first protein antitumor antibiotic, neocarzinostatin, at Tohoku University Medical School and subsequently obtained PhD and MD degrees in 1972. After spending several years at the Children's Hospital Cancer Center of Harvard (now the Dana Farber Cancer Center) in Boston, he became Professor at Kumamoto University Medical School until his retirement to move to Sojo University School of Pharmacy in 2004. He developed the first polymer conjugate drugs (SMANCS) in 1979 and SMANCS/Lipiodol therapy for hepatoma. The enhanced permeation and retention (EPR) effect was discovered in 1986 during his studies on many polymer–protein conjugates, which is currently one of the principle gold standards for tumor targeting.

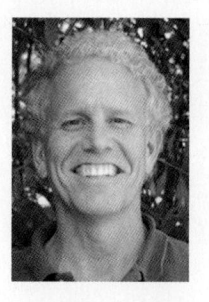

Kerri A. Massey received her PhD from the Department of Neuroscience at the University of California San Diego where she studied synapse development. She joined the Schnitzer lab in 2008, and now focuses on understanding the distinct biological processes that occur at the surface of vascular endothelial cells in different organs and how innate transport processes can be exploited to deliver drugs and imaging agents to single organs *in vivo*.

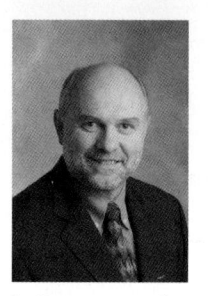

Lawrence D. Mayer is Founder, President, and Head of Research at Celator Pharmaceuticals. He received his BS in both Chemistry and Biology (1978), *summa cum laude*, from Wartburg College, and his PhD in Biochemistry (1983) from the University of Minnesota. He has played a lead role in the discovery and development of a number of drugs through phase II clinical trials, three of which eventually achieved market approval. He held senior management positions at The Canadian Liposome Company and QLT Inc. before joining the BC Cancer Agency, where he established and directed the Health Canada-accredited Investigational Drug Program. Celator was formed in 2000 as a spin-out of his laboratory at the BC Cancer Agency. He has authored more than 200 scientific publications and has more than 35 patents awarded or pending.

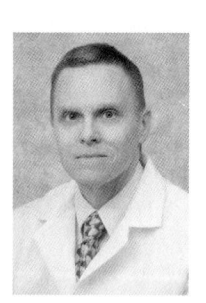

Michael R. McDevitt is an Associate Attending Radiochemist in the Departments of Medicine and Radiology at Memorial Hospital and an Associate Laboratory Member at Sloan-Kettering Institute. He specializes in the development of targeted radiolabeled drug constructs. Recently, he has been investigating the integration of nanomaterials such as carbon nanotubes into a drug design paradigm. After receiving his PhD degree in Chemistry from Case Western Reserve University in 1985, he worked in biotechnology and joined Memorial Sloan-Kettering Cancer Center in 1995. In 2004, he received a Master's degree in Chemical Engineering from The City University of New York. He is also a member of Memorial Sloan-Kettering Cancer Center's Brain Tumor Center and Nanotechnology Center.

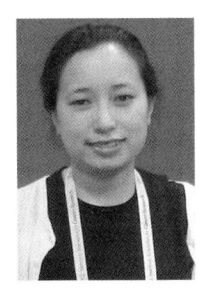

Shama Moktan received a BS in Biology with honors from the University of Mississippi in 2004. She entered the PhD program in Biochemistry at the University of Mississippi Medical Center in 2006. She then joined Dr. Drazen Raucher's laboratory in 2007. Her PhD work is focused on the development of elastin-like polypeptides for thermally targeted delivery of cell inhibitory peptides and small molecule drugs.

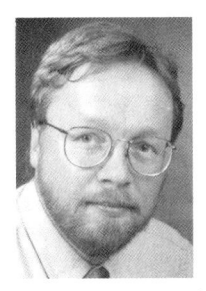

Klaus Mross graduated in Medicine from the University of Göttingen in 1985. He received his MD in 1985 and his thesis was published by Thieme Verlag. Subsequently, he carried out postdoctoral research during an EORTC fellowship at the Free University Amsterdam in the Department of Medical Oncology (Head Professor Dr. H. Pinedo) and worked on anthracyclines. He was board certified in Internal Medicine in 1993, and completed his habilitation 1994 and received the *Venia legendi* in Internal medicine. The habilitation was published by Zuckschwerdt Verlag in 1993. Since 1995, he has been Executive Physician of the Department of Medical Oncology in the Tumor Biology Center at the Albert Ludwigs University Freiburg and Head of the Clinical Trial Unit. In 1997, he became board certified in Hematology and Oncology. He is cofounder of the Central European Society of Anticancer Research (CESAR). His main topics in research are anthracyclines, pharmacokinetics and metabolism, imaging biomarkers, angiogenesis inhibitors, and phase I and II studies.

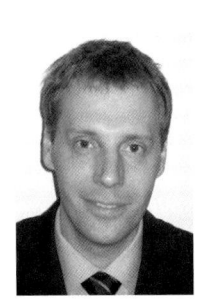

Pawel Mroz received his MD and PhD degrees from the Medical University of Warsaw, Poland. He joined the Wellman Center for Photomedicine at Massachusetts General Hospital, Harvard Medical School as a Postdoctoral Research Fellow in the laboratory of Dr. Michael R. Hamblin in 2005. In 2008 he was appointed as an Instructor at Harvard Medical School, and Assistant in Immunology at Massachusetts General Hospital and Wellman Center. He has been investigating the variety of antitumor immune responses after photodynamic therapy (PDT); in particular, he has been investigating the role of T-regulatory cells and tumor antigens in this process. Additionally, he has been involved in several projects evaluating the applications of new photosensitizers for PDT of cancer. He has received several awards for his research.

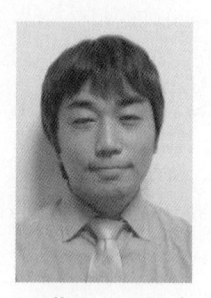

Nobuhiro Nishiyama received his PhD under the supervision of Professor K. Kataoka in Materials Engineering from the University of Tokyo in 2001. After a Postdoctoral Fellowship in the research group of Professor J. Kopecek at the University of Utah, he joined the research group of Professor K. Kataoka again in 2003 and has been an Associate Professor in the Division of Clinical Biotechnology, Graduate School of Medicine, University of Tokyo since 2009. His main interest concerns the biomedical applications of intelligent nanodevices for drug and gene delivery.

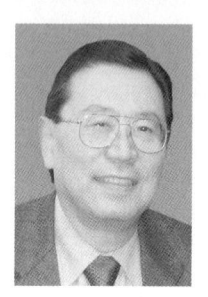

Iwao Ojima received his BS, MS, and PhD (1973) degrees from the University of Tokyo, Japan. He joined the Sagami Institute of Chemical Research and held a position of Senior Research Fellow until 1983. He joined the faculty at the Department of Chemistry, State University of New York at Stony Brook first as Associate Professor (1983), was promoted to Professor (1984), Leading Professor (1991), and then to Distinguished Professor (1995). He served as the Department Chairman from 1997 to 2003. He has been serving as the Founding Director for the Institute of Chemical Biology and Drug Discovery (ICB&DD) since 2003. He has a wide range of research interests in synthetic organic and medicinal chemistry as well as chemical biology, including discovery and development of anticancer agents and antimicrobials, targeted drug delivery, catalytic methodologies, and asymmetric synthesis. His awards and honors include the Arthur C. Cope Scholar Award (1994), E. B. Hershberg Award for Important Discoveries of Medicinally Active Substances (2001) from the American Chemical Society, Chemical Society of Japan Award (1999), and Outstanding Inventor Award (2002) from the Research Foundation of the State University of New York; Inductee of the Medicinal Chemistry Hall of Fame, American Chemical Society; and Fellow of J. S. Guggenheim Memorial Foundation, the American Association for the Advancement of Science, the New York Academy of Sciences, and the American Chemical Society.

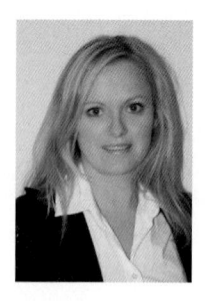

Melanie Ott graduated in Pharmacy from the University of Heidelberg, Germany in 1998. After an appointment as a Pharmacist in 1999 she worked in a public pharmacy. In 2001, she began research at the, Institute of Pharmacy and Molecular Biotechnology, University of Heidelberg, Germany, where she received her PhD in 2009. Since then she has worked as a Postdoctoral Research Scientist at the Institute. Her research interests are drug delivery, membrane transport proteins, and blood–central nervous system barriers.

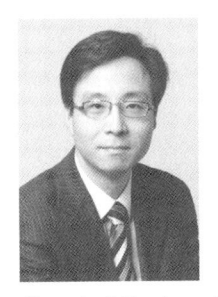

Jae Hyung Park received his PhD degree in Materials Science and Engineering under the supervision of Professor You Han Bae from Gwangju Institute of Science and Technology in 2002. He carried out a 2-year postdoctoral research at Korea Institute of Science and Technology under the supervision of Dr. Ick Chan Kwon. In 2004, he joined Professor Kinam Park's group at the School of Pharmacy, Purdue University, as an Associate Postdoctoral Researcher. Since 2005 he has been an Assistant Professor at the Department of Chemical Engineering, Kyung Hee University, South Korea. His current research interests include areas of: hydrogel nanoparticles for drug delivery and optical imaging; hydrotropic polymer conjugates for improving water solubility of poorly soluble drugs; biocompatible polymers bearing cyclodextrins for protein delivery; cationic polymers as a nonviral gene delivery system; and hybrid nanoparticles for theranostics. He has published more than 60 peer-reviewed articles and six book chapters.

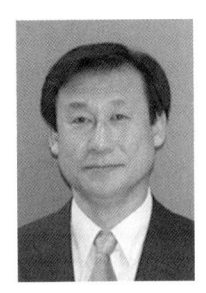

Kinam Park is Showalter Distinguished Professor of Biomedical Engineering and Professor of Pharmaceutics at Purdue University in West Lafayette, Indiana (USA). His research has been focused on the use of various polymers and hydrogels for controlled drug delivery. His current research includes nano/micro fabrication of particles, hydrotropic polymeric micelles, superporous hydrogels, fast-melting tablet formulations, and drug-eluting stents. He is currently the Editor-in-Chief of the *Journal of Controlled Release*.

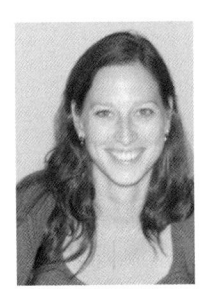

Dina Polyak is an MS student at Tel Aviv University under the supervision of Dr. Ronit Satchi-Fainaro. She investigates the implementation of polymer therapeutics targeting integrins on cancer cells and cancer vasculature. Following completion *cum laude* of her BPharm studies at Ben-Gurion University of the Negev, she practiced as a pharmacist at Hillel Yaffe Medical Center.

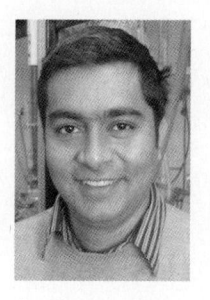

Mohiuddin Abdul Quadir received his PhD in Organic Chemistry in 2010 from the Free University of Berlin under the supervision of Professor Rainer Haag. His research topic focused on the delivery of drugs and bioactive molecules through the blood–brain barrier with dendritic polymer architectures. He is engaged at Dhaka University, Bangladesh as an Assistant Professor and is currently performing postdoctoral research in the Haag group in the Free University of Berlin, where he works on the development of functional dendritic architectures for the early diagnosis of diseases.

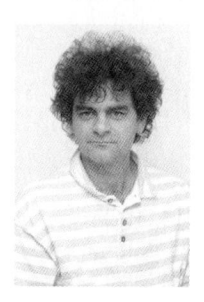

Drazen Raucher if Professor of Biochemistry and Associate member of the Cancer Institute at University of Mississippi Medical Center. He recived BS degree in Mathematics and Physics (1988), from University of Osijek, Croatia, and PhD in Molecular Biophysics (1995) from Institute of Molecular Biophysics, Florida State University. His research is focused on the development of thermally responsive biopolymer for targeted delivery of anti-cancer therapeutics to solid tumors.

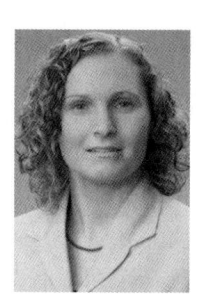

Valeska Reichel graduated in Pharmacy from the University of Kiel, Germany in 2002. After an appointment as a Pharmacist in 2003 she worked as a Research Scientist at the Institute of Pharmacy and Molecular Biotechnology, University of Heidelberg, Germany, where she received her PhD in 2006. Since then she has been employed as a Lecturer and Research Scientist at the Institute. Her research interests are drug delivery, membrane transport proteins, and blood–central nervous system barriers.

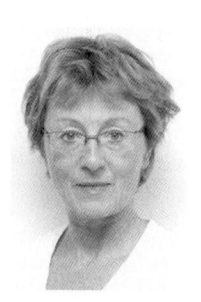

Inger Sandlie is Professor at the Department of Molecular Biosciences (IMBV), University of Oslo, Norway and Deputy Director of the Center for Immune Regulation at the Institute for Immunology. She trained in Biochemistry and obtained her PhD in 1981 at the University of Bergen on a problem related to DNA repair. She then did a postdoc with Lawrence Grossman at Johns Hopkins University in Baltimore, MD, USA – still on DNA repair. After her return to Norway in 1985, she focused on antibody engineering, and worked at The Norwegian Radium Hospital for 3 years before she joined the Faculty of the Biology Department in 1988 and IMBV in 2005. Her main published scientific achievements concern the function of the Fc region of antibodies, and in particular the role of the hinge region and isotype-specific amino acids for structure and function of IgG and IgD, the molecular requirements for polymerization and polyIg receptor interaction of IgA and IgM, as well as the development of "troybodies" and "vaccibodies." She has authored more than 80 scientific publications and holds seven patents. Her research is currently focused on two projects: (i) studies of the interaction between Fcγ receptors, in particular the neonatal Fc receptor, with IgG and albumin, and (ii) expression and engineering of soluble T-cell receptors (TCRs) and major histocompatibility complex (MHC) class II for the study of specific TCR–peptide–MHC complexes.

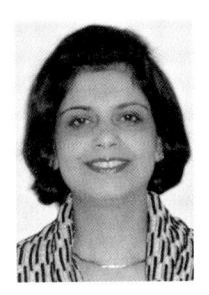

Puja Sapra received a Bachelors degree from the All India Institute of Medical Sciences, an MS in Pharmacology from the University of Strathclyde, UK, and a PhD in Pharmacology from the University of Alberta, Canada. During her PhD she developed several antibody-targeted liposomal anticancer drugs. In 2003, she joined Immunomedics as a Staff Scientist, where she was involved in the preclinical development of various antibody–drug/toxin conjugates, and also supported the preclinical and clinical pharmacology/toxicology programs of naked anti-CD22 mAb and anti-CD20 mAb. From 2005 to 2009, she worked at Enzon Pharmaceuticals, where she led the pharmacology group, and developed PEGylated drug conjugates and locked nucleic acid-based antisense oligonucleotides, including PEG-SN-38 and survivin antisense oligonucleotide that are undergoing clinical trials. In 2009, she joined the Bioconjugates group at Wyeth Discovery Research Oncology as Associate Director. In 2010, after the acquisition of Wyeth by Pfizer, she was promoted to Director, Center of Integrative Biology and Biotherapeutics (CIBB), Pfizer and currently oversees all ADC therapeutic programs at CIBB, Pfizer. She is a British Chevening Scholar and an Alberta Foundation Researcher, and an author of more than 30 scientific publications, book chapters, or patents.

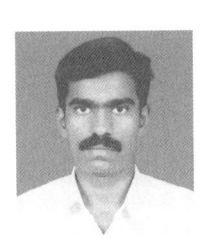

Gurusamy Saravanakumar received his Master's degree in Applied Chemistry from Madurai Kamaraj University, India in 2003 under the guidance of Professor Alagunambi Ramasubbu. He is currently pursuing his PhD degree at Kyung Hee University, South Korea under the guidance of Professor Jae Hyung Park. His primary research interests focus on the development of novel polymeric nanoparticle-based carriers for cancer therapeutics and imaging applications.

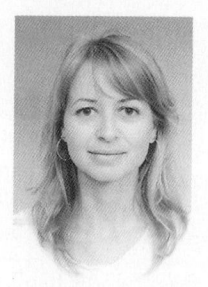

Ronit Satchi-Fainaro received her Bachelor of Pharmacy from the Hebrew University, Israel (1995) and her PhD from the University of London, UK (1999). Together with Professor Ruth Duncan, she developed PDEPT (polymer-directed enzyme prodrug therapy) – a novel two-step approach to target cancer. She then completed a 2-year postdoctoral appointment at Tel Aviv University working on protein biochemistry, for which she holds several patents. She spent 2 years as a Fulbright and Rothschild Scholar at Harvard University and Children's Hospital Boston working with Dr. Judah Folkman on novel polymer-conjugated angiogenesis inhibitors to target tumor vasculature. In 2002, she was appointed Instructor at Boston Children's Hospital and Harvard Medical School. Since October 2005, she has been a Senior Lecturer at the Department of Physiology and Pharmacology at the Sackler School of Medicine at Tel Aviv University and a Visiting Associate Professor at Harvard Medical School and Children's Hospital Boston. Her research interests include investigations relating to tumor and vascular biology, tumor dormancy, mechanism of action of angiogenesis inhibitors, self-assembly of polymeric architectures, and novel approaches to target cancer. She is the recipient of the 2010 Juludan Prize for the Advancement of Technology in Medicine.

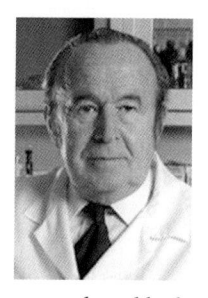

Andrew V. Schally PhD, MDHC received his training in England, Canada, Sweden, and the United States. During the period from 1954 to 1977 he worked in the field of neuroendocrinology. His group was responsible for the isolation and elucidation of the structure of hypothalamic luteinizing hormone-releasing hormone. He was awarded the Nobel Prize in Medicine and Physiology in 1977 for his pioneering work on hypothalamic peptides. Grasping the therapeutic potential of hypothalamic hormones, he switched to cancer research and he became an endocrine oncologist. He is a world leader on targeting hormone-related cancers, and is largely responsible for the field of hormone ablation for the treatment of prostate and other cancers. Various classes of anticancer peptides including targeted to analogs peptide receptors on tumors were developed in his laboratory and are in clinical trials. He is the Distinguished Leonard M. Miller Professor of Pathology and Professor in the Division of Hematology/Oncology of the Department of Medicine at the University of Miami Miller School of Medicine. He is also Chief of the Endocrine, Polypeptide Cancer Institute at the Veterans Affairs Medical Center, Miami, and Distinguished Medical Research Scientist, US Department of Veterans Affairs. He has more than 2300 publications to his credit.

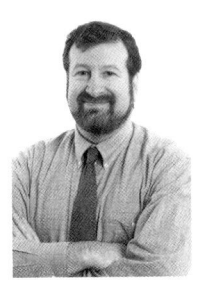

David A. Scheinberg received his MD and PhD at the Johns Hopkins University School of Medicine, and trained in Medical Oncology at Memorial Sloan-Kettering Cancer Center. For 30 years his research interests have been in the development of, and principles for practice of, monoclonal antibody-based therapeutics with a particular interest in radioimmunotherapy and α-particle therapy. He is currently Chairman of the Molecular Pharmacology and Chemistry Program, the Experimental Therapeutics Center and the Nanotechnology Center at Memorial Sloan-Kettering Cancer Center.

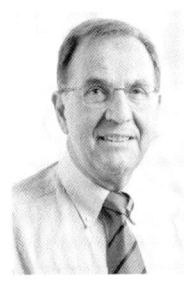

Peter M. Schlag graduated in Medicine at Düsseldorf University (Germany). He performed his postdoctoral research and medical specialization at the University of Ulm (Germany), the MD Anderson Cancer Center, the National Institutes of Health, and the Washington Cancer Center, Washington DC. He was then promoted to the position of Associate Professor and Head of the Section of Surgical Oncology at the Surgical Department of the University of Heidelberg (Germany). He was Visiting Professor at the Roswell Park Memorial Cancer Center, Buffalo, NY. Since 1992, he has been a Full Professor at the Humboldt University Berlin (Germany), heading the Department for Surgery and Surgical Oncology, Charité, and since 2001 Medical Director of the Robert-Rössle Cancer Center, Berlin. Since 2008 he has been Director of the Charité Comprehensive Cancer Center, Berlin. His research focus is on tumor metastasis and progression, on the development of new diagnostic tools and therapies for detection and management of metastases, as well as prediction signatures for tumor therapy response. In particular, the molecular mechanisms of tumor metastasis and responsible genes are investigated with an emphasis on translation into clinical applications.

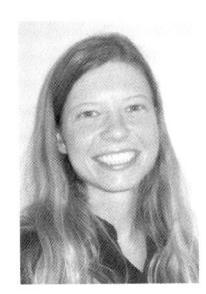

Jan E. Schnitzer received an MD from the University of Pittsburgh Medical School. He did his postdoctoral training at Yale University School of Medicine in the Department of Cell Biology under the mentorship of Nobel laureate Dr. George Palade. From 1999 to 2009, he was Professor of Molecular and Cellular Biology at the Sidney Kimmel Cancer Center. In 2009, he became Director of the Proteogenomics Research Institute for Systems Medicine. His research has historically focused on capillary permeability, transvascular transport, and the vascular endothelium. More recently, his group has focused on understanding the role of the vascular endothelium and its surface proteins and transport vesicles in normal and pathological processes, and how the restrictive endothelial cell barrier can be overcome to deliver drugs, imaging agents, nanoparticles, and even gene vectors *in vivo*.

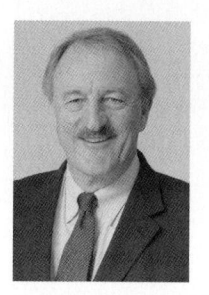

Markus Schwaiger MD received his medical training at the Medical School of the Free University of Berlin, Germany, and completed a Fellowship at the Division of Nuclear Medicine, UCLA School of Medicine, Los Angeles, CA, USA. He worked as Assistant Professor of Radiological Sciences, Division of Nuclear Medicine, UCLA School of Medicine, Professor of Medicine, Division of Nuclear Medicine, University of Michigan, and professor and Director, Department of Nuclear Medicine, Technical University in Munich, Germany. He was Dean of the School of Medicine, Technical University in Munich, Germany from 2002 to 2010. He has published 622 peer-reviewed publications in international scientific journals, 96 book chapters and 866 abstracts, and has been invited to give 511 presentations.

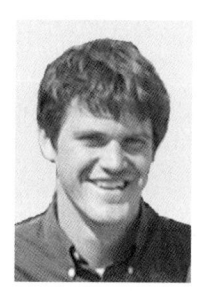

Joshua D. Seitz began his undergraduate research at the University of Vermont, working with Dr. A. Paul Krapcho in the synthesis of bis-phenanthroline-based ligands as G-Quadruplex-stabilizing agents. After graduating with a BS in Chemistry in 2007, he came to Stony Brook University for its Graduate Chemistry Program. He joined the Ojima Research Laboratory in 2009 for his PhD research. He is currently engaged in the design, synthesis, and biological evaluation of novel taxane-based drug conjugates for tumor-targeted cancer chemotherapy.

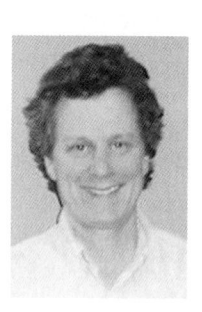

Peter D. Senter earned his PhD in Chemistry from the University of Illinois in Urbana and then carried out postdoctoral research at the Max Planck Institute in Göttingen, Germany. After various positions at the Dana Farber Cancer Institute, Bristol-Myers Squibb, and Cytokine Networks, he joined Seattle Genetics in 1998, and initiated research programs that led to the technology used for SGN-35 and other promising antibody–drug conjugates.

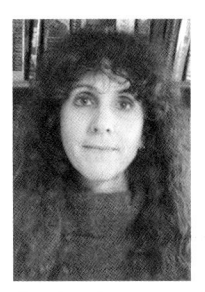

Rita E. Serda received her PhD in Biomedical Sciences from the University of New Mexico in 2006. Her postdoctoral research was done in the laboratory of Mauro Ferrari in the Department of Nanomedicine and Biomedical Engineering at the University of Texas Health Science Center at Houston. In 2010, she was promoted to Assistant Professor and Co-Director of the nBME Scholarly Project Concentration for medical students. In October 2010, she joined the Methodist Hospital Research Institute and is continuing research on the development of nanocarriers for drug delivery.

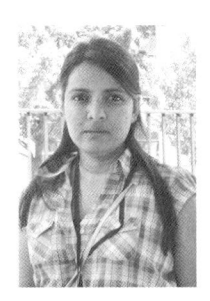

Sulbha K. Sharma is a Research Technologist at the Wellman Center for Photomedicine, Massachusetts General Hospital, Boston, USA She developed her interest in photodynamic therapy during her PhD during when she evaluated the photodynamic effects of some of the chlorophyll derivatives both *in vitro* and *in vivo*. Recently, her studies are focused on the effects of low-level light therapy with special interest in primary cortical neurons and also on the photodynamic effects of functionalized fullerenes.

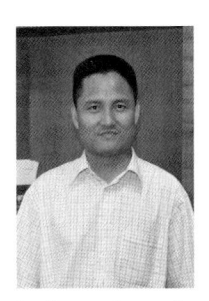

Haifa Shen received his Bachelor's degree from Zhejiang University Medical School (China) in 1985 and his PhD degree from the University of Texas–Houston in 1993. He then carried out postdoctoral research at the National Cancer Institute. After 8 years in the pharmaceutical industry working on cancer drug development, he returned to the University of Texas–Houston in February 2010 as an Assistant Professor. In October 2010, he joined the Methodist Hospital Research Institute in Houston where his research is focused on developing nanotherapeutics for personalized therapy of human cancers.

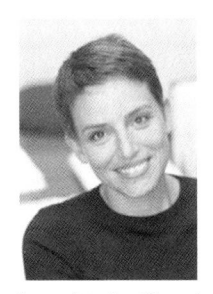

Stavroula Sofou is an Associate Professor in the Departments of Biomedical Engineering and Chemical and Biochemical Engineering at Rutgers University. Previously, she was an Assistant Professor in the Department of Chemical and Biological Engineering at the Polytechnic Institute of New York University, and an Associate Director of the Center for Drug Delivery Research at Poly-SUNY/Downstate Medical Center. She received her Diploma in Chemical Engineering from the National Technical University of Athens, Greece, and her PhD in Chemical Engineering from Columbia University with a distinction for her thesis. She was a Postdoctoral Research Fellow at the Memorial Sloan-Kettering Cancer Center in Medical Physics/Experimental Therapeutics. In September 2004, she established the Laboratory for Biomembranes and Drug Delivery Systems. Her research goal is to understand the role of intermolecular and interfacial interactions of self-assembling materials with the biological milieu, and to combine this knowledge with engineering principles to design successful devices to promote human health. Translational research on testing and optimization of these devices as diagnostics and therapeutics for medical applications is of special significance to her goals.

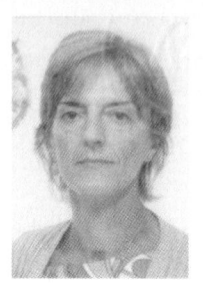

Giuseppina Di Stefano graduated in Biological Sciences in 1988 from the University of Bologna. In 1995, she obtained her PhD in Biology and Physiology of the Cell. Since 2005, she has been Associate Professor of General Pathology at the School of Medicine, University of Bologna. Her research activity has largely addressed the study of liver targeting of antiviral and antineoplastic drugs mediated by the hepatic receptor for asialoglycoproteins.

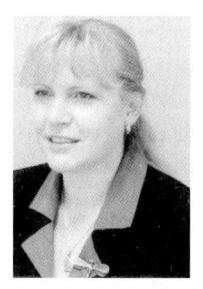

Ulrike Stein graduated in Biochemistry and in Biochemical Medicine. She completed her PhD thesis in Biochemistry at the Humboldt University, Berlin. She was a visiting scientist as an Alexander von Humboldt Fellow at the National Cancer Institute, Frederick, MD, and was invited as a guest consultant several times during the following years. She is group leader of the Tumor Metastasis and Therapy Response Group at the Max Delbrück Center (1996–2000), at the Robert Rössle Tumor Clinic, Charité University Medicine (2000–2006), and since 2007 at the Experimental and Clinical Research Center, Charité University Medicine, Berlin, as part of the Surgical Oncology department. She received her Habilitation in Biochemistry in 2003. In 2009 she was appointed Professor at the Charité University Medicine, Berlin.

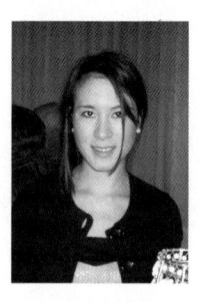

Agathe K. Streiff graduated in Anatomy and Cell Biology from McGill University in Montreal, Canada in 2009. She is currently a second-year medical student at the University of Texas Medical School at Houston with an interest in clinical applications of nanoparticles in drug delivery.

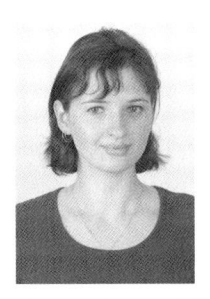

Julia Suhorutšenko is a PhD student at the University of Tartu and a Research Fellow at the Institute of Technology, Department of Science and Technology. Her research interests focus on the application of CPPs in nucleic acid delivery and tumor targeting. She was born and grew up in Estonia. She received her Master's degree in Gene technology at the University of Tartu in 2008 and continued as a Researcher at Ülo Langel's group. She has worked as a specialist in the Estonian Biocenter and in the Competence Center for Cancer Research in Estonia on the Immunotherapy Project. She is a member of Estonian Society for Immunology and Allergology, and also a member of Estonian Society of Human Genetics. She has published three research papers in molecular biotechnology and biomedicine.

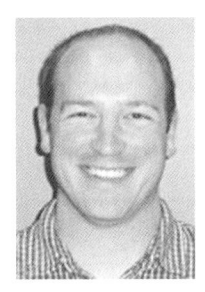

Django Sussman earned his PhD from the University of California, Santa Cruz, in Molecular, Cellular, and Developmental Biology in 2000. He then became an American Cancer Society Postdoctoral Fellow at the Fred Hutchinson Cancer Research Center where he studied the structure–function relationship in endonucleases leading to rational and computational redesigns for altered specificity. Since 2007, he has led the antibody engineering efforts at Seattle Genetics, focusing on antibody humanization and improving the pharmacokinetics, efficacy, and tolerability of antibody–drug conjugates.

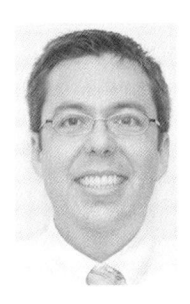

Patrick D. Sutphin MD, PhD received his medical and graduate degrees at Stanford University School of Medicine in 2007. He completed his PhD studies in the lab of Amato J. Giaccia where he focused on the development of drugs to specifically target renal cell carcinoma through synthetic lethality. Currently, he is a Third-Year Resident in the Diagnostic Radiology Residency Program at Massachusetts General Hospital with an interest in the diagnostic and therapeutic applications of magnetic nanoparticles.

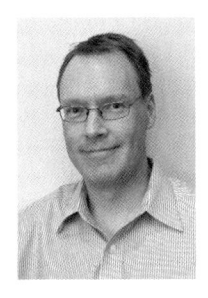

Paul G. Tardi is Director (Preformulation) at Celator Pharmaceuticals. He received his PhD from the University of Manitoba. He has 15 years experience in the pharmaceutical industry with specific experience in the area of liposomal formulation development. He worked at Inex Pharmaceuticals for 5 years where he was involved in the liposomal formulation of various cytotoxics as well as mRNA. As Director of Preformulation at Celator for 10 years he has successfully formulated four liposomal drug combinations and one nanoparticle drug combination. For two of these drug combinations he was involved in the research, process development, and clinical manufacturing of the liposomal drug products. He has authored 35 publications and has 15 patents either awarded or under review.

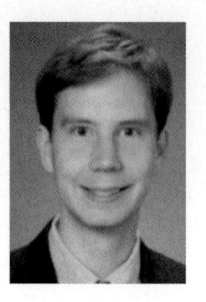

Benjamin A. Teply received his AB in Chemistry and Physics from Harvard University, MS in Biomedical Engineering from the University of Michigan, and MD from the University of Nebraska. He researched biomaterials, including aptamer-targeted drug delivery systems, in the laboratories of Professor Robert Langer and Professor Omid Farokhzad.

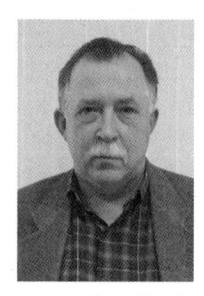

Vladimir P. Torchilin PhD, DSc is a Distinguished Professor of Pharmaceutical Sciences and Director, Center for Pharmaceutical Biotechnology and Nanomedicine, Northeastern University, Boston, MA. He graduated from Moscow University with a MS in Chemistry, and also obtained his PhD and DSc in Polymer Chemistry, Chemical Kinetics and Catalysis, and Chemistry of Physiologically Active Compounds in 1971 and 1980, respectively, from Moscow University. In 1991, he joined the Massachusetts General Hospital and Harvard Medical School as the Head of the Chemistry Program, Center for Imaging and Pharmaceutical Research, and Associate Professor of Radiology. Since 1998, he has been with Northeastern University. He was the Chair of the Department of Pharmaceutical Sciences in 1998–2008. His research interests have focused on biomedical polymers, polymeric drugs, immobilized medicinal enzymes, drug delivery and targeting, pharmaceutical nanocarriers for diagnostic and therapeutic agents, and experimental cancer immunology. He has published more than 300 original papers, more than 100 reviews and book chapters, wrote and edited 10 books, including *Immobilized Enzymes in Medicine, The Handbook on Targeted Delivery of Imaging Agents, Liposomes: A Practical Approach, Nanoparticulates as Pharmaceutical Carriers, Multifunctional Pharmaceutical Nanocarriers, Biomedical Aspects of Drug Targeting*, and *Delivery of Protein and Peptide Drugs in Cancer*, and holds more that 40 patents. He is Editor-in-Chief of *Current Drug Discovery Technologies*, Co-Editor-in-Chief of *Drug Delivery*, and on the Editorial Boards of many leading journals in the field, including *Journal of Controlled Release* (Review Editor), *Bioconjugate Chemistry, Advanced Drug Delivery Reviews, European Journal of Pharmaceutics and Biopharmaceutics, Journal of Drug Targeting, Molecular Pharmaceutics, Journal of Biomedical Nanotechnology*, and others. Among his many awards, he was the recipient of the 1982 Lenin Prize in Science and Technology (the highest scientific award in the former USSR). He was elected as a Member of European

Academy of Sciences. He is also a Fellow of the American Institute of Medical and Biological Engineering and of the American Association of Pharmaceutical Scientists (AAPS), and received the 2005 Research Achievements in Pharmaceutics and Drug Delivery Award from the AAPS, 2007 Research Achievements Award from the Pharmaceutical Sciences World Congress, 2009 AAPS Journal Award, 2009 International Journal of Nanomedicine Distinguished Scientist Award, and 2010 Controlled Release Society Founders Award. In 2005–2006, he served as a President of the Controlled Release Society.

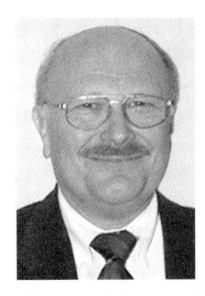

Peter Vaupel became Professor Emeritus at the University Medical Center in Mainz, Germany in October 2008. Before that he was Professor and Chairman of the Institute of Physiology and Pathophysiology at the University of Mainz, a position he assumed in 1989. In October 2008, he additionally took on the post of Affiliate Professor at the Department of Radiation Therapy and Radiological Oncology, Klinikum rechts der Isar, Technical University, Munich and at the Department of Radiooncology and Radiation Therapy, University Medical Center in Mainz. On completion of his Dr. med. thesis, he trained in General Medicine and Physiology. Following promotion to Associate Professor of Physiology in 1975, he was appointed Full Professor of Physiology in 1977. In 1984, he became Head of the Department of Applied Physiology at the University of Mainz, and later in 1987, he took up the newly established Andrew Werk Cook Professorship of Radiation Biology/Tumor Biology/Physiology at Harvard Medical School in Boston, MA. In 1996, he became a Full Member of the Academy of Science and Literature at Mainz. His research interests include the oxygenation status, blood flow, microcirculation, pH distribution, bioenergetics of malignant tumor and hypoxia-induced malignant progression, acquired treatment resistance, and pathophysiology of localized hyperthermia. He has published 475 original research articles, review papers, and book chapters. He is an Associate Editor of several peer-reviewed journals, and has received numerous scientific awards and honors.

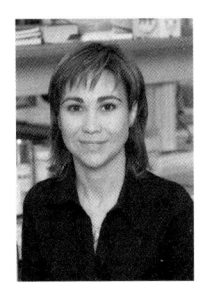

María J. Vicent received her PhD degree in 2001 in Chemistry on Solid Supports from University Jaume I Castellón after several scientific stays in Professor Fréchet's laboratory at the University California, Berkeley (USA). She then moved to more biomedically oriented research, initially with a the Spanish company Instituto Biomar SA and subsequently at the Center for Polymer Therapeutics with Professor R. Duncan after the award of a Marie Curie Postdoctoral Fellowship in 2002. In 2004, she joined the Centro de Investigación Príncipe Felipe (CIPF) as a Research Associate through a Marie Curie Reintegration contract and was promoted to her current position, Head of the Polymer

Therapeutics Laboratory at CIPF, in 2006. Her research group focused on the development of novel nanopharmaceuticals for different therapeutic applications, and has been funded by national and European grants (several acting as coordinator). She received the Fourth Idea Award on Basic Sciences from "Fundación de las Artes y las Ciencias," coauthored more than 45 peer-reviewed papers and four patents, and supervised six PhD theses. She is the Spanish President of the Spanish–Portuguese Chapter of the Controlled Release Society and Chair of key conferences on the nanomedicine field, such as the International Symposium on Polymer Therapeutics: From Laboratory to Clinical Practice.

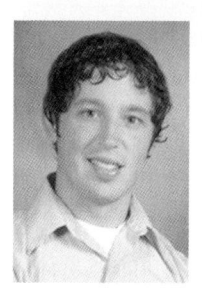

Carlos H. Villa is a MD PhD candidate at the Weill Cornell/Rockefeller/Sloan-Kettering Tri-Institutional Program. He received a BSE from Tulane University in Chemical Engineering. His current research interests are in the development of novel self-assembling nanomaterials for therapeutic applications.

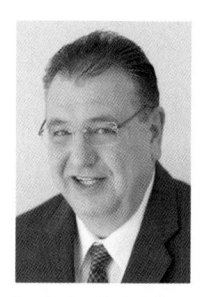

Iontcho R. Vlahov was born and raised in Sofia, Bulgaria. After graduating with a Diploma in Organic Chemistry from the University of Sofia, he obtained his PhD degree (Dr. rer. nat.) from Ruhr University, Bochum, Germany under the guidance of Professor G. Snatzke. In 1985 he joined the Bulgarian Academy of Sciences and in 1990 moved to the University of Konstanz, Germany as an Alexander von Humboldt Fellow. There he worked with Professor R.R. Schmidt on the synthesis of complex carbohydrates. In 1994 he joined Professor Linhardt's group at the University of Iowa, USA. In 1996 he accepted a position as a Head of Discovery Chemistry at Ivax (Miami, FL) and 1999 joined Endocyte (West Lafayette, IN), where he is currently Vice President, Discovery Chemistry. His work has led to over 50 articles, numerous patents, and three targeted drugs that are currently undergoing clinical trials.

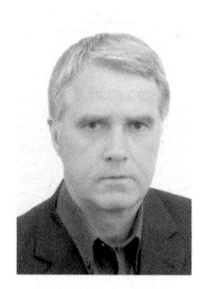

Wolfgang Walther graduated in Biochemistry and received his PhD at the Academy of Sciences, Berlin. He did his postgraduate research at the Imperial Cancer Research Fund, London and as visiting scientist at Glasgow and Strathclyde University, UK. He developed regulable conditional vector systems for gene therapy as an Alexander von Humboldt Fellow at the National Cancer Institute, Frederick, MD. Since 2007 he has been group leader of the Experimental and Clinical

Gene Therapy Group at the Experimental and Clinical Research Center, Charité, University Medicine Berlin at the Max-Delbrück-Center for Molecular Medicine, Berlin. His research is focused on nonviral cancer gene therapy for the treatment of solid tumors with an emphasis on translation to clinical applications.

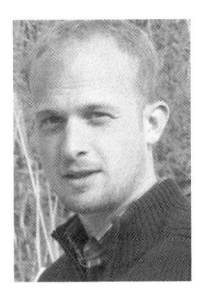

André Warnecke studied Chemistry at the Universities of Clausthal and Freiburg. In 1997, he received his Diploma in the field of Metallocene Chemistry. Under the supervision of Professor R. Mülhaupt, he prepared his PhD thesis on albumin-binding prodrugs of anticancer agents that he finished in 2001. He then started to work as a Research Fellow in the group of F. Kratz at the Tumor Biology Center. Currently, he is developing suitable chemical architectures for innovative drug release strategies.

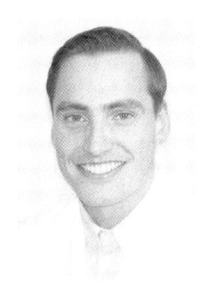

Jürgen K. Willmann MD is an Assistant Professor of Radiology in the Department of Radiology at Stanford University School of Medicine, Head of the Translational Molecular Imaging Laboratory, and member of the Molecular Imaging Program at Stanford). He received his MD from the Albert-Ludwigs-University in Freiburg, Germany in 1998, did his Radiology residence training at the University Hospital in Zurich, Switzerland, and received the *Venia Legendi* in Diagnostic Radiology from the University of Zurich in 2005. He has authored over 80 scientific peer-reviewed publications and book chapters focusing on novel anatomical/morphological, functional, and molecular imaging strategies in cancer and cardiovascular diseases, and serves as an editor and reviewer for numerous scientific journals.

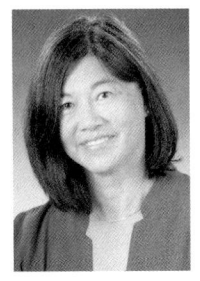

Anna M. Wu received her PhD in Molecular Biophysics and Biochemistry from Yale University. Following postdoctoral studies at Yale University and the University of California, San Francisco, she joined the research staff at the Beckman Research Institute of the City of Hope in Duarte, CA, where for many years she headed the Antibody Engineering Group. Since 2002, she has been a professor in the Department of Molecular and Medical Pharmacology at the David Geffen School of Medicine at UCLA. Her research focuses on engineering antibodies for imaging and therapeutic applications in cancer.

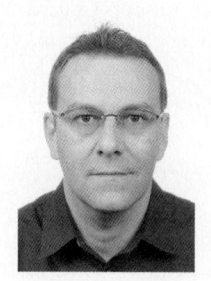

Andreas Wunder graduated in Biology (Diploma) in 1992 and was awarded as "Doctor of Natural Sciences" in 1997, both from the University of Kaiserslautern. Thereafter, he obtained his Postdoctoral Lecture Qualification ("Habilitation") from the University of Heidelberg in 2001. From 1992 until 2002, he researched at the German Cancer Research Center (DKFZ) in Heidelberg on the field of targeted drug delivery in cancer and rheumatoid arthritis. From 2002 to 2004, he was a Research Scientist at the Center for Molecular Imaging Research in Boston. After 1 year at the University of Regensburg, he continued his work on specific imaging of biological processes using noninvasive imaging techniques at the Charité Hospital in Berlin. Since 2005, he has been Group Leader at the Department Neurology and the Center for Stroke Research, Berlin. Since 2010 he heads the Small Animal Imaging Center of the Charité Hospital at the CVK.

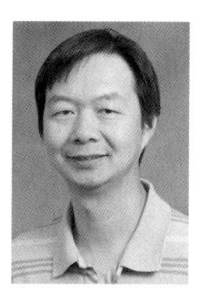

Kai Xiao is a Postdoctoral Fellow in the Department of Biochemistry and Molecular Medicine, UC Davis School of Medicine. In 2003, he received his MD from West China University of Medical Science, Chengdu, China. In 2009, he received his PhD in Pharmacology and Toxicology from Sichuan University, Chengdu, China. Then, he started his postdoctoral training in Dr. Kit S. Lam's lab at UC Davis Medical Center. His research interest is focused on the development of cancer-targeting ligands and drug delivery system for targeted imaging and therapy of cancer.

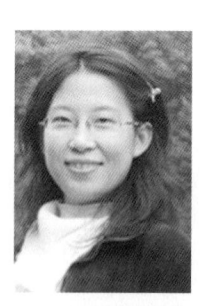

Zeyu Xiao received her Bachelor in Pharmacy from Peking University (China) in 2003. She received her PhD in Chemical Biology from the Joint Research Programme between the Chinese Academy of Sciences (China) and University of Florida (USA) in 2008. Since then, she has started joint postdoctoral research at Professor Omid Farokhzad's Laboratory at Brigham and Women's Hospital and at Professor Robert Langer's Laboratory in MIT. Her research is focused on internalizing aptamer selection and aptamer-based targeted nanoparticle delivery for *in vivo* applications.

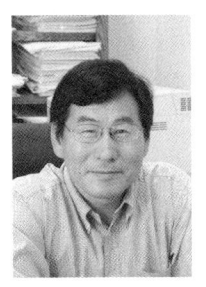

Haiqing Yin received his BS and PhD in Chemistry from Peking University, China. Currently, he is working as a Research Associate at the Department of Pharmaceutics and Pharmaceutical Chemistry of the University of Utah. His interest focuses on pH-responsive polymeric nanocarriers for delivery of therapeutic anticancer drugs, including the design and synthesis of novel multifunctional biopolymers, fabrication and physicochemical characterization of nanocarriers for anticancer drug delivery, and *in vitro/vivo* testing of the therapeutic effect of the formulations. He has authored 15 scientific publications and one patent application.

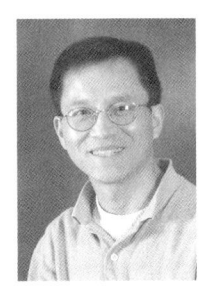

Fei You is a Synthetic Organic Chemist in the Discovery Chemistry Department at Endocyte; he has been working on the synthesis of cytotoxic compounds and their folate conjugates. He received his PhD in Organic Chemistry from Brown University. At Brown, he did research on the synthesis of *C*-glycoside ravidomycin and HIV reverse transcriptase inhibitors with Professor Kathlyn A. Parker. Then he did his postdoctoral research on metal-mediated reactions with Professor W. Dean Harman at the University of Virginia. Before coming to the United States, he received his BS in Chemistry from Nanjing University in China. He also did research on opto-electronic functional coordination compounds with Professor Xiaozeng You at Nanjing University.

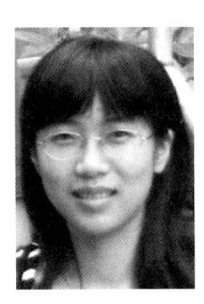

Yuan Zhang received her Master degree in the Department of Pharmaceutics, School of Pharmaceutical Sciences in Peking University (Beijing, China) in 2009. She then carried out her PhD studies in the Division of Molecular Pharmaceutics in the Eshelman School of Pharmacy, University of North Carolina at Chapel Hill till now. Her research areas are ligand targeted nonviral vector drug delivery systems. She is currently working on LCP nanoparticles encapsulating chemotherapeutics and gene drugs for lung tumor therapy.

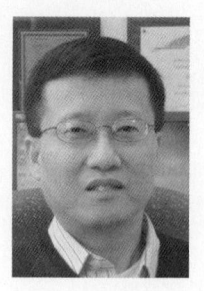

Hong Zhao received his PhD in Organic Chemistry from Rutgers University (New Brunswick, NJ) in 1997. He then joined Enzon Pharmaceuticals Inc. to study drug delivery technologies with Dr. Richard Greenwald. His research interest is to expand the application of PEGylation technology to various types of drug molecules, including small molecules, peptides, and oligonucleotides, by developing novel linker technologies. Since 2004, he has led the Organic and Medicinal Chemistry group at Enzon to advance PEGylation technology to address drug delivery needs mainly in the oncology field.

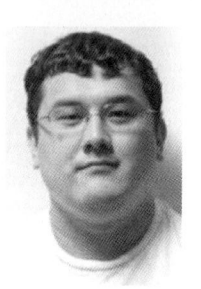

Timur Zhiyentayev graduated from Lomonosov Moscow State University (Russia) in 2009 where he worked the under supervision of Dr. Nickolay Melik-Nubarov. He joined the group of Dr. Michael R. Hamblin at Massachusetts General Hospital (Boston, USA) as a Research Intern in 2008. He started his PhD study in Chemistry at Massachusetts Institute of Technology (Cambridge, USA) in 2009. In 2010 he moved to California Institute of Technology (Pasadena, USA) where he is working with Dr. Long Cai on the development and application of super-resolution strategies in fluorescent microscopy.

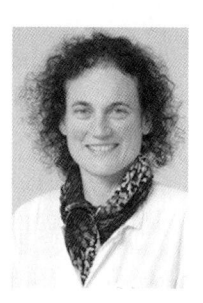

Sibylle Ziegler received her PhD in Physics from the University of Mainz, Germany in 1989. After a Postdoctoral Fellowship at the German Cancer Center in Heidelberg and the Hammersmith Hospital in London, UK she joined the Nuclear Medicine Department at the Technical University in Munich in 1993. Her research is focused on nuclear medical instrumentation and data analysis with an emphasis on multimodal imaging.

Drug Delivery in Oncology – Challenges and Perspectives

Felix Kratz

Summary

To date, none of the approximately 60 anticancer dugs used in conventional chemotherapy exhibits a selective uptake in tumor tissue and generally only a very small fraction of the administered dose reaches the tumor site. If surgery or radiotherapy is not effective, cure rates are in the range of 10% and, as a consequence, 90% of chemotherapeutic agents are administered in the palliative setting to stabilize the disease or to improve the quality of life. With such a low rate of drug accumulation in the tumor it is in fact surprising that tumor remissions can be attained; admittedly, these are achieved in the fast-growing tumors where cytostatic agents alone or in combination therapy are most effective in killing the rapidly dividing tumor cells by inhibiting different specific targets of the tumor cell that are responsible for tumor proliferation. Generally, however, tumor doubling times are slow, the tumor cells are in different stages of their cell cycles, and vascularization in the tumors is heterogeneous with necrotic and hypoxic areas being present that respond poorly to anticancer agents. Last, but not least, late-stage tumors have mostly formed micro- and macrometastases that are characterized by the multidrug resistance phenotype that includes changes in the cellular target of the respective drug, alterations in enzymatic activation and detoxification mechanisms, defective apoptotic pathways, membrane changes as well as elimination of the drug from the tumor cell through the action of drug efflux pumps. For treating metastatic cancer, chemotherapy regimens applied alone or in combination with hormones or novel agents such as monoclonal antibodies and signal transduction inhibitors are to date the best option of inhibiting or reducing the size of the primary tumor and/or metastases. However, treatment is basically palliative and improvement in overall survival through the introduction of novel drugs has generally not been more than a few months. Anticancer agents have steep dose–response curves, which has the consequence that a critical toxic concentration of the drug must be exposed to the tumor cell for a sufficient time to induce cell killing. The dilemma of conventional chemotherapy as well as with low-molecular-weight targeted therapeutics is that due to an unfavorable biodistribution and a lack of accumulation in tumor tissue, they exhibit poor therapeutic indices and tumor remissions are often not achieved. It is here where the potential of drug delivery in oncology resides. Any means of transporting and delivering anticancer drugs in higher concentrations to the tumor over a long period of time whilst sparing healthy tissue is a step to a more effective cancer chemotherapy. This goal has been pursued for approximately 60 years, and has encompassed encapsulating or conjugating drugs with vitamins, lipids, peptides, oligonucleotides, antibodies, serum proteins, synthetic or natural polymers, liposomes, or protein- or polymer-based nano- or microparticles. Aided by the advent of sophisticated diagnostic tumor imaging and analytical tools that have enabled a far more precise understanding of the biochemical and physiological characteristics of tumor cells and tissue, as well as the expression of tumor-associated receptors and antigens, scientists have more opportunities than ever for designing and validating new drug delivery systems. During this process, we are also learning that similar to the translation of targeted therapies into the clinic, drug delivery systems are probably most effective in the form of a personalized medicine and in combination with established chemotherapeutic regimens. This three-volume state-of-the art book gives an account of the different anticancer drug delivery systems realized to date, the products that have reached the clinical setting or have obtained market approval, and the challenges that lie ahead in translational research in the area of cancer drug delivery.

Introduction

> Alle Ding' sind Gift, und nichts ohn' Gift; allein die Dosis macht, daß ein Ding kein Gift ist [All things are poison and nothing is without poison, only the dose permits something not to be poisonous]

When Paracelsus, a pioneer in the application of chemicals and minerals in medicine, wrote this theorem in the sixteenth century, he addressed a fundamental principle that the practicing oncologist faces every day: "How can I treat and hopefully cure a cancer patient with a drug at a nontoxic or acceptable dose without the risk of conversely overdosing and risking severe side-effects or even the death of my patient?"

Paracelsus (1493–1541; true name was Phillippus Aureolus Theophrastus Bombastus von Hohenheim) (Figure 1) went on to summarize his own views on drug development: "Many have said of Alchemy, that it is for the making of gold and silver. For me such is not the aim, but to consider only what virtue and power may lie in medicines" [1].

Scientists over the past 60 years have developed around 60 clinically established cytostatic agents, which are classified into alkylating agents, antimetabolites, anthracyclines, plant alkaloids, microtubule inhibitors or modulators, topoisomerase inhibitors, and other antitumor agents. Their modes of action are diverse and

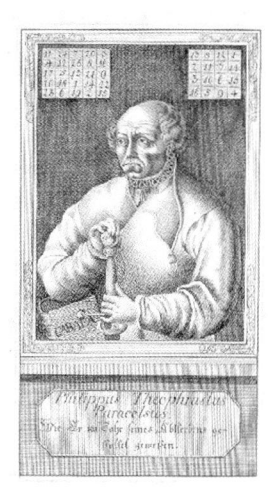

Drug Delivery in Oncology – Challenges and Perspectives | LXI

Figure 1 Paracelsus (Phillippus Aureolus Theophrastus Bombastus von Hohenheim, 1493–1541). "Paracelsus," meaning "equal to or greater than Celsus," refers to the Roman encyclopedist Aulus Cornelius Celsus from the first century, known for his tract on medicine. Paracelsus is also credited with giving zinc its name, calling it *zincum*, and is regarded as the first systematic botanist.

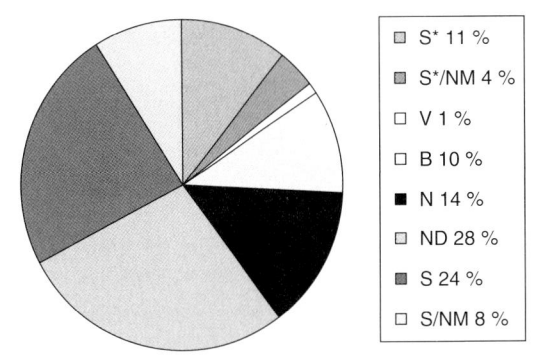

Figure 2 All available anticancer drugs, 1940s to June 2006, by source ($N = 175$). The major categories: B = biological, usually a large (greater than 45 residues) peptide or protein either isolated from an organism/cell line or produced by biotechnological means; N = natural product; ND = derived from a natural product and is usually a semisynthetic modification; NM = natural product mimic; S = totally synthetic drug, often found by random screening/modification of an existing agent; S* = made by total synthesis, but the pharmacophore is/was from a natural product; V = vaccine. (Adapted from [2].)

manifold, and sometimes overlap, resulting in cytotoxic and/or cytostatic effects by affecting cell division, DNA synthesis, or apoptosis.

The era of cancer chemotherapy started with a great deal of optimism in the 1950s after alkylating agents, antimetabolites, and platinum complexes proved to be highly effective in the treatment of hematological malignancies and certain solid tumors. Often the word *chemo*therapy conjures fears in cancer patients due to the notion that they are being treated with toxic and synthetically designed chemicals. Without intending to play down the side-effects of anticancer therapy in any way, 60–70% of anticancer chemotherapeutic agents are in fact natural products or derived from them (Figure 2, as analyzed in depth by Newman and Cragg [2]).

Tumors that respond best to cytostatic or cytotoxic agents are those with fast doubling times of the order of a few days. These include chorioncarcinomas, lymphomas, leukemias, rhabdosarcomas, and testicular cancers. The response rates of the most common solid tumors (i.e., breast, lung, prostate, ovarian, liver, colorectal, gastric, and colorectal cancer) were far less encouraging. From around 1965 onwards, the mostly empirical approach of combining cytostatic agents improved the response rate, the overall survival, and the quality of life for many solid tumors. However, cure rates for the most common metastatic cancers (i.e., lung cancer, colon cancer, breast cancer, and prostate cancer) remained low, and the response rate for many cancers such as renal cell carcinoma, pancreatic carcinoma, gastric carcinoma, hepatocellular carcinoma, glioblastoma, and sarcoma was disappointingly poor.

Although oncologists were well aware of the narrow therapeutic windows of cytostatic agents, there was a continuing hope for many years that by using screening programs, improved preclinical animal models, and optimized combination therapies, new cytotoxic or cytostatic agents would emerge for treating solid tumors more effectively and eventually result in higher cure rates with side-effects being the price that had to be paid.

Despite several novel and effective cytostatic agents being discovered or developed in the past two decades, the advances in molecular and tumor biology from the 1980s onwards, which allowed a progressive elucidation of the genetic, cellular, subcellular as well as physiological mechanisms underlying cancer, continually made scientists working in drug development realize that cancer posed challenges that were not comparable to other fields of chemotherapy where major breakthroughs had been achieved, such as in the treatment of antibacterial, antifungal, or antiprotozoal diseases. Basically, two insights into the characteristics of malignant cells and tissue accounted for this recognition (see Chapter 1):

(i) Cancer cells essentially do not express any molecular targets, neither intra- nor extracellularly, that are unique and not present in healthy tissue.
(ii) The biochemical, cellular, and physiological nature of angiogenesis, proliferation, and invasion of cancer cells as well as the intricate steps involved in the formation of metastases results in tumors that hinder the penetration of therapeutic agents, and in addition a hostile microenvironment develops within the tumor characterized by necrotic, hypoxic, and acidic areas promoting chemoresistance.

In the following section the complexity and heterogeneity of malignant diseases is addressed, as well as the mechanisms of how tumor cells evade the cell-killing effect of drugs on a cellular, subcellular as well as physiological level and the challenges that lie ahead for improving the therapy of this worldwide disease, which according to the World Health Organization accounted for approximately 7.9 million deaths in 2010.

Dilemma and Challenge of Treating Malignant Diseases

A tumor is a neoplasm characterized by a failure in the regulation of tissue growth. The term "tumor" is not synonymous with cancer. A tumor can be benign, premalignant, or malignant, whereas cancer is by definition malignant. The abnormal proliferation of tissues is caused by mutations of genes that fall into two categories: oncogenes that promote cell growth and reproduction, and tumor suppressor genes that inhibit cell division and survival. Cancer develops through the formation of novel oncogenes, the overexpression of normal oncogenes, or the malfunction of tumor suppressor genes. Typically, changes in many genes are required to transform a normal cell into a cancer cell.

The transformation of normal cells into cancer has often been compared to a slow-starting chain reaction caused by initial genetic errors that progressively allow the cells to escape the controls that limit normal tissue growth until the formed cell cluster drives progression toward more invasive stages (Figure 3a). In order to do so, the cancer cell population must form new blood vessels – a process called angiogenesis – to satisfy their growing need for oxygen and nutrients. This is induced when proangiogenic molecules outweigh the effects of molecules with antiangiogenic activities. A so-called angiogenic switch takes place that can already occur when the malignant cell cluster reaches a size of merely 100–200 µm, and cancer cells, endothelial cells, stromal cells, and inflammatory cells secrete growth factors, permeability regulating factors, migration stimulators, proteolytic enzymes, extracellular matrix molecules, and adhesion molecules. The growth factors can be vascular-specific, such as the vascular endothelial growth factors (VEGFs) and their receptors, the angiopoietin family (Ang), Tie receptors, and the ephrins. Nonspecific molecules include platelet-derived growth factor (PDGF), basic fibroblast growth factors (bFGFs), transforming growth factor (TGF)-β, tumor necrosis factor-α (TNF)-α, and epidermal growth factor (EGF).

The process of angiogenesis is extremely complex and requires a series of steps in the "angiogenic cascade," including (Figure 3b):

- Dilation of existing vessels.
- Activation, migration, and proliferation of endothelial cells.
- Hyperpermeability of postcapillary venules and vessel destabilization.
- Localized degradation of basement membrane by proteases such as matrix metalloproteases, cathepsins, urokinase, and plasmin.
- Extracellular matrix remodeling.
- Tube and sprout formation of vessels, and recruitment of pericytes and smooth muscle cells and vessel maturation.

Angiogenesis is not only a prerequisite for the transformation from a small, often dormant cluster of cancer cells to a solid tumor, but is also required for the spread of a tumor – the formation of metastases (the word originating from the Greek "angeion", which means vessel, and "genesis", which means birth). For metastases to form, a complex series of steps in which cancer cells leave the original tumor site and migrate to other parts of the body via the bloodstream or the lymphatic

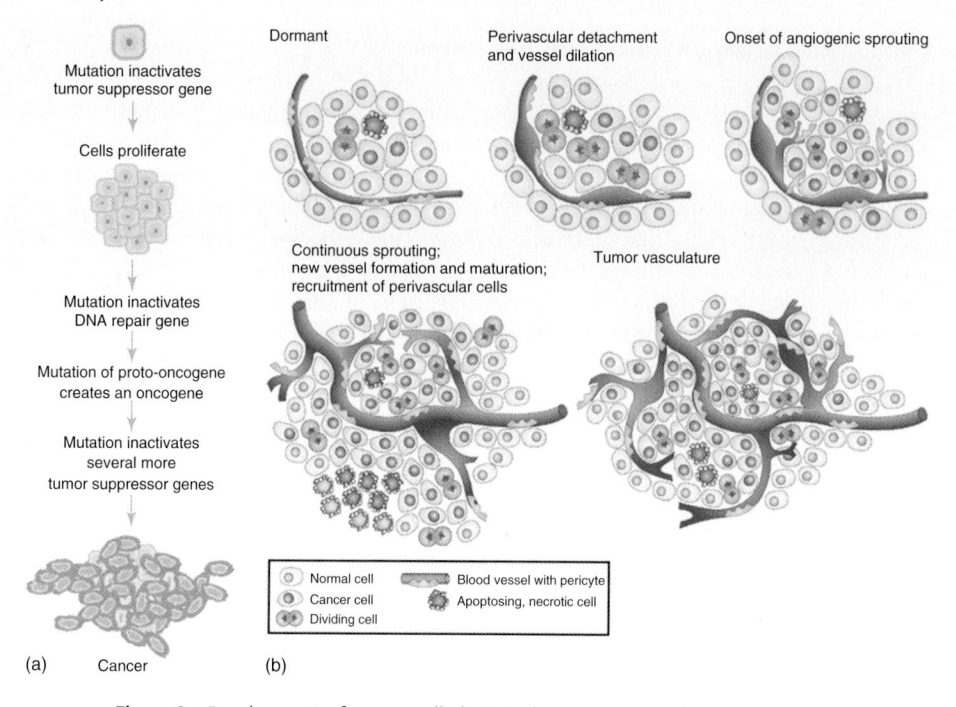

Figure 3 Development of cancer cell clusters due to a series of mutations in oncogenes or tumor suppressor genes (http://en.wikipedia.org/wiki/Cancer), and (b) growth of the solid tumor due to tumor angiogenesis – the formation of blood vessels that supply the cancer cells with oxygen and essential nutrients (modified from [3], with permission).

system have to take place. New evidence suggests that is not only the properties of the metastatic cancer cells, but also of the endothelial progenitor cells that allow single cancer cells to break away from a primary tumor and enter the blood vessels. This mosaicity of endothelial cells and tumor cells together with the secretion of proteases that degrade proteins of the extracellular matrix of the primary tumor allows for substantial shedding of tumor cells into the vasculature. Although the numbers of cells that leave a primary tumor can be of the order of many millions per day, the process of metastasis formation is in fact a very inefficient process because only a small fraction of the cells that leave a tumor are able to survive in the blood or lymphatic vessels, and only a few will have the intrinsic property to find a suitable location to settle and re-enter the tissues and form new tumors. Nevertheless, the formation of metastatic tumors is very common in the late stages of cancer due to the increasing number of tumor cells that are shed from the growing primary tumor. The most common places for the metastases to occur are the lungs, liver, brain, bones, and peritoneal or pleural cavities (see Figure 4 as an example of liver metastases originating from a pancreatic cancer).

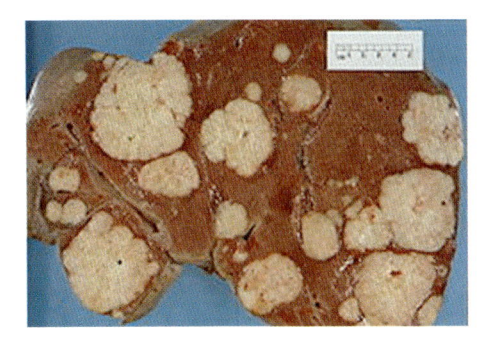

Figure 4 Dissection (surface cut) of a liver showing multiple metastatic nodules originating from a pancreatic cancer (http://en.wikipedia.org/wiki/Metastasis).

The successful treatment of metastases represents such a vital challenge because they are responsible for approximately 90% of cancer-related deaths as well as for the many devastating symptoms that emerge and progress rapidly. In contrast, a primary tumor, such as a prostate cancer, can grow extremely slowly for many years without causing any symptoms at all.

Narrow Therapeutic Window of Cytostatic Agents

One of the main dilemmas of treating solid tumors is that they are not detected early enough and once diagnosed have often formed metastases. If they cannot be treated by surgery in combination with radiotherapy or neoadjuvant chemotherapy, the prognosis for curing the patient, mostly expressed in the literature as at least a 5-year tumor-free interval, remains highly unsatisfactory. Current chemotherapy regimens applied alone or in combination with hormones or novel agents such as monoclonal antibodies and signal transduction inhibitors are to date the best option for inhibiting or reducing the size of the primary tumor and/or metastases. Chemotherapy regimens are generally applied intravenously in cycles (ranging from a 1- to 4-week interval), with the frequency and duration of treatments limited by the toxicity to the patient. Most commonly, chemotherapy acts by killing cells that divide actively – one of the main properties of most cancer cells. As a consequence, cytostatic agents also harm cells that divide rapidly under normal circumstances, such as cells in the bone marrow, digestive tract, and hair follicles, producing side-effects in these organs. In most cases the cytostatic agents have distinct toxicity profiles, such as neurotoxicity, nephrotoxicity, dermatotoxicity, ototoxicity, and cardiotoxicity. These can be difficult to treat, are often dose-limiting, and in some cases are irreversible.

Despite these drawbacks, it is obligatory that repeated and optimized chemotherapy cycles be administered in order to obtain the best therapeutic outcome and to continuously reduce the size of the tumors or metastases. Only a fraction of the cells in a tumor die with each treatment cycle. This principle is known as the *log-cell-kill hypothesis*, which is a generally accepted hypothesis for hematological cancers that states that during every cycle of chemotherapy the same fraction of tumor cells is killed, but not the same number. When mice with leukemia are treated with constant doses of anticancer agents, the number of leukemia cells diminishes logarithmically; if, for example, 99% of leukemia cells are killed after the first administration, this is equivalent to a decrease of 10^9–10^7 cells, which corresponds to 2 orders of magnitude (two log steps). A second administration will also result in a 99% cell kill, but the number of tumor cells is only reduced from 10^7 to 10^5, which is only 10 million cells compared to the billion cells in the first cycle. In other words, in this idealized model, the fraction of cells that are killed remains constant, but the number of cells killed over time constantly decreases.

Transferring the log-cell-kill hypothesis to solid tumors is not as straightforward as it appears at first glance (Figure 5). With modern diagnostics, a tumor is detectable when it reaches a size of 1 cm³ after 30 doubling cycles, which

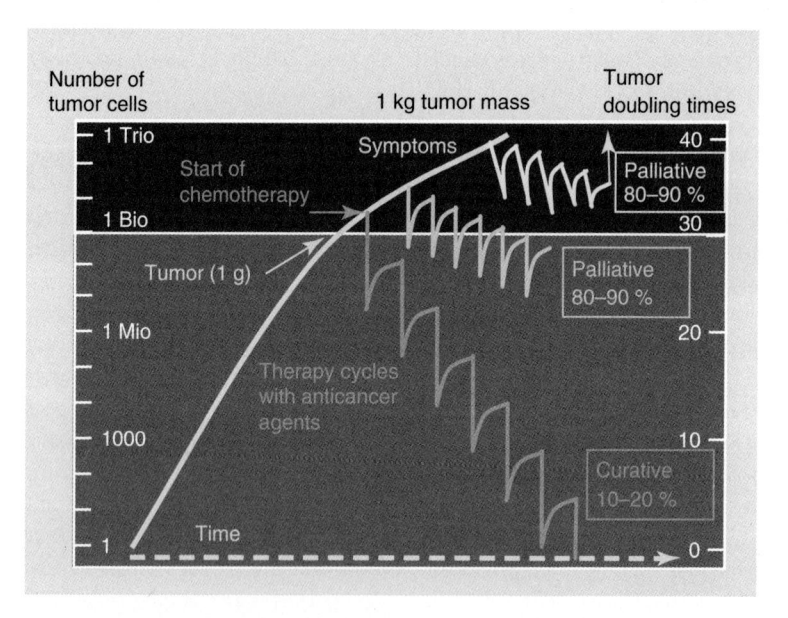

Figure 5 Tumor growth curve of a solid tumor. Once the tumor comprises approximately 1 billion tumor cells, its size is around 1 cm³ (1 g) and it becomes detectable. The initial tumor cell has to perform 30 doubling steps to reach this size (which can take months to years considering that the tumor doubling times for human tumors lies in the range of 5–200 days), and merely further 10 doublings are needed to reach a mass of 1 kg assuming tumor growth occurs exponentially. This generally does take place because of an insufficient growing vasculature in large tumors leading to a lack of supply of nutrients and tumor necrosis. Of note is that according to the log-cell-kill hypothesis many cycles of chemotherapy are necessary to eliminate all of the tumor cells and only in 10–20% of cases are cures achieved. Palliative treatment is particularly disappointing with large tumors where only a relatively small fraction of tumor cells respond to anticancer agents.

corresponds to 1 g (i.e., 10^9 cancer cells). Only 10 further doubling steps are necessary for the tumor to reach a size of 1 kg (i.e., 10^{12} cancer cells). In this time interval, tumor symptoms start emerging.

These insights are the reason why during curative, adjuvant, or palliative chemotherapy the doses and cycles of anticancer agents should not be reduced or discontinued even if the tumor or tumor lesions are no longer detectable, assuming that the treatment is tolerated by the patient. The log-cell-kill hypothesis can additionally be viewed as a theoretical basis for further treating patients for longer periods even though a complete remission has apparently been achieved.

However, the log-cell-kill hypothesis is strictly valid only for solid tumors, if at all, and only for those that are fast growing; however, in most cases the effect of cytostatic or cytotoxic agents on tumor growth can be described by the so-called Gompertz growth curve. This implies that tumor growth diminishes with increasing size of the tumor, which is noted in the semilogarithmic plot by a decreasing slope of the tumor growth curve as depicted in Figure 5. With increasing tumor size, many tumor cells remain in the G phase (quiescent phase) of the cell cycle because of an insufficient growing vasculature leading to a lack of supply of nutrients and tumor necrosis. In this phase, the response to treatment with anticancer agents is significantly reduced and the initial cycle of chemotherapy only manages to kill a fraction of the tumor cells, mostly those proliferating in the periphery of the tumor. As a consequence, the tumor mass is reduced, and quiescent cells are reactivated to enter the cell cycle and multiply. This is the reason why the response in the second or third cycle of palliative treatment is often better than in the first cycle because a higher percentage of tumor cells are killed.

Unfortunately, in this advanced stage of the disease further reduction of tumor size is seldom achieved because a population of tumor cells that has developed chemoresistance and/or micrometastases has already formed. Intrinsic or acquired chemoresistance is a major problem in cancer therapy. In the majority of cases the cancer cells develop resistance against a spectrum of anticancer agents – a phenomenon called multidrug resistance (MDR). A number of biochemical mechanisms have been described that are responsible for the MDR phenotype, which include changes in the cellular target of the respective drug, alterations in enzymatic activation and detoxification mechanisms, defective apoptotic pathways, membrane changes as well as elimination of the drug from the tumor cell through the action of drug efflux pumps such as P-glycoprotein, multiple resistance protein (MRP), and breast cancer resistance protein (BCRP), which belong to the ATP-binding cassette (ABC) transporter family. Hence, the concentration of the anticancer agent in tumor cells remains too low and cannot counterbalance the diverse mechanisms of chemoresistance. In addition, there are a number of physiological mechanisms that are responsible for resistance to chemotherapy as well as an impaired accessibility of anticancer drugs and drug delivery systems to all parts of the malignant tissue due to the heterogeneity of the tumor mass, as will be described below (for details, see Chapter 2).

Heterogeneity of Solid Tumors: Abnormal Blood Vessel Networks, Tumor Physiology, and Tumor Environment

Once a tumor cell cluster, whether in its initial stage as a primary tumor or in later stages when forming metastases, induces an angiogenic switch, its vasculature and microenvironment change dramatically, and an abnormal cellular organization, vessel structure, and physiological function develops. As an example, in contrast to the unbranched, nearly parallel vessels of healthy tissue (Figure 6A, right) of a murine brain, the vasculature of a brain tumor is dense, chaotic, and highly branched (Figure 6A, left).

The new tumor vessels formed during angiogenesis differ markedly from those of normal tissue and the neovasculature is characterized by an irregular shape, high density, and heterogeneity (Figure 6B). In addition, the endothelial cells are poorly aligned or disorganized with large fenestrations (Figure 6C, b–c). Other differences affect the perivascular cells, the basement membrane, and the smooth muscle layer that are frequently absent or abnormal. As a consequence, solid tumors are heterogeneous and form a complex society of cells in different microenvironments that can hinder the penetration not only of low-molecular-weight anticancer compounds, but also of macromolecular drug delivery systems through the same or different mechanisms.

These pathophysiological properties of tumors that influence the delivery of drugs to tumor tissue include (for details, see Chapter 2):

(i) **Abnormal structure of tumor vasculature.** The variable vascular density restricts the anticancer drug from reaching all parts within the tumor. This is due to the abnormal branching patterns and intercapillary distances in growing tumors. Tumor vessels are dilated, tortuous, and heterogeneous in their

Figure 6 (A–C) Differences in the architecture of microvessels and endothelial cells between healthy and tumor tissue. (A) Normal vasculature in the brain of a mouse (right) is very orderly, compared with the extremely branched vasculature of a mammary brain tumor (left). (B) Scanning electron microscopy (SEM) imaging of a polymer cast of normal microvasculature (vasa vasorum of rat carotid sinus, left) and tumor microvasculature (xenograft of a human head and neck cancer of a nude mouse, right). Marked differences are found in the degree of organization and an apparent lack of conventional hierarchy of blood vessels in the tumor sample. (C) SEM images of the luminal surface of healthy blood vessels (mammary gland, left) and tumor (MCa-IV mouse mammary carcinoma, right) blood vessels. While the healthy vessels are smooth and have tight endothelial junctions, the tumor vessels show widened intercellular spaces, overlapping endothelial cells, and other abnormalities. SEM images: (a) luminal surface of normal blood vessel, which is smooth and has tight endothelial junctions (arrowheads, mouse mammary gland); (b) tumor blood vessel, which has widened intercellular spaces, overlapping endothelial cells, multiple cellular processes, and other abnormalities (arrowheads, MCa-IV mouse mammary carcinoma); and (c) high magnification of a hole in the endothelium (arrows) showing the underlying basement membrane filaments (arrowheads). Scale bar: 5 μm in (a); 2 μm in (b); 0.5 μm in (c). (Reproduced kind permission of M. Konerding, University of Mainz, modified from [4].)

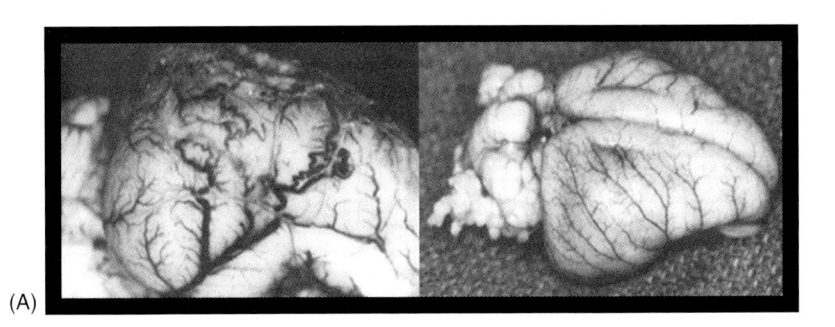

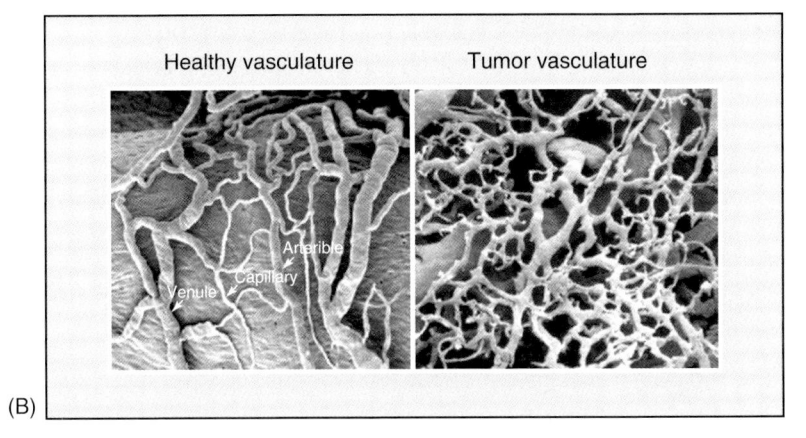

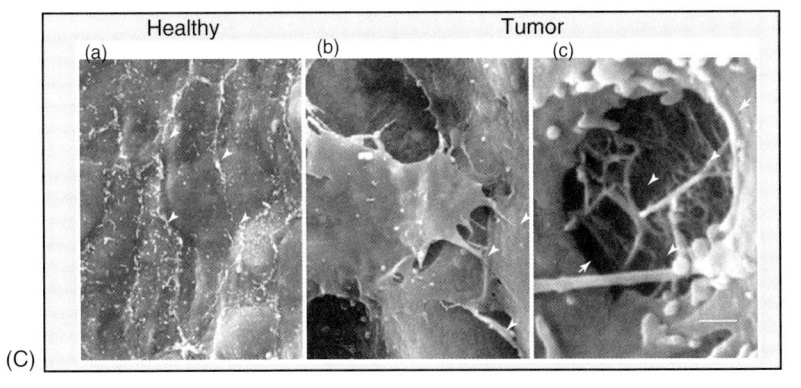

Drug Delivery in Oncology – Challenges and Perspectives | **LXIX**

(A)

(B) Healthy vasculature   Tumor vasculature

(C) Healthy   Tumor
(a)   (b)   (c)

spatial distribution. Intervessel distances in solid tumors can vary between 10 and 1000 μm, and thus many viable tumor cells are not exposed to detectable concentrations of low-molecular-weight drugs following a single injection. In these tumor regions the anticancer drugs do not achieve sufficient concentrations to kill all of the cancer cells. In addition, the concentrations of essential nutrients in these tumor regions are also low, leading to hypoxic, acidic, and necrotic areas that can partially or completely reduce the cytotoxicity of the anticancer agent.

(ii) **Abnormal blood flow in tumors.** Blood flow rates in many tumors are generally lower than those in many normal tissues and can vary considerably, ranging from around 0.01 to around 3.0 ml/g/min. The heterogeneity of tumor blood flow directly hinders the delivery of therapeutic agents to tumors and additionally causes interstitial pressure that in turn compromises the effectiveness of various therapies, and selects for more aggressive and metastatic cancer cells.

(iii) **Interstitial fluid pressure in tumors.** The interstitial compartment of tumors is significantly different to that of normal tissues. Primarily, as a result of vessel leakiness and hyperpermeablity with a concomitant bulk flow of free fluid into the interstitial space that cannot be removed effectively due to a lack of functional lymphatics, most solid tumors have an increased interstitial fluid pressure. Increased interstitial fluid pressure within solid tumors above all inhibits the extravascular transport of larger molecules and nanoparticles because they rely more heavily on convection as opposed to simple transport by diffusion of low-molecular-weight drugs; exceptions being the transport into the core of the tumor through receptors expressed on the tumor endothelium by transcytosis such as for albumin (see Chapters 4 and 35).

The interstitial fluid pressure can, however, also hamper the efficacy of low-molecular-weight anticancer drugs because, although it is fairly uniform within the center regions of the tumor, the interstitial fluid pressure is significantly reduced at the tumor periphery, and interstitial fluid oozes out of the tumor and subsequently removes anticancer agents from the tumor tissue.

(iv) **Pathophysiological tumor microenvironment as an obstacle in tumor therapy.** As mentioned above, abnormal blood vessels are formed during tumor growth and blood flow in these vessels is heterogeneous, thus the intermittent blood supply leaves portions of the tumor with regions where the oxygen concentration is significantly lower than in healthy tissues. As a consequence, the lack of oxygen promotes an anaerobic metabolism of tumor cells and an extracellular acidosis in tumor tissue in the range of pH 6.0–6.8 prevails, primarily due to excessive production of lactic acid and CO_2. The hypoxic tumor cells as well as acidosis present in many solid tumors manifest a pathophysiological microenvironment that is often resistant to radiotherapy and chemotherapy. On the one hand, the mode of action of several anticancer agents (e.g., cyclophosphamide, methotrexate, 5-fluorouracil (5-FU), etoposide, carboplatin, bleomycin, and anthracyclines) is oxygen-dependent and thus hypoxia protects tumor cells from damage by chemotherapy. On the other hand, extracellular acidosis in tumors reduces the tissue and cellular uptake of weakly basic drugs such as anthracyclines, bleomycin, mitoxantrone, and vinca alkaloids because their cellular uptake by diffusion is primarily efficient only for the nonionized form of the molecule. In addition, various mechanisms may additionally be involved in the acidosis-induced resistance to anticancer drugs, including an increased efflux of drugs, resistance to apoptosis, and an increased activity of DNA repair enzymes. That regions of hypoxic, acidic, and necrotic influence tissue penetration of a drug such as doxorubicin is shown impressively for three different preclinical tumors in mice in Figure 7. The immunofluorescence images after administration show the blood vessels in red, hypoxic areas in green, and doxorubicin in blue. The penetration lengths for doxorubicin

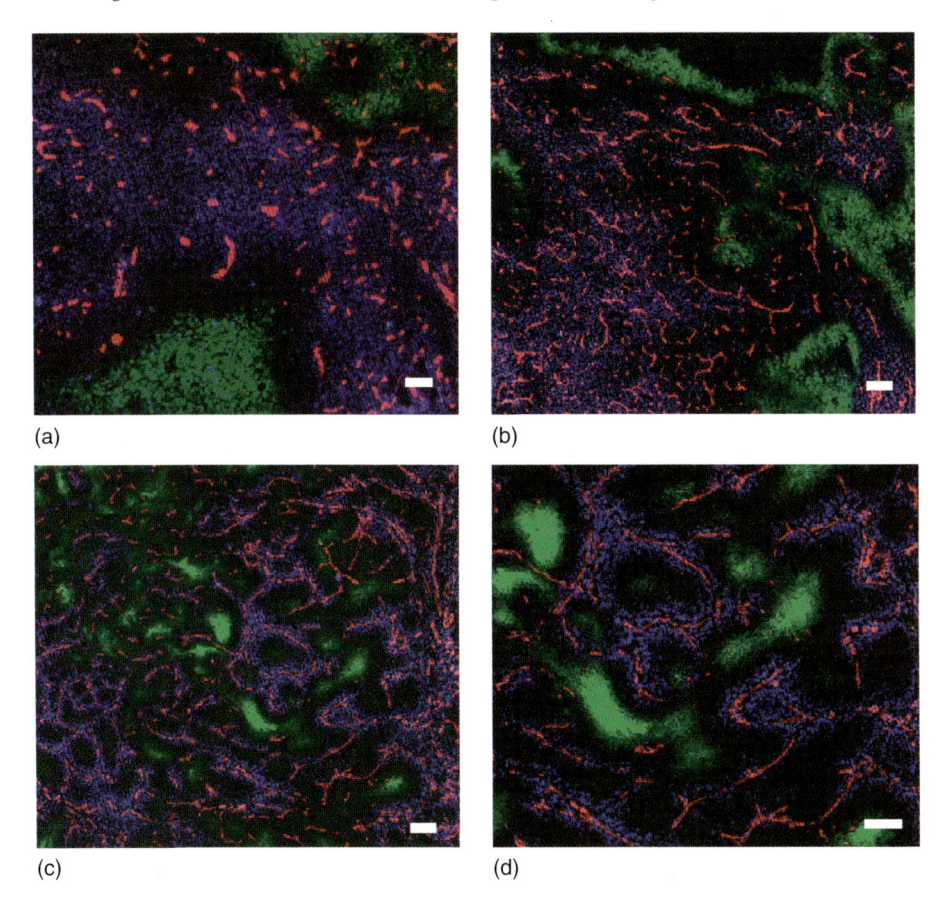

Figure 7 Representative three-color composite images showing the perivascular distribution of doxorubicin (blue) in relation to blood vessels (red) and hypoxic regions (green) in three different tumors growing in the right flank of mice: (a) human prostate PC-3 carcinoma, (b) mouse mammary sarcoma EMT-6, and (c and d) 16/C mammary carcinoma. Bar: 100 µm. (From [5].)

from the nearest blood vessels vary considerably within a 100 µm range and doxorubicin is unable to accumulate in hypoxic areas.

Drug Treatment for Cancer Diseases: State-of-the-Art

Current drug treatment for cancer diseases is based on therapy with cytostatic agents, hormones, cytokines, targeted therapeutics (monoclonal antibodies, tyrosine kinase inhibitors, proteasome inhibitors, histone deacetylase (HDAC) inhibitors), drug delivery systems (liposomes, albumin nanoparticles), and supportive care (pain therapy, hematopoietic growth factors, alternative therapies). Figure 8 gives a historic overview of the major classes of drugs and representative examples of the global cancer market. Sales for cancer-treating drugs increased by 10–14% in the past 3 years and is predicted to expand to approximately US$100 billion by 2012.

It is apparent when interpreting Figure 8 that the largest number of new drugs belong to so-called *targeted therapy*, which is defined as a medication that blocks the growth of cancer cells by interfering with specific intra- or extracellular molecular targets needed for carcinogenesis and tumor growth rather than by simply interfering with rapidly dividing cells. This term is somewhat misleading because most cytostatic agents used in chemotherapy also act on one or several molecular targets. The major difference is that many of the drugs that act as cytostatic agents were discovered by serendipity or in screening programs of natural products against a panel of tumor cell lines and were at the time often developed without any notion of their mode of action or cellular targets. In contrast, a new generation of targeted therapeutics was designed with an isolated target in hand, allowing for the generation of rationally designed drugs that had predetermined modes of activity. These agents were often derived using such techniques as high-throughput screening, molecular modeling, and structure-based design.

From the 1980s onwards this was a logically consistent step to take. Molecular and genetic approaches uncovered entirely new signaling networks of intra- and extracellular kinases, growth factor receptors, and antigens that regulate activities of tumor cells and tumor tissue, such as their epigenetic nature, their proliferation and survival as well as angiogenesis. As a result, the pharmaceutical and biotech industry invested heavily into the generation of targeted therapeutics.

When examining Figure 8, it is logical to ask whether the development of these new drugs in the past decade has translated into a reduction in cancer mortality or 5-year relative survival. In developed countries, approximately one in four deaths are due to cancer. If we take the American Cancer Society's *Cancer Facts & Figures* report of 2010 for the United States as a guideline, the 5-year survival rate for all cancers diagnosed from 1999 to 2005 in the United States was 68%, up from 50% in 1975–1977. This improvement is primarily due to earlier diagnosis and conventional chemotherapy, but above all due to the refinement in surgery and radiotherapy, which have for many indications reached an optimal technical endpoint.

Drug Delivery in Oncology – Challenges and Perspectives | LXXIII

	Cytostatic agents				Cytokines	Targeted therapeutics		Drug delivery systems
1950	Alkylating agents							
1955	Antimetabolites							
1960		Hormones						
1965	N-mustards	Tamoxifen®, Toremifen®						
1970	Platinum complexes	Estrogenes: Fosfesterol®						
1975								
1980	Anthracyclines							
1985	Vinca-alcaloids							
1990		Flutamid® Bicalutamid						
1995	Taxanes	Cytadren® Letrozol® Ananstrozol®			Interleukin-2			Liposomes: Doxil®, Daunsosome®, Myocet®
2000	Camptothecins				Interferon-α			Drug polymer conjugate: SMANCS®
2005	Xeloda®, a 5-FU prodrug					Antibodies	Small molecules	Albumin taxol Nanoparticle: Abraxane®
2010	Epithilones					Herceptin® Campath® Rituxan® Avastin® Erbitux®	Gleevec® Iressa®, Tarceva® Velcade® Virinostat®	

Figure 8 Major classes of drugs for treating cancer since 1950 and representative examples.

Table 1 Cancer incidence and 5-year prevalence trend from 2005 to 2009 in the United States[a].

Year	Cancer incidence	Five-year prevalence trend
2005	1372910	4519388
2007	1444920	4665096
2008	1437180	4540106
2009	1479350	4774257

[a] http/www.cancer.org.com.

In contrast, as shown in Table 1, an analysis of the cancer incidence and 5-year prevalence trend from 2005 to 2009 reveals that the overall 5-year-survival rate increased by merely around 5.7%, with the number of new cases increasing from 1 372 910 in 2005 to 1 437 180 in 2009 owing basically to an aging population.

It should be emphasized that nearly all targeted therapeutics, whether antibodies or small molecules, are used in combination with conventional chemotherapy and it is largely these combination protocols that account for the increase in overall survival rates for cancer patients. This analysis is not in any way meant to discredit the efforts and successes that have been achieved with so-called targeted therapy, and R&D in this field should certainly be continued. Rather, the analysis shows how difficult it is to treat cancer even with rationally designed drugs with defined targets. In many cases the actual therapeutic advantages gained were suboptimal. This underscores how progress in cancer treatment is achieved in small steps.

If there is room for criticism, it is that the scientific community, the cancer funding organizations as well as the pharmaceutical industry are prone to follow new trends and easily forget that an empirical as opposed to a rational approach in drug design can be equally successful. For example, cisplatin has made testicular cancer in young men a curable cancer. The drug is a metal complex discovered fortuitously by Barnett Rosenberg when he noticed that that during an electrolysis experiment with platinum electrodes the growth of the common bacteria *Escherichia coli* was inhibited. In contrast, Gleevec® is a selective inhibitor of an aberrant, constitutively active enzyme, the BCR–ABL tyrosine kinase, that was developed by rational drug design and screening chemical libraries with subsequent lead optimization. The drug is highly effective in treating chronic myelogenous leukemia and gastrointestinal stromal tumors, and is currently being investigated in other tumor indications. Rational design of targeted therapeutics can even take a paradox turn. Although sorafenib (marketed as Nexavar® by Bayer) was developed as a specific kinase type II inhibitor against Raf kinase, it was subsequently found to inhibit a variety of kinase receptors, including VEGF, EGF, and PDGF receptors. As it turned out, sorafenib was not approved in tumors with high Raf kinase expression such as melanoma or colorectal cancer, but is now approved as a multikinase inhibitor for advanced renal cell carcinoma and advanced hepatocellular carcinoma, (i.e., tumor indications for which it was never originally intended). Conversely,

Figure 9

```
┌─────────────────────┐  ┌─────────────────────┐  ┌─────────────────────┐
│ Micro- and macro-   │  │ Macromolecular      │  │ Low-molecular weight│
│ particulate drug    │  │ drug conjugates     │  │ drug conjugates     │
│ delivery systems    │  │                     │  │                     │
└─────────────────────┘  └─────────────────────┘  └─────────────────────┘
```

- Liposomes
- Nanoparticles
- Hydrogels
- Micelles

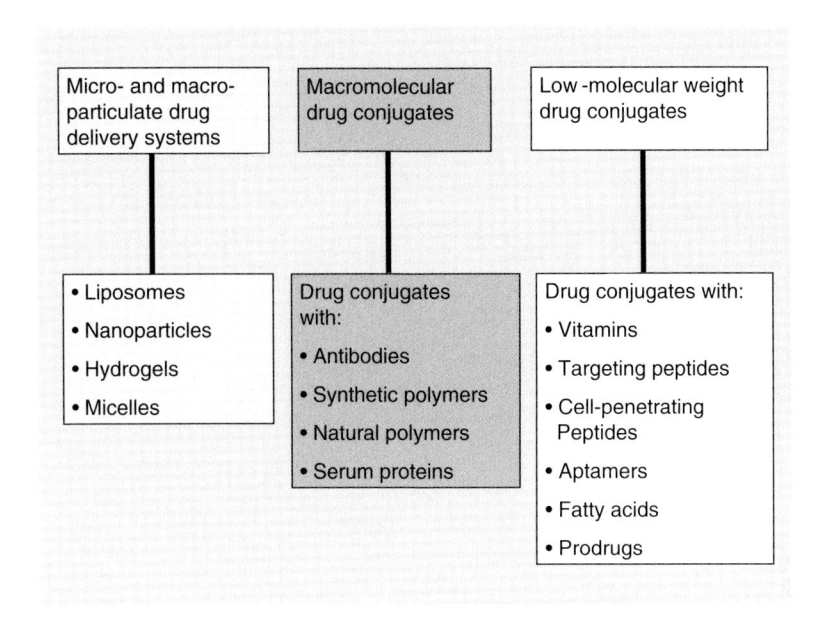

Drug conjugates with:
- Antibodies
- Synthetic polymers
- Natural polymers
- Serum proteins

Drug conjugates with:
- Vitamins
- Targeting peptides
- Cell-penetrating Peptides
- Aptamers
- Fatty acids
- Prodrugs

Figure 9 Classification of drug delivery systems.

even after intensive investigations and thousands of publications on this topic, we still do not know why cisplatin is so highly effective against testicular cancer and not against other solid tumors.

Principles of Tumor Targeting

Drug delivery systems can be classified as micro- and macroparticulate drug delivery systems, macromolecular drug conjugates, and low-molecular-weight drug conjugates (Figure 9).

Whereas the drug is physically encapsulated in liposomes, nanoparticles, hydrogels, or micelles, it is covalently bound to the diverse low- and high-molecular weight drug carriers when developing drug conjugates. Transporting the drug cargo to the tumor site relies on two principles – defined as active and passive targeting, which are described below.

Active Targeting: Receptors and Antigens on Tumor Cells

Active targeting is based on cellular differences between normal and cancer tissue. From 1975 onwards the field of drug targeting received an important impetus with the development of monoclonal antibodies by Köhler and Milstein. Using this technology, it was now possible to derive pure antibodies that bound specifically to targets that were overexpressed on tumor cells. Thus, it seemed that the realization

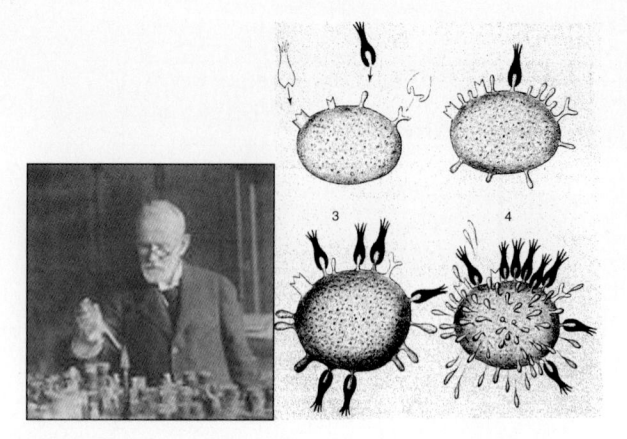

Figure 10 Hand drawing by Paul Ehrlich (1854–1915) illustrating his concept of receptor–ligand interaction. (Thanks to Professor Gerd Folkers of the ETH, Zurich, Switzerland for supplying this drawing.)

of Paul Ehrlich's early twentieth century vision of "the magic bullet" was at hand (Figure 10).

Although Paul Ehrlich is often regarded as the father of chemotherapy and drug targeting that is based on the concept of affinity, he was not involved in the concepts of drug delivery as is often mistakenly cited in the literature [6]. The concept of cancer drug delivery implies transporting the anticancer drug to the tumor tissue and cells with subsequent release, either intra- or extracellularly. Drug conjugates developed for active targeting comprise mostly high-molecular weight carriers, but low-molecular weight compounds are also used. A suitable carrier combines optimal loading and release properties, long-term circulation, low toxicity, and high affinity for the receptor or antigen without increasing drug levels in healthy tissue.

The elucidation of suitable membrane-associated targets and the subsequent targeting properties of carriers and validation in preclinical models in the clinic have been expedited by the advances in immunohistochemistry, fluorescence-activated cell sorting analysis, and ultimately the refinement of tumor imaging techniques that can be routinely applied in the preclinical as well as clinical setting (see Chapters 7, 8, 9, and 15).

Selected cellular targets together with appropriate carriers that have been investigated for active targeting in cancer therapy are shown in Table 2.

Passive Targeting and the Enhanced and Permeation Effect in Relation to Tumor Targeting

In same year as Köhler and Milstein reported on their pioneering work on the production of monoclonal antibodies, Helmut Ringsdorf proposed a general scheme of designing a drug delivery system using synthetic polymers for low-molecular

Table 2 Examples of membrane-associated targets and drug carriers for active targeting.

Receptors	Representative drug carrier
Vascular receptors Integrins ($\alpha_v\beta_3$, $\alpha_v\beta_5$), Nucleolin, Aminopeptidase N, Endoglin, VEGF receptor (VEGF1–4)	linear peptides, cyclic peptides, antibodies, immunoliposomes
Receptors of plasma proteins, Low-density lipoprotein receptor, Transferrin receptor, Albondin (gp60)	lipoproteins, transferrin, albumin antibodies
Peptide receptors, Somatostatin receptor, Bombesin receptor, Neuropeptide Y receptors, Luteinizing hormone receptor	linear peptides
Receptors for growth factors and vitamins, Folate receptors, EGF receptors (e.g., EGF1, EGF2, HER2), TGF receptor, FGF receptors	folic acid, antibodies
Carbohydrate recognizing receptors, Asialoglycoprotein receptor, Galectins (e.g., galectin 1, galectin 3), Selectins (e.g., E-selectin, P-selectin), Hyaluronic acid receptors (CD44, glucose uptake transporters	lactosaminated albumin, gylocoside clusters, natural polymers, sugars
Antigens Cluster of differentiation (e.g., CD20, CD33), Carcinoembryonic antigen, Blood group carbohydrates, Mucin-type glycoproteins (MUC1, CanAg), Lewis Y, Lewis X Cancer testis antigens (CT7, MAGE-A3), Prostate-specific membrane antigen	antibodies, immunoliposomes

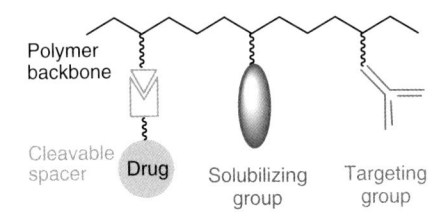

Figure 11 Ringsdorf's model for a polymeric drug containing the drug, solubilizing groups, and targeting groups bound to a linear polymer backbone.

weight drugs (Figure 11). One to several drug molecules are bound to a polymeric backbone through a spacer that incorporates a predetermined breaking point to ensure release of the drug before or after cellular uptake of the conjugate. The system can also contain solubilizing groups or targeting moieties that render water solubility and targeting properties to the carrier.

Ringsdorf's visionary model for developing drug delivery systems was basically ignored for many years, and it was not until Hiroshi Maeda laid the foundations for

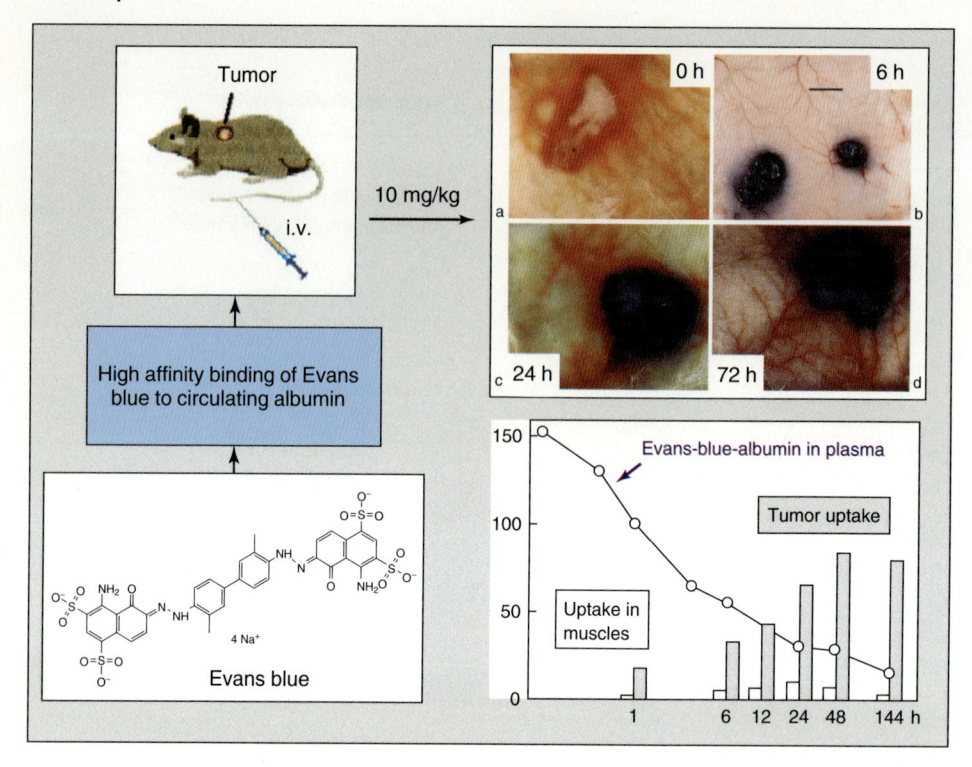

Figure 12 After injection of Evans blue into mice. The dye binds selectively and tightly to circulating albumin, and due to the leaky vasculature and defective lymphatic drainage system in subcutaneously growing tumors is retained in tumor tissue. Hiroshi Maeda coined the term "enhanced permeation and retention effect" for this mechanism of passive tumor targeting for macromolecules.

passive targeting in 1986 that drug conjugates with synthetic polymers were intensively synthesized and evaluated for their antitumor efficacy. In 1986, he reported on a simple animal experiment. He intravenously injected the albumin-binding dye Evans blue into mice bearing subcutaneously growing tumors and to his surprise found that the Evans blue–albumin complex accumulated within tumors very efficiently (Figure 12). As an explanation for this phenomenon, Hiroshi Maeda coined the expression "enhanced permeability and retention" in relation to passive tumor targeting – the so-called EPR effect. In contrast to active targeting that proceeds on a cellular level focusing on the specific molecular interactions with tumor-associated cell receptors or antigens, passive targeting represents a more universal strategy of tumor targeting that exploits anomalies of malignant tissue resulting from the tumor's pathophysiology. As described above, blood vessels differ markedly from those of normal tissue, characterized by an irregular shape and the endothelial cells are poorly aligned or disorganized with large fenestrations having diameters in the range of around 100–500 nm. These anatomical features make the vasculature

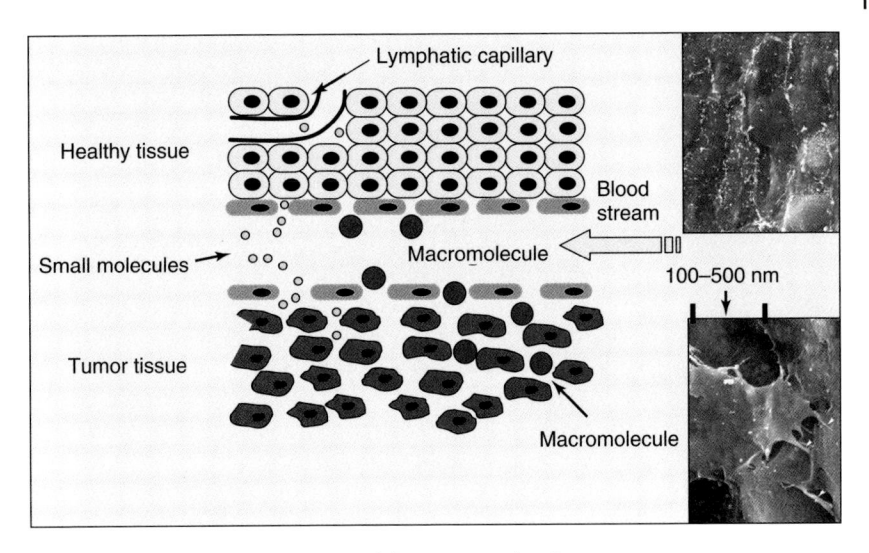

Figure 13 Schematic representation of the anatomical and physiological characteristics of normal and tumor tissue with respect to the vascular permeability and retention of small and large molecules (EPR effect).

of tumor tissue permeable for macromolecules such as albumin or even larger nano-sized particles. Once the macromolecules have permeated into the tumor bed, a second effect is responsible for their tumor accumulation. Whereas smaller molecules are rapidly cleared from the tumor interstitium, large molecules are retained due to an impaired or absent lymphatic system (Figure 13).

A number of factors influence the EPR effect in preclinical animal models: the size and type of the tumor, and the tumor model (subcutaneously growing, intramuscular growing, spontaneously growing, orthotopically implanted, or chemically induced) all affect vascularization and the extent of hypoxic and necrotic areas. Indeed, techniques such as intravital imaging have provided a detailed insight into the tumor microcirculation and microenvironment confirming hyperpermeability, a heterogeneous and compromised blood flow, and an absence of functional lymphatic vessels resulting in elevated interstitial fluid pressure that hinder the delivery of therapeutic agents to tumors. It is therefore likely that although the EPR effect is universal to all tumors, the extent of the EPR effect can vary considerably within the tumor. Interestingly, there are a number of strategies emerging that enhance the EPR effect, including raising blood pressure or coadministering drugs that act as vascular mediators and release nitric oxide (see Chapter 3 for details).

In summary, the EPR effect has laid the foundation for developing a spectrum of drug delivery systems ranging from micro- and macroparticles, liposomes, drug conjugates with synthetic polymers to serum proteins.

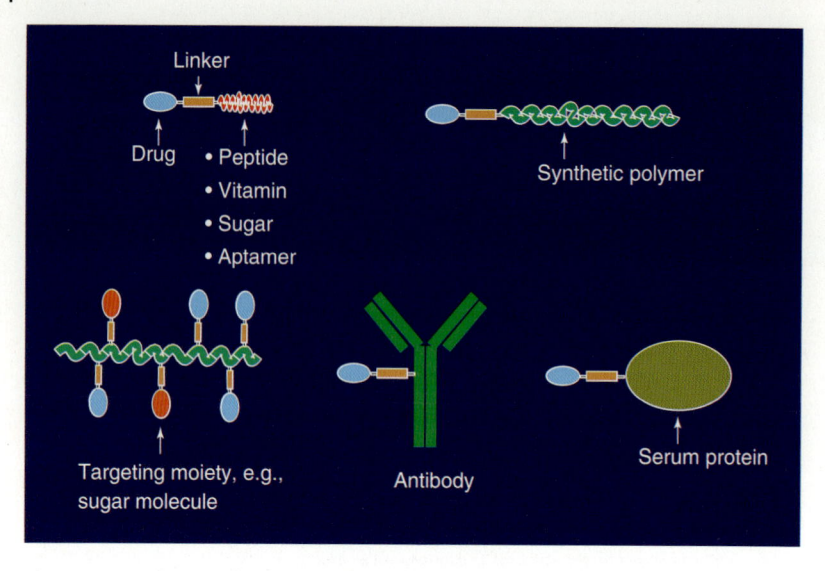

Figure 14 Examples of low- and high-molecular weight drug conjugates. In the vast majority of drug conjugates the drugs are bound through predetermined breaking points to the carrier (see Chapters 10, 12, 17–24, 37, 38, 40, 41).

Design and Development of Drug Delivery Systems

The principle structures of drug delivery systems that have been developed during the past six decades are depicted in Figures 14 and 15. While the drug conjugates with different carriers illustrated in Figure 14 can be small molecules as well as macromolecular drug delivery systems usually between 5 and 20 nm in size, the micro- and macroparticulate drug delivery systems are by nature all large particles with diameters exceeding 50 nm. These drug delivery systems encompass encapsulating or conjugating drugs with vitamins, lipids, peptides, aptamers, antibodies, synthetic or natural polymers, liposomes, or protein- or polymer-based nano- or microparticles. Related approaches have also been realized for the drug delivery of DNA and RNA as illustrated in Figure 16.

Both the covalent coupling of a drug or the physical encapsulation of a drug inside a carrier allow active or passive targeting drug delivery strategies to be realized. When designing drug delivery systems, the drug bound to the carrier should have sufficient stability in the bloodstream, but allow the drug to be released effectively at the tumor site by enzymatic cleavage, by reduction, or in a pH-dependent manner. Release of the free drug can occur extra- and/or intracellularly. Low- and high-molecular weight drug delivery systems that interact with a tumor-associated antigen or receptor are taken up by the tumor cell through antigen- or receptor-mediated endocytosis, drug delivery systems that follow a passive targeting approach by adsorptive or fluid-phase endocytosis. As depicted in

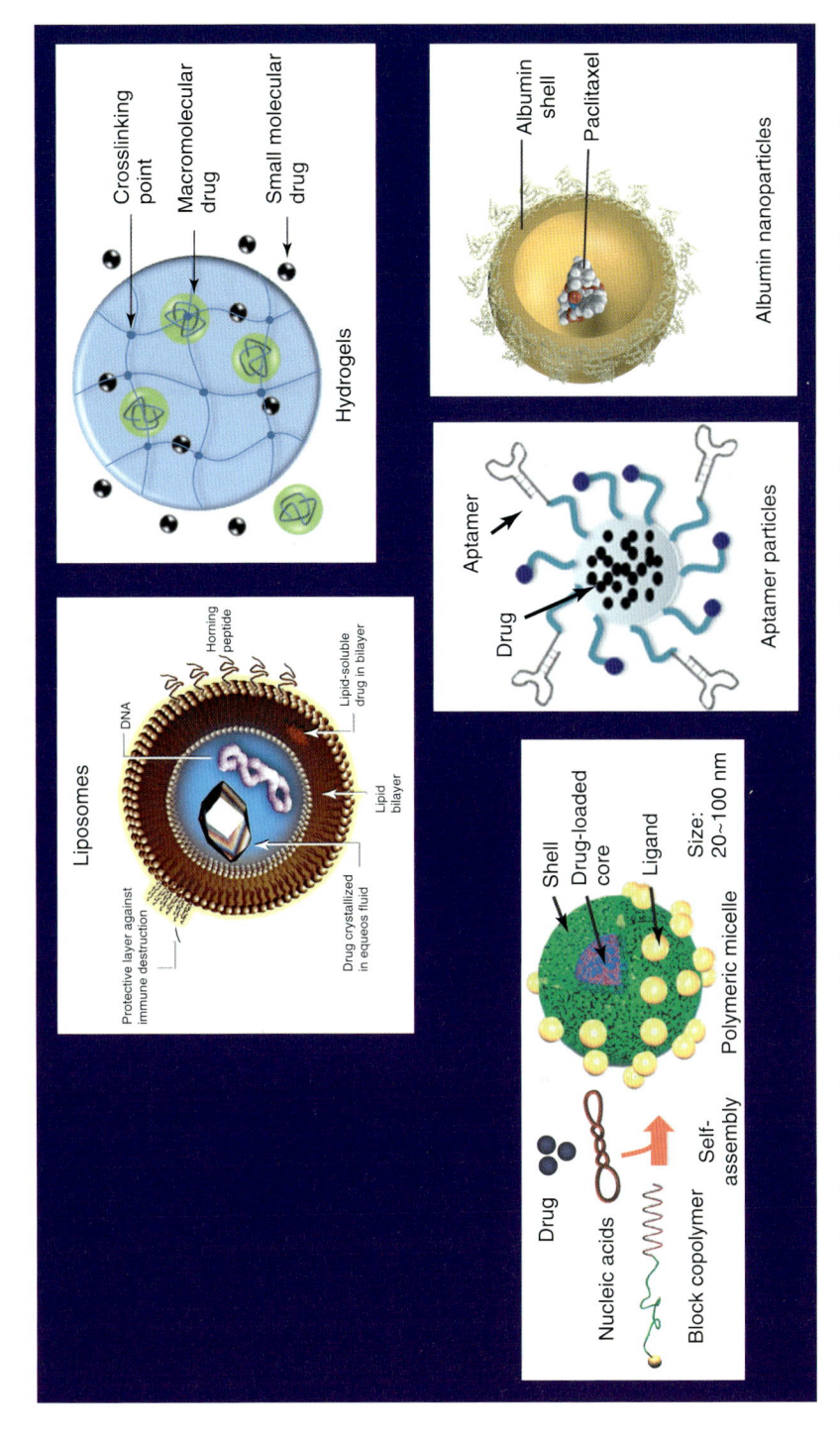

Figure 15 Examples of micro- and macroparticulate systems ranging from liposomes (*http://en.wikipedia.org/wiki/Liposome*), hydrogels (see Chapter 33), micelles (*http://en.wikipedia.org/wiki/Micelle* and Chapters 32 and 34), apatmer nanoparticles (see Chapter 39), and albumin–drug nanoparticles (see Chapter 35).

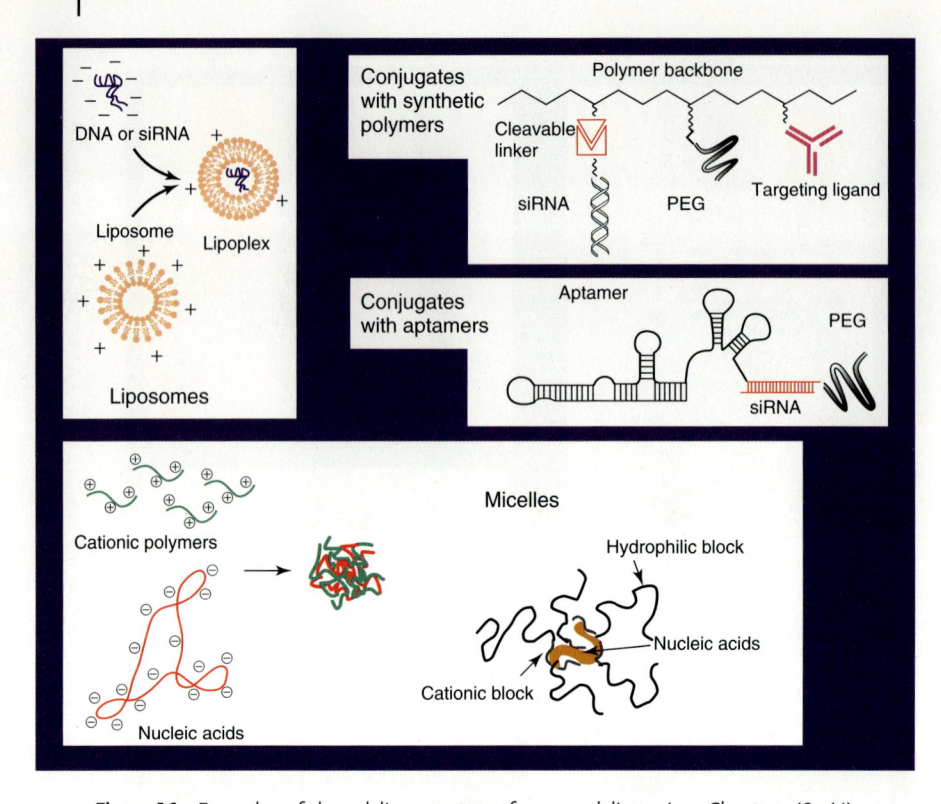

Figure 16 Examples of drug delivery systems for gene delivery (see Chapters 42–44).

Figure 17, invaginations occur at the cell surface during endocytosis and endosomes are formed that migrate into the cytoplasm. Depending on the drug carrier and the kind of endocytosis process involved, a series of sorting steps take place in which the endosome is either transported to certain cell organelles (e.g., the Golgi apparatus), returns to the cell surface (recycling), or forms primary and secondary lysosomes, respectively. The pH drop during endocytosis is considerable – from 7.2 to 7.4 in the extracellular space to pH 6.5–5.0 in the endosomes and to around pH 4.5–4.0 in primary and secondary lysosomes. In the lysosomes a large number of enzymes such as esterases, proteases, or lipases become active.

There has been considerable research toward developing tailor-made cleavable linkers that exploit the endosomal/lysosomal pathways for prodrug activation. Additional efforts include extracellular cleavage of carrier-linked prodrugs that is mediated through the activity of proteases that are secreted by the tumor cells.

A further option for releasing the conjugated or encapsulated drug in the tumor tissue or tumor cells is by hydrolysis or diffusion.

Major challenges in the development of drug delivery systems include designing tailor-made cleavable linkers and defining the precise chemical modification of the drug, isolating and purifying macromolecular drug delivery systems from unbound

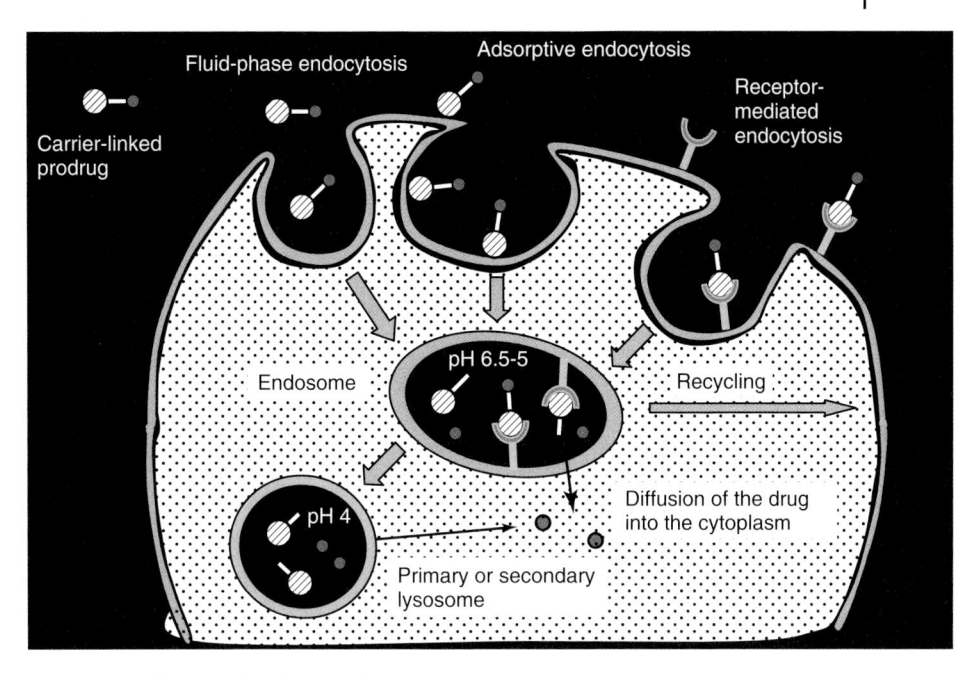

Figure 17 Cellular uptake of drug delivery systems as illustrated for carrier-linked prodrugs by either fluid-phase, adsorptive, or receptor-mediated endocytosis.

drug, achieving a stable and efficient encapsulation, and finally manufacturing the drug delivery systems and preparing sterile clinical trial samples. Also of critical importance is the precise characterization of the drug delivery system. Although this does not pose an obstacle for low-molecular-weight drug conjugates such as drug conjugates with vitamins, peptides, or fatty acids, the physicochemical characterization of macromolecular and nano-sized drug delivery systems can be cumbersome. In contrast to low-molecular-weight prodrugs, macromolecular drug delivery systems are not uniform, having molecular weight dispersities, charge distributions, and a range of drug loading ratios. While the heterogeneity of macromolecular drug delivery systems, which include drug conjugates with antibodies, synthetic polymers or liposomes, and nanoparticles and microparticles, creates additional complexities with respect to reproducibility and analytical characterization, the technology has been put into place to address these issues.

For the vast majority of drug delivery systems that are described by the authors in this book, technical and manufacturing issues have been solved and convincing *in vivo* proof of concepts have been obtained in tumor-bearing animal models. Although only a few drug delivery systems have reached market approval, such as liposomes (Doxil®, Daunosome®, Myocet®), the albumin taxol nanoparticle Abraxane®, a drug–polymer conjugate SMANCS (a conjugate of poly(styrene-*co*-maleic acid/anhydride) and the antitumor agent neocarzinostatin)

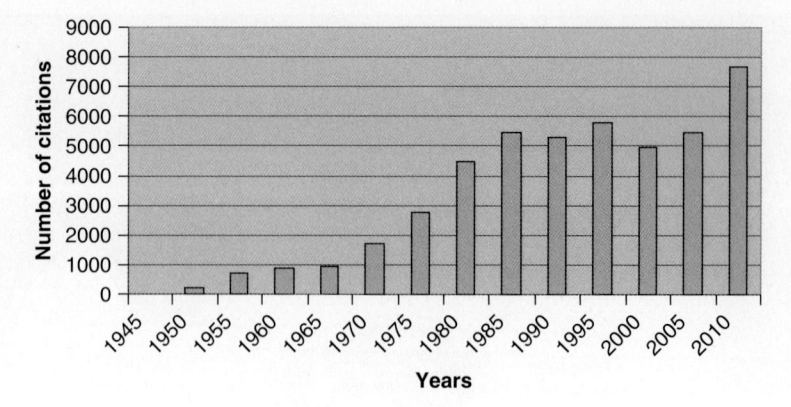

Figure 18 Number of citations in PubMed combining the key word "cancer" with "drug delivery" from 1945 to 2010 over respective 5-year periods.

(Figure 8), phase I–III trials have been performed with the majority of drug delivery approaches. These translational efforts are vital steps in the development of drug delivery systems in oncology and provide important clinical information, including efficacy, toxicity issues, biodistribution, tumor targeting, and pharmacokinetics. These clinical data together with further preclinical R&D will guide us through the challenges that lie ahead of adding new drug delivery systems to the routine treatment of cancer diseases and will help to answer pivotal questions such as:

- Which drug delivery systems are suitable for which tumor indication?
- How can we avoid the uptake of macromolecular drug delivery systems in the reticuloendothelial system (macrophages, liver, and spleen)?
- What are the optimal dosing schedules for the individual drug delivery systems?
- How can potential cumulative toxicity be avoided?
- Which drug combinations with drug delivery systems are most effective?
- At what stage of cancer should we begin with administering drug delivery systems?

The development of drug delivery systems is a relatively new field of research compared to conventional chemotherapy. However, interest in this area is greatly expanding, as can be seen by the continual increase in publications on drug delivery concepts and cancer since 1945 (Figure 18).

With nearly 8000 publications appearing between 2005 and 2010, and the clinical experience achieved to date, there is reason for optimism that drug delivery systems will play a significant role in clinical cancer medicine. In addition, there is now considerable evidence that these systems can be combined with conventional therapies and add to the repertoire of agents used for cancer chemotherapy. It is highly likely that many of the new macromolecular-based approaches described in this book will eventually lead to approved drugs that will make differences in the lives of patients suffering from cancer.

References

1. Holmyard, E.J. (1990) *Alchemy*, Dover, New York, p. 170.
2. Newman, D.J. and Cragg, G.M. (2007) Natural products as sources of new drugs over the last 25 years. *J. Nat. Prod.*, **70**, 461–477.
3. Bergers, G. and Benjamin, L.E. (2003) Tumorigenesis and the angiogenic switch. *Nat. Rev. Cancer*, **3**, 401–410.
4. Vaupel, P. (2004) Tumor microenvironmental physiology and its implications for radiation oncology. *Semin. Radiat. Oncol.*, **14**, 198–206.
5. Primeau, A.J., Rendon, A., Hedley, D., Lilge, L., and Tannock, I.F. (2005) The distribution of the anticancer drug doxorubicin in relation to blood vessels in solid tumors. *Clin. Cancer Res.*, **11**, 8782–8788.
6. Bäumler, E. (2001) *Paul Ehrlich. Forscher für das Leben*, 3rd edn, Minerva, Wissen.

Part I
Principles of Tumor Targeting

1
Limits of Conventional Cancer Chemotherapy
Klaus Mross and Felix Kratz

1.1
Introduction: The Era of Cancer Chemotherapy

The first effective anticancer drug that was developed was not worked out theoretically in a research laboratory, but took its beginning due to a tragic incidence during World War II. A German air raid in Bari, Italy led to the exposure and deaths of more than 1000 people to mustard gas (Figure 1.1).

The autopsies of the victims that Dr. Stewart Francis Alexander, an expert in chemical warfare, was subsequently deployed to investigate suggested that profound lymphoid and myeloid suppression had occurred after exposure. Dr. Alexander intuitively realized that since mustard gas primarily stopped the division of those types of somatic cells whose nature it was to divide fast, mustard gas should also potentially suppress the division of certain types of cancerous cells, which he noted in his report [1].

With this information in hand, two pharmacologists, Dr. Louis S. Goodman and Dr. Alfred Gilman, reasoned that mustard gas derivatives could be used to treat lymphoma, since lymphoma is a tumor of lymphoid cells. After setting up an animal model for lymphomas in mice, they were able to demonstrate that they could treat the tumor-bearing mice effectively with mustard agents. In a one-patient trial, they injected a related agent, the prototype nitrogen mustard anticancer chemotherapeutic, mustine, into a patient with non-Hodgkin's lymphoma and observed a dramatic reduction in the patient's tumor masses. Although this effect lasted only a few weeks, it was probably the first well-documented experimental trial that a cancer patient could be treated by a cytotoxic pharmacological agent, which has been in use under the brand name Mustargen® [2].

Shortly after World War II, Sidney Farber's work at the Harvard Medical School paved the way for the first rational design of an anticancer drug that earned him the name as the father of modern cancer chemotherapy (Figure 1.2). Farber had appreciated the work by Lucy Wills who had shown that folic acid seemed to stimulate the proliferation of acute lymphoblastic leukemia (ALL) cells when administered to children with this cancer. In collaboration with chemists at Lederle Laboratories, Farber probed folate analogs as antiproliferative agents

1 Limits of Conventional Cancer Chemotherapy

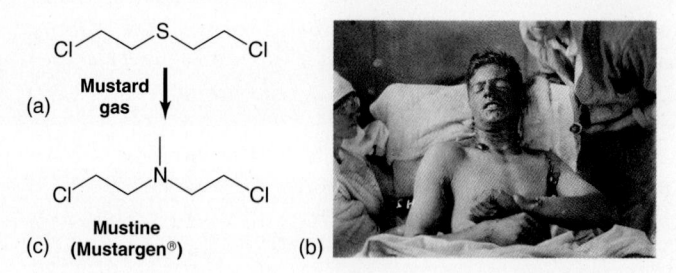

Figure 1.1 (a) Structure of mustard gas (1,5-dichloro-3-thiapentane), a highly toxic alkylating agent used as a vesicant warfare agent during World War I and II that produces severe burns and damage to the bone marrow and lymphoid system; (b) unidentified Canadian soldier with burns caused by mustard gas, ca. 1916–1918; (c) the structure of mustine (Mustargen), the first prototype of an alkylating agent, which has been used for treating Hodgkin's and non-Hodgkin's disease.

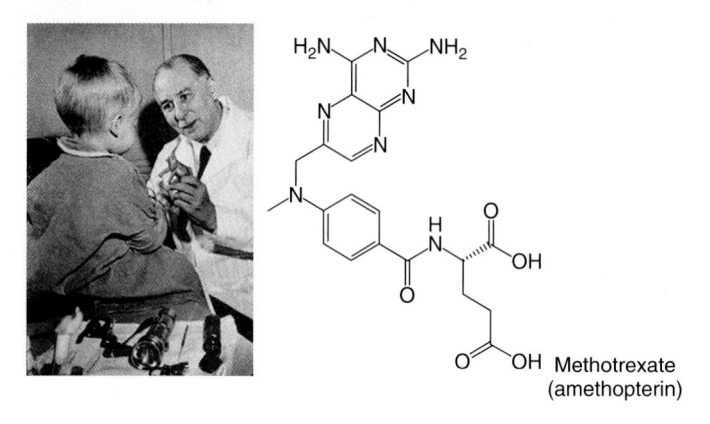

Figure 1.2 Sidney Farber discovers the first rationally designed anticancer agent, methotrexate, an inhibitor of the enzyme dihydrofolate reductase, which was successfully used to treat ALL and subsequently to successfully cure chorioncarcinomas (fast-growing solid tumors).

and discovered that certain analogs – first aminopterin and then amethopterin (now methotrexate) – were antagonists of folic acid and blocked the function of folate-requiring enzymes. In 1948, these agents became the first drugs to induce remissions in children with ALL. Although remissions were not long-lasting, the principle was clear – antifolates could suppress proliferation of malignant cells. It is somewhat surprising and in some ways bizarre that although Paul Ehrlich had set firm grounds with Salvarsan®, an arsenic-containing complex to treat syphilis successfully nearly 40 years earlier despite heavy protests from influential members of the scientific community, Farber met resistance once again to conducting his studies with a chemotherapeutic principle at a time when the commonly held medical belief was that leukemia was incurable and that the children should be allowed to die in peace. Even after Farber's 1948 report in the *New England Journal of Medicine* it was met with sarcasm and conspicuous astonishment [3].

As a deserved compensation, a decade later at the National Cancer Institute (NCI), Roy Hertz and Min Chiu Li discovered that the same methotrexate treatment alone could cure chorioncarcinoma (1958) – the first solid tumor to be cured by chemotherapy [4].

From the mid-1950s onwards, further progress in cancer chemotherapy was characterized primarily by four features: (i) further synthetic development of alkylating agents, antimetabolites, and platinum complexes, (ii) a federal initiative by the NCI that developed the methodologies and screening tools (e.g., cell line panels and animal models) for fostering a drug discovery program with a strong focus on identifying active natural products, (iii) establishment of standardized combination regimens that would prove to be more efficacious than single-agent therapy in several tumor indications, and (iv) clinical proof that adjuvant chemotherapy (i.e., treatment with anticancer agents after complete surgical resection of the tumor burden) significantly extended survival in several tumors indications, including those in a more advanced stage.

As a result, approximately 60–70% of anticancer chemotherapeutic agents are natural products or derived from them (Figure 1.3), as analyzed in depth by Newman and Cragg [5]. In their review article of 2007, they assessed the influence of natural products and their mimics as leads to anticancer drugs. By using data from the US Food and Drug Administration listings of antitumor drugs, coupled with previous data sources and with help from Japanese colleagues, they could show that over the whole category of anticancer drugs that entered clinical trials, these could be categorized as follows: biological "B" (18; 10%), natural product "N" (25; 14%), derived from a natural product "ND" (48; 28%), totally synthetic drug "S" (42; 24%), S/NM (14; 8%), made by total synthesis, but the pharmacophore is/was from a natural product "S*" (20; 11%), S*/NM (6; 4%), and vaccine "V"

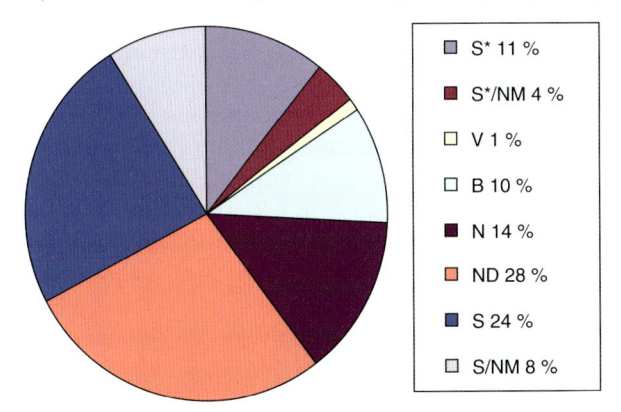

Figure 1.3 All available anticancer drugs, 1940s to June 2006, by source (N = 175). The major categories: B, biological; usually a large (more than 45 residues) peptide or protein either isolated from an organism/cell line or produced by biotechnological means; N, natural product; ND, derived from a natural product and is usually a semisynthetic modification; NM, natural product mimic; S, totally synthetic drug, often found by random screening/modification of an existing agent; S*, made by total synthesis, but the pharmacophore is/was from a natural product; V, vaccine. (Modified from [5].)

(2; 1%). If one removes the biologicals and vaccines, reducing the overall number to 155 (100%), the number of naturally inspired agents (i.e., N, ND, S/NM, S*, S*/NM) is 113 (72.9%).

Although chemotherapeutic anticancer agents are classified into alkylating agents, antimetabolites, anthracyclines, plant alkaloids, microtubule inhibitors or modulators, topoisomerase inhibitors, and other antitumor agents, the modes of action can be diverse and manifold, resulting finally in a cytotoxic and/or cytostatic effect by affecting cell division, DNA synthesis and function, or apoptosis (programmed cell death). Some typical representatives of the different classes of antineoplastic agents are depicted in Figure 1.4.

With a few exceptions, these antitumor agents are delivered intravenously (melphalan, busulfan, and capecitabine can be administered orally). In some cases, isolated limb perfusion (used in melanoma and soft-tissue sarcoma), or isolated infusion of chemotherapy into the liver or the lung have been used. The main purpose of these approaches is to deliver a very high dose of chemotherapy to tumor sites without causing overwhelming systemic damage. Depending on the patient, cancer, stage of cancer, type of chemotherapy, and dosage, intravenous chemotherapy may be given on either an inpatient or an outpatient basis. For continuous, frequent, or prolonged intravenous chemotherapy administration, various systems may be surgically inserted into the vasculature to maintain access. Commonly used systems are the Hickman line, the Port-a-Cath®, or the PICC (peripherally inserted central catheter) line. These have a lower infection risk, are much less prone to phlebitis or extravasation, and abolish the need for repeated insertion of peripheral cannulae.

Tumors that responded best to cytostatic or cytotoxic agents were those with a fast doubling time of the order of a few days that include chorioncarcinoma, lymphoma, leukemia, rhabdosarcoma, and testicular cancers.

The response rates of the most common solid tumors – breast, lung, prostate, ovarian, liver, colorectal, gastric, and colorectal cancer – were far less encouraging. Over the past two decades, chemotherapy of these tumors has gradually but consistently been improved by the use of new developed drugs and optimized combinations of chemotherapeutic agents. An illustrative example is colon cancer. When only 5-Fluorouracil (5-FU) was available in the 1980s and early 1990s, the mean survival time was 12 months, which was even better than best supportive care (that had a survival time of 6 months). With the development of oxaliplatin and irinotecan, and optimizing the schedule of the combinations with 5-FU and folinic acid, the mean survival time has increased to more than 18 months. With the development of the two monoclonal antibodies (monoclonal antibody mAbs) cetuximab (Erbitux®) and bevacizumab (Avastin®) the mean survival time has reached 24 months or more for some subtypes. The rationale for using a combination of drugs is manifold. (i) By combining the drugs below their respective maximum tolerated dose as single agents, the overall systemic toxicity for the patient during chemotherapy cycles can be reduced. (ii) The individual tumor cells are in different stages of the cell cycle (G_2, S, M, G_1, G_0), such that some are proliferating, differentiating, or resting (quiescent) (Figure 1.5 and Table 1.1). As anticancer agents

ALKYLATING AGENTS

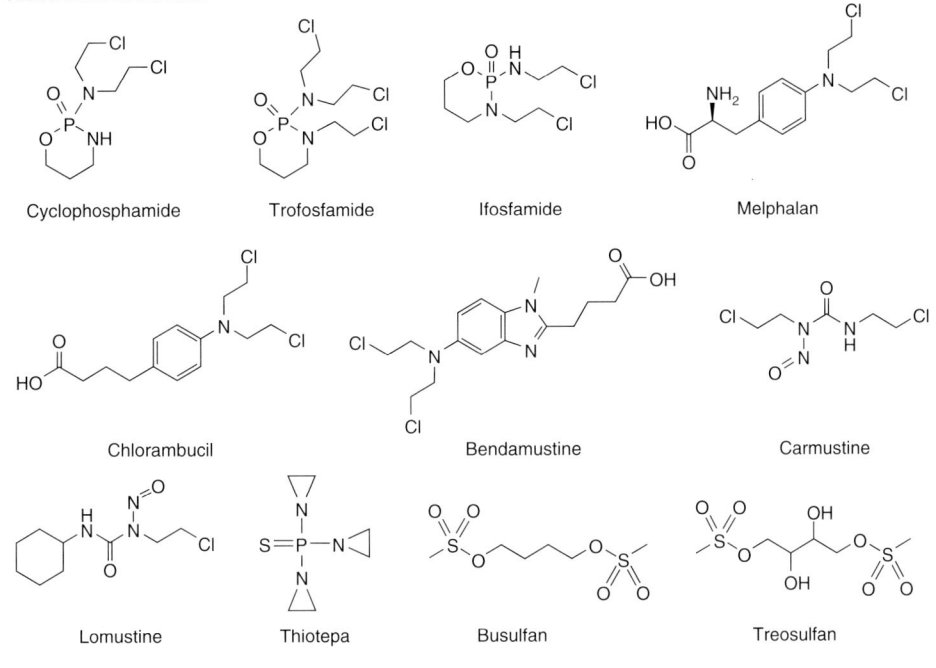

Cyclophosphamide Trofosfamide Ifosfamide Melphalan

Chlorambucil Bendamustine Carmustine

Lomustine Thiotepa Busulfan Treosulfan

PLATINUM COMPLEXES

Cisplatin Carboplatin Oxaliplatin

ANTIMETABOLITES
Folic acid antagonists

Methotrexate Raltitrexed

Figure 1.4 Chemical structures of the major representative classes of conventional anticancer agents used routinely in cancer chemotherapy.

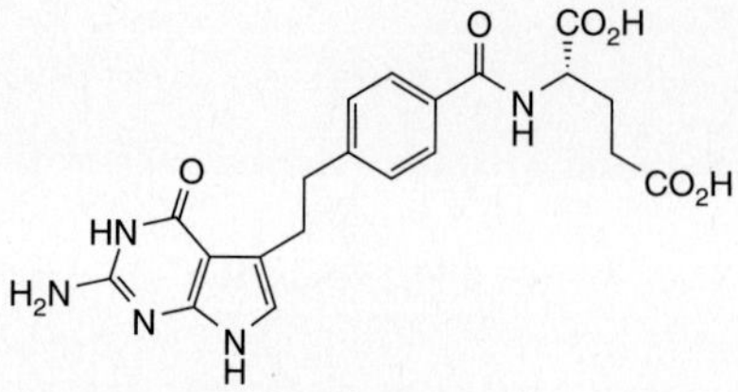

Permetrexed

Purine analogs

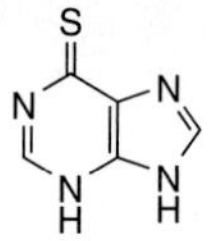

Mercaptopurine 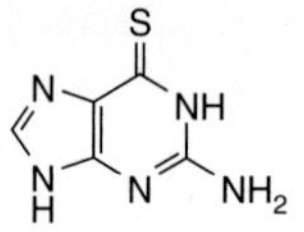 Thioguanine 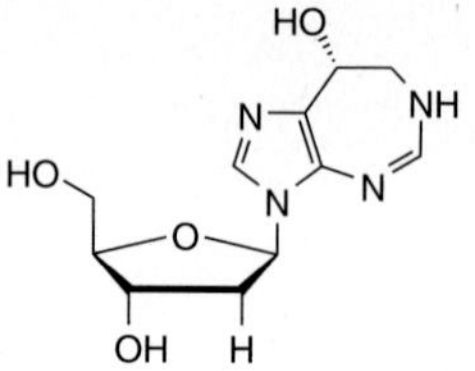 Pentostatin

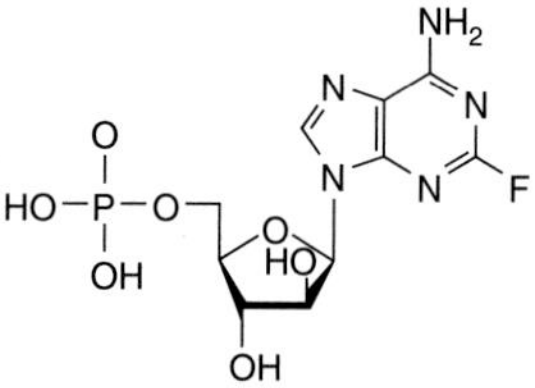

Fludarinbinphosphate 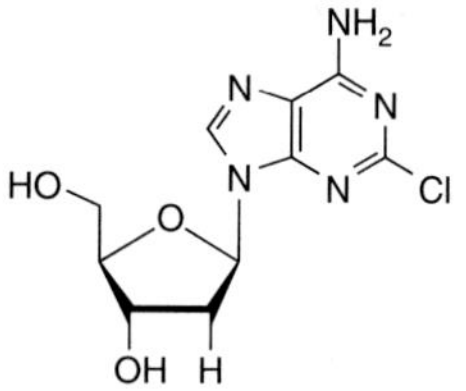 Cladribin

Pyrimidine analogs

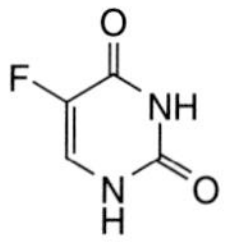

5-Fluorouracil 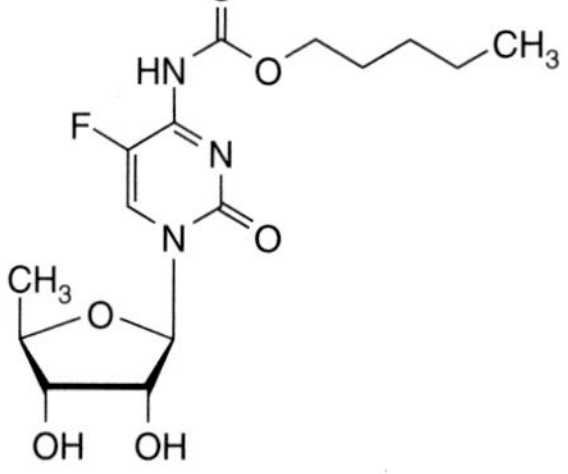 Capecitabine 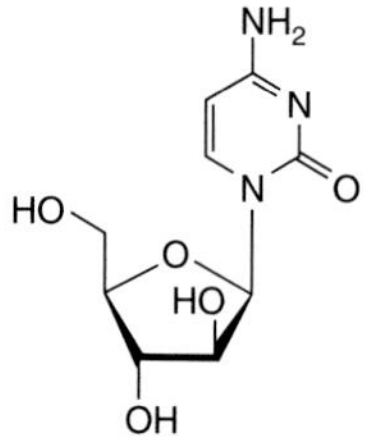 Cytarabine 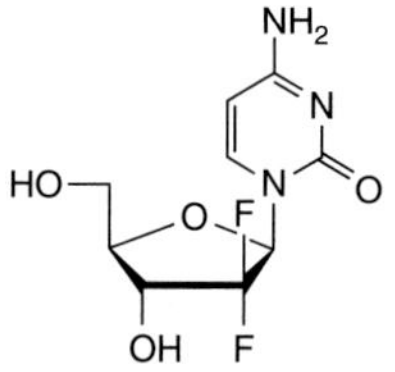 Gemcitabine

MICROTUBULE INHIBITORS
Vinca alkaloids

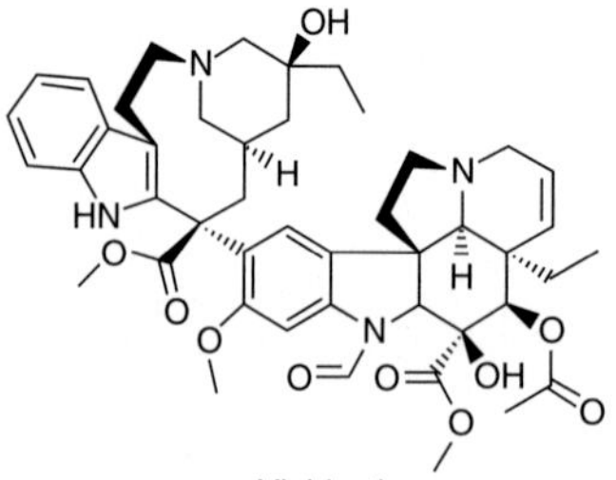

Vinblastine 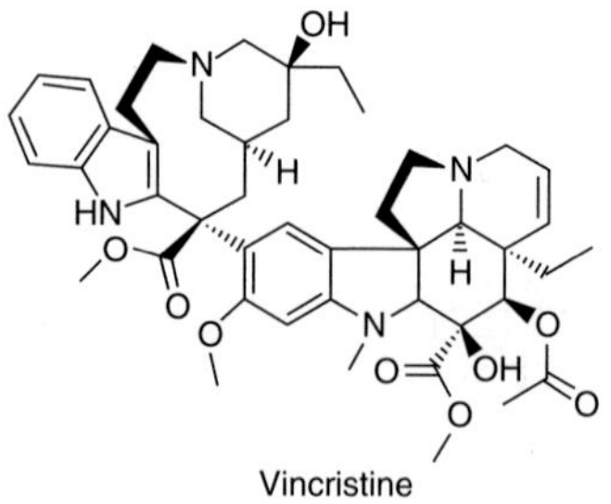 Vincristine

Figure 1.4 (continued)

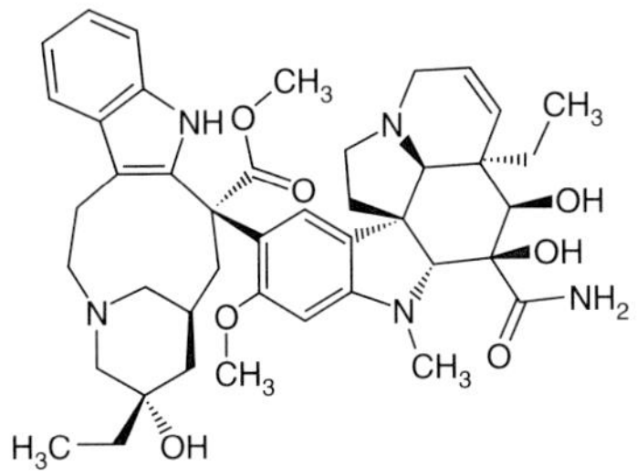

1.1 Introduction: The Era of Cancer Chemotherapy | 9

Vindesine

Taxanes

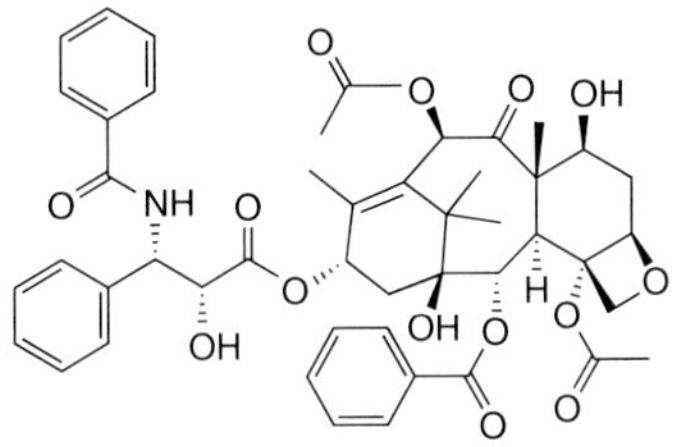

Paclitaxel

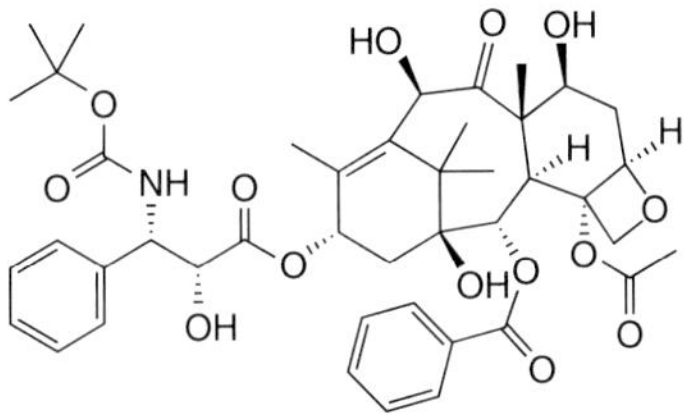

Docetaxel

TOPOISOMERASE I AND II INHIBITORS

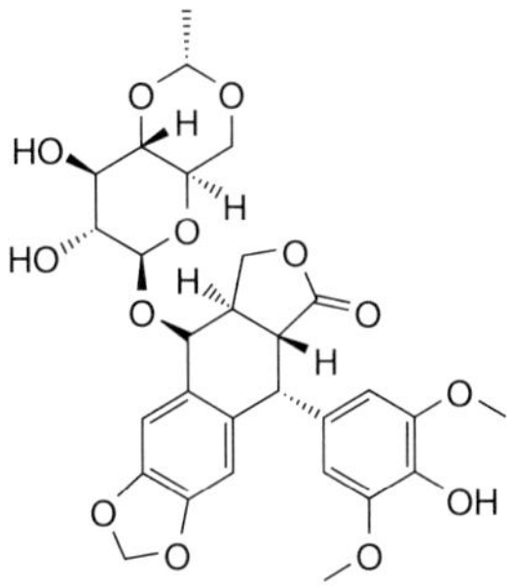

Etoposide

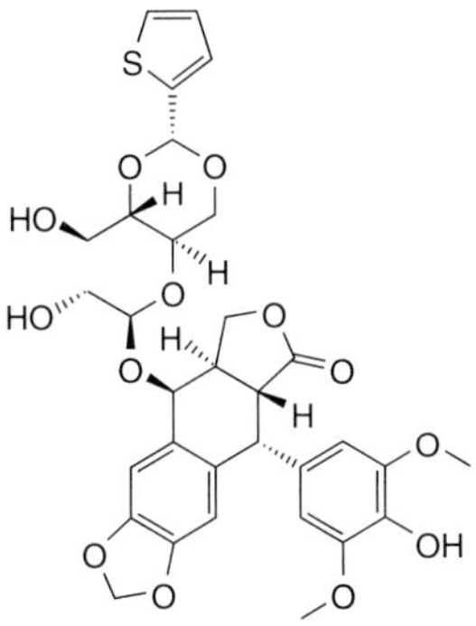

Teniposide

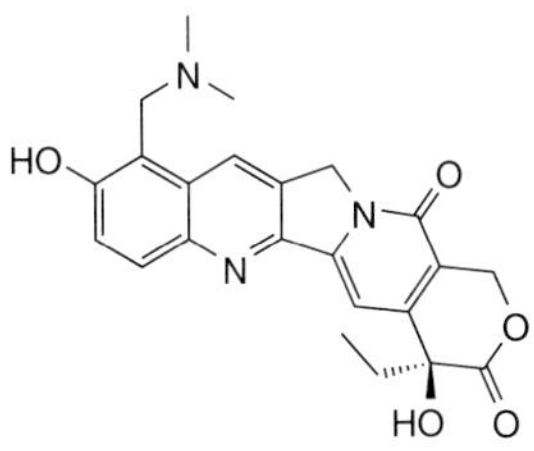

Topotecan

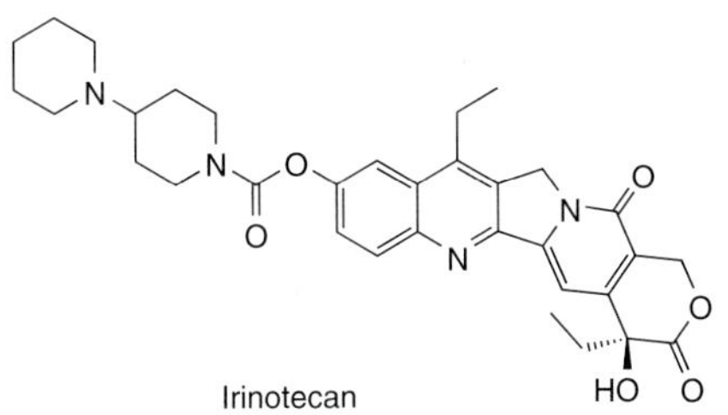

Irinotecan

Figure 1.4 (continued)

CYTOSTATIC ANTIBIOTICS

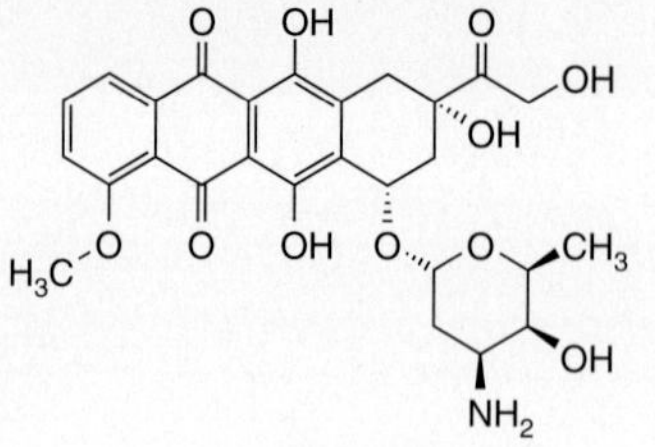

Doxorubicin

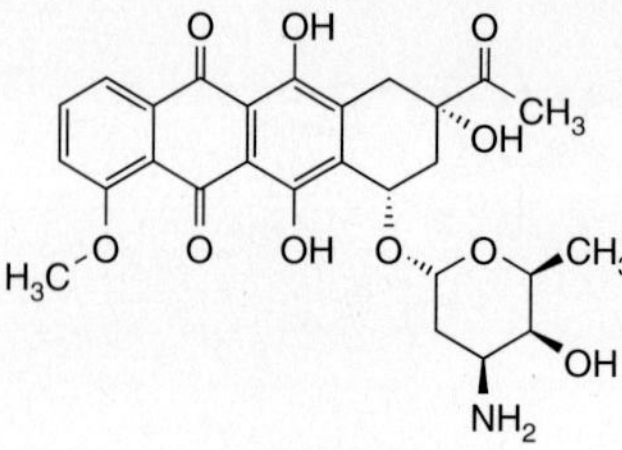

Daunorubicin

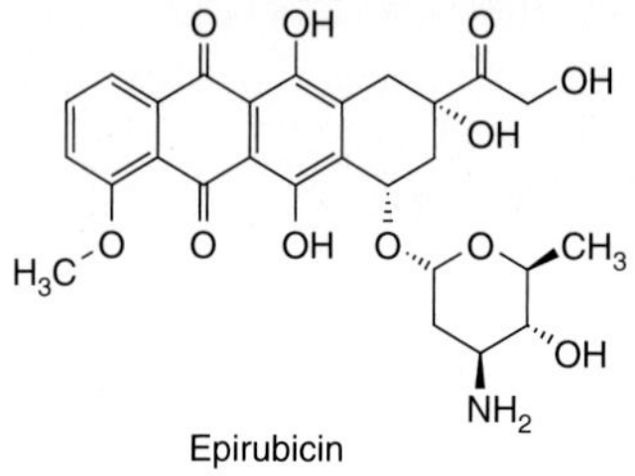

Epirubicin

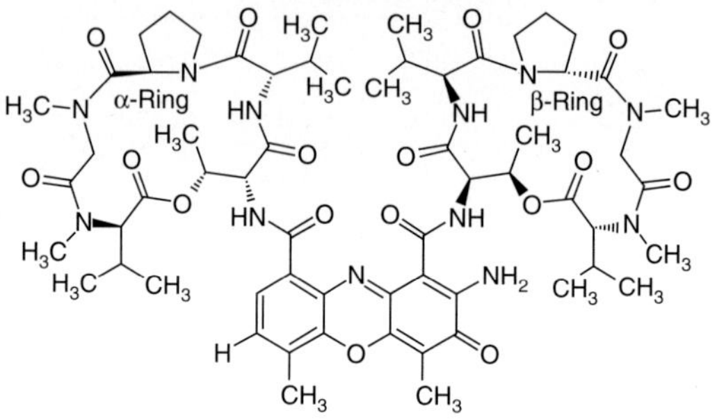

Dactinomycin

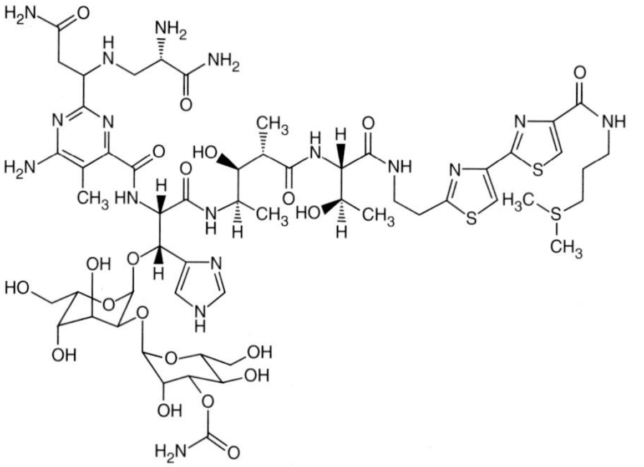

Bleomycin

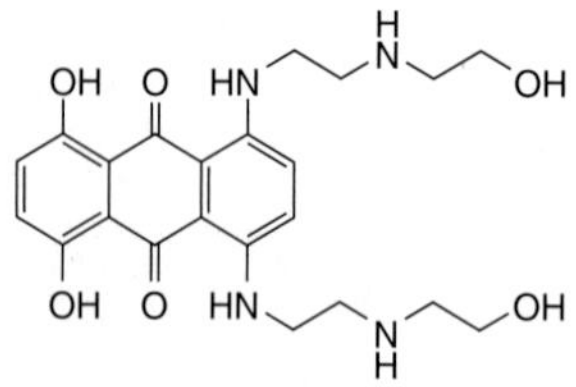

Mitoxantrone

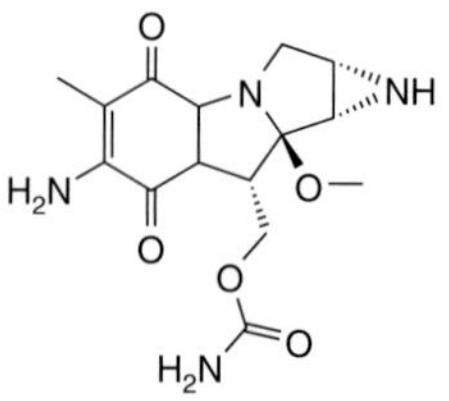

Mitomycin C

Figure 1.4 (continued)

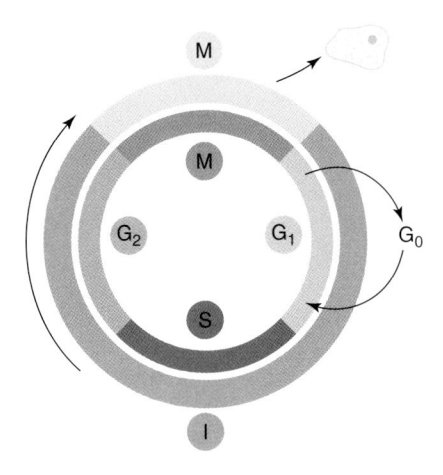

Figure 1.5 Schematic of the cell cycle. Outer ring: I = interphase, M = mitosis; inner ring: M = mitosis, G_1 = gap 1, G_2 = gap 2, S = synthesis; not in ring: G_0 = gap 0/resting. The duration of mitosis in relation to the other phases has been exaggerated in this diagram. Also see Table 1.1. (Adapted from *en.wikipedia.org/wiki/Cell_cycle*.)

Table 1.1 Phases of the cell cycle (also see Figure 1.5).

Phase	Abbreviation	Description
Gap 0	G_0	a resting phase where the cell has left the cycle and has stopped dividing.
Gap 1	G_1	cells increase in size in gap 1 and G_1 checkpoint control mechanisms make preparations for DNA synthesis
Synthesis	S	DNA replication occurs during this phase
Gap 2	G_2	during the gap between DNA synthesis and mitosis, the cell will continue to grow; the G_2 checkpoint control mechanism ensures that everything is ready to enter the M (mitosis) phase and divide.
Mitosis	M	cell growth stops at this stage and cellular energy is focused on the orderly division into two daughter cells; a checkpoint in the middle of mitosis (metaphase checkpoint) ensures that the cell is ready to complete cell division

Adapted from *en.wikipedia.org/wiki/Cell_cycle*.

inhibit tumor growth at different stages of the cell cycle, it is logical to assume that a combination of selected anticancer drugs acting at different stages of the cell cycle will result in an overall improved cell kill of the heterogeneous tumor cell population that on the whole is asynchronous with respect to tumor proliferation. (iii) Tumor cells become resistant to a single agent, thus by using different drugs (phase-specific, phase-unspecific, as well as cycle-specific) concurrently it would be easier to target and kill individual tumor cells at their respective checkpoints, and the likelihood of the tumor developing resistance to the combination would be suppressed by applying several anticancer drugs simultaneously.

The major breakthrough for this approach was achieved around 1965 when James Holland, Emil Freireich, and Emil Frei rationalized that cancer chemotherapy should follow the strategy of antibiotic therapy of using combinations of drugs, each with a different mechanism of action, to inhibit the tumor cell population in the different stages of their cell cycle and also to prevent the emergence of resistance. Holland, Freireich, and Frei simultaneously administered methotrexate (an antifolate), vincristine (a vinca alkaloid), 6-mercaptopurine (6-MP), and prednisone – together referred to as the POMP regimen – and induced long-term remissions in children with ALL. With subsequent incremental refinements of these original protocols in the United Kingdom and Germany, ALL in children has become a largely curable disease and was extended to lymphomas where a combination of a nitrogen mustard, vincristine, procarbazine, and prednisone – known as the MOPP regimen – can cure patients with Hodgkin's and non-Hodgkin's lymphoma.

Currently, nearly all successful cancer chemotherapy regimens use this paradigm of multiple drugs given simultaneously, mainly in curative chemotherapy protocols (R-CHOP, BEACOPP, ABVD, COPP-ABVD, FAC, BEP, etc.), but also first-line and second-line chemotherapy regimens in palliative settings (solid tumors with metastases) generally include combinations with two or three drugs for maximizing the therapeutic effect (e.g., FOLFOX, FOLFIRI, ECF, DCF, FLOT, CDDP/GEM, CDDP/VP-16, CBDCA/PAC, IFO/DOX, etc.) (Table 1.2).

Despite the relatively slow progress in treating the most common solid tumors, especially once metastasized, another important strategy for the use of chemotherapy emerged – adjuvant therapy. If the tumor could be removed or the tumor burden reduced by surgery, then anticancer agents should be able to destroy any remaining malignant cells or micrometastases post-therapy, thus reducing the probability of tumor remission and/or the formation of metastases. This notion was nourished by the observation in animal models that anticancer drugs were most effective in eliminating tumors of smaller volume. It was again Emil Frei who first demonstrated this effect – high doses of methotrexate prevented the recurrence of osteosarcoma following surgical removal of the primary tumor [6]. Similarly, 5-FU was later shown to improve survival in colon cancer stage II and III (above all in stage III with lymph node metastasis) when used as an adjuvant to surgery in treating patients with colon cancer, and Gianni Bonadonna at the Istituto Nazionale Tumori di Milano, Italy, demonstrated that adjuvant chemotherapy after complete surgical resection of breast tumors significantly extended survival with CMF (cyclophosphamide/methotrexate/5-FU) even in more advanced cancer [7]. In subsequent years, adjuvant chemotherapy for treating breast cancer relied on an anthracycline-based regimen (FAC (5-FU/doxorubicin (adriamycin)/cyclophosphamide) or AC (doxorubicin (adriamycin)/cyclophosphamide)) followed by taxanes (docetaxel or paclitaxel) with or without trastuzumab (Herceptin®) in HER2/*neu*-positive tumors [8].

Table 1.2 Examples of commonly used cancer chemotherapy regimens in first-line, second-line, and palliative treatment.

Abbreviation for the combination protocol	Drugs used in the regimen	Tumor indication
FOLFOX	folinic acid 5-FU oxaliplatin	colon cancer
FOLFIRI	folinic acid 5-FU irinotecan	colon cancer
ECF	epirubicin cisplatin 5-FU	gastric cancer
DCF	docetaxel cisplatin 5-FU	gastric cancer
FLOT	5-FU leucovorin (folinic acid) oxaliplatin taxotere (docetaxel)	gastric cancer
R-CHOP	rituximab cyclophosphamide hydroxy-daunomycin (doxorubicin) oncovin (vincristine) prednisone (cortisone)	non-Hodgkin's lymphoma
FAC	5-FU adriamycin (doxorubicin) cyclophosphamide	breast cancer
BEP	bleomycin etoposide cisplatin	testicular cancer
BEACOPP	bleomycin etoposide adriamycin cyclophosphamide oncovine (vincristine) procarbacin prednisolone (cortisone)	Hodgkin's lymphoma
ABVD	adriamycin (doxorubicin) bleomycin vinblastine decarbacin	Hodgkin's lymphoma

1.2
Dilemma and Challenge of Treating Malignant Diseases

One of the main dilemmas of treating solid tumors is that they are not detected early enough and once diagnosed have often formed metastases. If they cannot be treated by surgery in combination with radiotherapy or neoadjuvant chemotherapy, the prognosis for curing the patient, mostly expressed in the literature as at least a 5-year tumor-free interval, remains highly unsatisfactory. Current chemotherapy regimens applied alone or in combination with novel agents such as mAbs and signal transduction inhibitors are to date the best option of inhibiting or reducing the size of the primary tumor and/or metastases. Chemotherapy regimens are generally applied in cycles (ranging from a 1- to 4-week interval), with the frequency and duration of treatments limited by toxicity to the patient. Most commonly, chemotherapy acts by killing cells that divide actively – one of the main properties of most cancer cells. This means that they also harm cells that divide rapidly under normal circumstances, such as cells in the bone marrow, digestive tract, and hair follicles (see Section 1.3).

It is instructive to understand the rationale for repeated doses that must be administered to continue to inhibit tumor growth or reduce the size of the tumor. As only a fraction of the cells in a tumor die with each treatment, it is obligatory that repeated and optimized chemotherapy cycles must be administered to obtain the best therapeutic outcome.

This principle is known as "log cell kill," often also referred to as "fractional cell kill," and is a generally accepted hypothesis for hematological cancers that states that during every cycle of chemotherapy or radiotherapy the same fraction of tumor cells is killed, but not the same number.

Howard E. Skipper laid the foundation for the log cell kill hypothesis in 1964 when carrying out experiments with mice suffering from leukemia [9]. Leukemia cells that grow exponentially result in a straight line when plotted on a semilogarithmic scale over time, reflecting the doubling of tumor cells. When the mice were treated with constant doses of anticancer agents, it was observed that the number of leukemia cells diminished logarithmically; if, for example, 99% of leukemia cells were killed after the first administration, this is equivalent to a decrease from 10^9 to 10^7 cells, which corresponds to 2 orders of magnitude (log steps). A second administration will also result in a 99% cell kill, but the number of tumor cells is only reduced from 10^7 to 10^5, which is only 10 million cells compared to the 1 billion cells in the first cycle. In other words, in this idealized model, the fraction of cells that are killed remains constant, but the number of cells killed over time constantly decreases.

Transferring the log cell kill hypothesis to solid tumors is not as straightforward as it appears at first glance (Figure 1.6).

With modern diagnostics, a tumor is detectable when it reaches a size of $1\,cm^3$ after 30 doubling cycles, which corresponds to $1\,g$ and 10^9 cancer cells. Only 10 further doubling steps are necessary for the tumor to reach a size of $1\,kg$ (10^{12} cancer cells). In this time interval tumor symptoms start emerging.

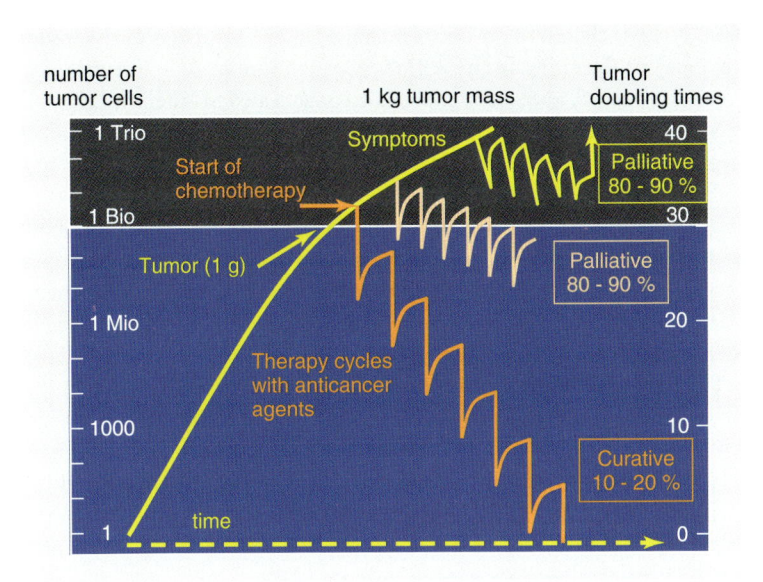

Figure 1.6 Tumor growth curve of a solid tumor. Once the tumor comprises approximately 1 billion tumor cells, its size is around 1 cm³ (1 g) and it becomes detectable. The initial tumor cell has to perform 30 doubling steps to reach this size (which can take months to years considering that the tumor doubling times for human tumors lies in the range of 5–200 days), and a mere 10 further doublings are needed to reach a mass of 1 kg assuming tumor growth occurs exponentially. This generally does not take place because of an insufficient growing vasculature in large tumors, leading to a lack of supply of nutrients and tumor necrosis. Of note is that according to the log cell kill hypothesis many cycles of chemotherapy are necessary to eliminate all of the tumor cells and only in 10–20% of cases are cures achieved. Palliative treatment is particularly disappointing with large tumors where only a relatively small fraction of tumor cells respond to anticancer agents.

These insights are the reason why during curative, adjuvant, or palliative chemotherapy the doses and cycles of anticancer agents should not be reduced or discontinued even if the tumor or tumor lesions are no longer detectable (assuming that the schedule is tolerated by the patient). The log cell kill hypothesis can additionally be viewed as a theoretical basis for further treating patients for longer periods although diagnostically a complete remission has been achieved.

However, the log cell kill hypothesis is not strictly valid for solid tumors, if at all, only for those that are fast growing, but in most cases the effect of cytostatic or cytotoxic agents on tumor growth can be described by the so-called Gompertz growth curve. This implies that tumor growth diminishes with increasing size of the tumor, which is noted in the semilogarithmic plot by a decreasing slope of the tumor growth curve. With increasing tumor size many tumor cells remain in the G_0 phase (quiescent phase) of the cell cycle because of an insufficient growing vasculature leading to a lack of supply of nutrients and tumor necrosis. In this phase, the response to treatment with anticancer agents is significantly reduced and the initial cycle of chemotherapy only manages to kill a fraction of the tumor cells, mostly those proliferating in the periphery of the tumor. As a consequence, the tumor mass is reduced, and quiescent cells are reactivated to enter the cell cycle and multiply. This is the reason why the response in the second or third cycle of palliative treatment is often better than in the first one because a higher percentage of tumor cells are killed.

Unfortunately, in this advanced stage of the disease further reduction of tumor size is seldom achieved because a population of tumor cells has developed chemoresistance. Intrinsic or acquired chemoresistance is a major problem in cancer therapy. In the majority of cases the cancer cells develop resistance against a spectrum of anticancer agents, a phenomenon called multidrug resistance (MDR). A number of biochemical mechanisms have been described that are responsible for the MDR phenotype, including changes in the cellular target of the respective drug, alterations in enzymatic activation and detoxification mechanisms, defective apoptotic pathways, membrane changes as well as elimination of the drug from the tumor cell through the action of drug efflux pumps, such as P-glycoprotein, multiple resistance protein (MRP), and breast cancer resistance protein (BCRP), which belong to the ATP-binding cassette transporter family [10].

In addition, tissue penetration into necrotic areas of the tumor is hampered. Solid tumors are heterogeneous and form a complex society of cells in different microenvironments. This includes variable vascular density, different intratumoral blood pressure, and regions of hypoxic, acidic, and necrotic areas. These factors have an influence on the tissue penetration of drug as shown for the anticancer drug in Figure 1.7, which is shown for three different preclinical tumors in mice with regard to the intratumoral distribution of doxorubicin [11]. The immunofluorescence images after administration show the blood vessels in red, hypoxic areas in green, and doxorubicin in blue. The penetration length for doxorubicin from the nearest blood vessels varies considerably within a 100 µm range and doxorubicin is unable to accumulate in hypoxic areas.

1.3
Adverse Effects

The side-effects associated with cancer chemotherapy can be classified as acute toxicities (patient-felt toxicities, which appear directly after administration or delayed after a few hours or days, e.g., nausea, vomiting, gastrointestinal symptoms, dyspnea, fever, skin reactions), cycle-dependent toxicities (e.g., bone marrow toxicities, stomatitis, mucositis, alopecia), or long-term or cumulative toxicities (e.g., cardiotoxicity, nephrotoxicity, neurotoxicity).

All the above anticancer chemotherapeutics are essentially cytotoxic regardless of whether they are of synthetic or of natural origin. Patients receiving these agents experience severe side-effects that limit the doses that can be administered and hence limit the beneficial effects. The therapeutic window is in general narrow due to the fact that the cytotoxic agents used are low-molecular-weight compounds

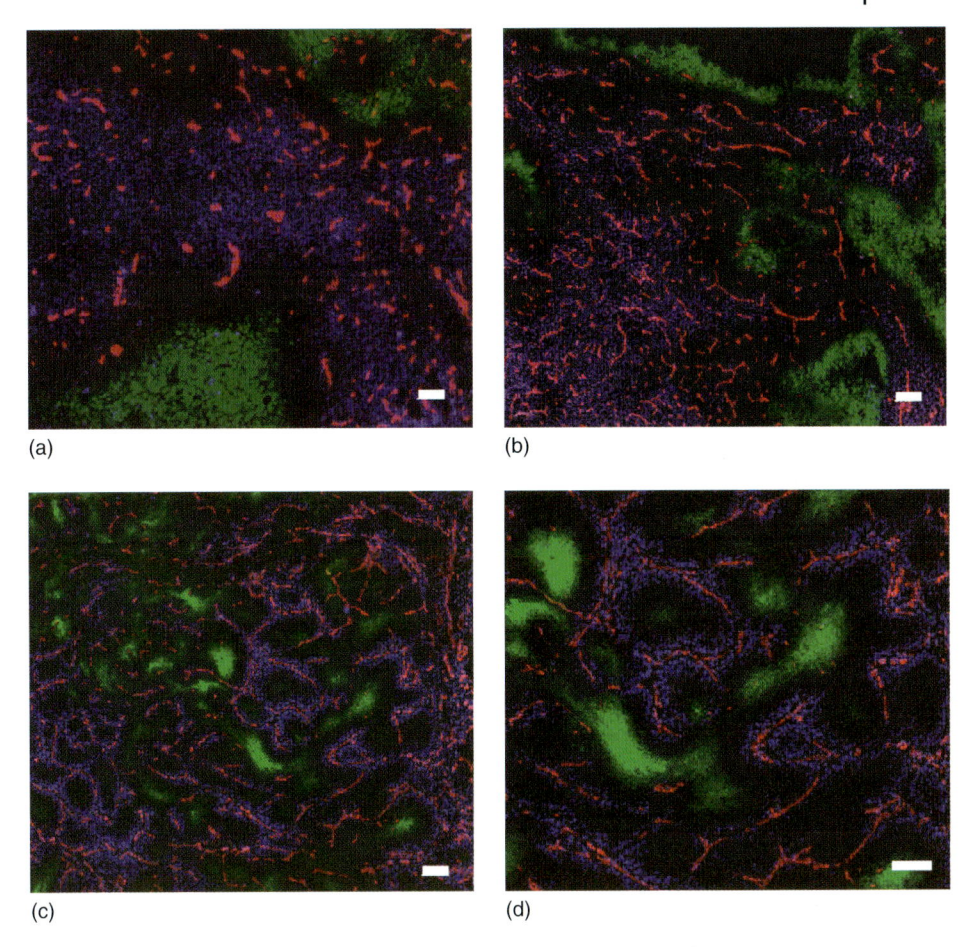

Figure 1.7 Representative three-color composite images showing the perivascular distribution of doxorubicin (blue) in relation to blood vessels (red) and hypoxic regions (green) in three different tumors growing in the right flank of mice: (a) human prostate PC-3 carcinoma, (b) mouse mammary sarcoma EMT6, and (c) and (d) 16/C mammary carcinoma. Bar: 100 μm. (Reproduced with permission from [11].)

(typically smaller than 1000 Da) that diffuse rapidly into healthy tissues with relatively small amounts of the drug reaching the target site. They are characterized by a rapid clearance, basically being eliminated from the circulation within minutes or hours, metabolized in the liver, and excreted via the bile duct or the kidneys.

Most commonly, chemotherapy acts by killing cells that are dividing – one of the main properties of most cancer cells, but not of all. The growth fraction can vary between 5 and 100%. The grading of a tumor depends on the behavior of the growth fraction, which can be roughly estimated by the Ki-67-positive fraction – an antigen that can be used as a proliferation marker for cancer cells. This means that cytostatic/cytotoxic agents also harm cells that divide rapidly under normal circumstances, in particular cells in the bone marrow, digestive tract, and hair follicles; this results in the most common side-effects of chemotherapy – myelosuppression (decreased production of blood cells), mucositis (inflammation of the lining of the digestive tract), and alopecia (hair loss).

Clinical investigators realized that the ability to manage these toxicities was crucial to the success of cancer chemotherapy. Most chemotherapeutic agents cause profound suppression of the bone marrow. This is reversible, but takes time to recover. Support with platelet and red cell transfusions as well as broad-spectrum antibiotics in the case of infection during this period is crucial to allow the patient to recover. The success of chemotherapy depends heavily on additional supportive care. This is independent from normal-dose chemotherapy or high-dose chemotherapies, including hematopoietic stem cell support (either autologous or allogeneic). Supportive care is a necessary part of a chemotherapy plan.

1.3.1
Common Side-Effects

Cancer chemotherapy has a broad range of side-effects that depend on the type of medications used. The most common side-effects are described below:

1.3.1.1 Depression of the Immune System
Virtually all chemotherapeutic regimens can cause depression of the immune system, often by affecting the bone marrow – a compartment with a very strong proliferation – subsequently leading to a decrease of white blood cells, red blood cells, and platelets. The latter two, when they occur, are improved with blood or platelet transfusion. Neutropenia (a decrease of the neutrophil granulocyte count below $0.5 \times 10^9/l$) can be improved with synthetic granulocyte colony-stimulating factor (G-CSF; e.g., filgrastim, lenograstim). The prophylactic use of G-CSF depends on the risk estimation for fever and infection. In cases where the risk estimation is greater than 10% (variables: age, chemotherapeutic drug, dosage, pretreatment, etc.), a prophylactic treatment with G-CSF is justified. More important in cases of fever of unknown origin is the early use of antibiotics. The therapeutic use of G-CSF in cases of neutropenia or neutropenic fever is less validated.

Depression of the immune system can result in potentially fatal infections. Although patients are encouraged to wash their hands, avoid people with infections, and to take other infection-reducing steps, about 85% of infections are due to naturally occurring microorganisms in the patient's own gut and skin. This may manifest as systemic infections (e.g., sepsis) or as localized outbreaks (e.g., shingles). Sometimes, chemotherapy treatments are postponed because the immune system is suppressed to a critically low level.

In very severe myelosuppression, which occurs in some regimens, almost all the bone marrow stem cells (cells that produce white and red blood cells) are destroyed and allogenic or autologous bone marrow cell transplants are necessary. In autologous bone marrow cell transplants the cells are removed from the patient before the treatment, multiplied, and then reinjected afterwards; in allogenic bone marrow cell transplants the source is a donor. The initial tremendously high mortality in the early days of an allogeneic hematopoietic cell transplantation has been successfully decreased during recent years.

In Japan, the government has approved the use of some medicinal mushrooms (e.g., *Trametes versicolor*) to counteract depression of the immune system in patients undergoing chemotherapy (*http://www.cancer.org/docroot/ETO/content/ETO_5_3X_Coriolous_Versicolor.asp*).

The United States' top-ranked hospital, the University of Texas MD Anderson Cancer Center, has reported that polysaccharide-K (PSK; an extract from *T. versicolor*) is a "promising candidate for chemoprevention due to the multiple effects on the malignant process, limited side effects, and safety of daily oral doses for extended periods of time" (*http://cancer.ucsd.edu/Outreach/PublicEducation/CAMs/coriolusversicolor.asp*). PSK is already used in pharmaceuticals designed to complement chemotherapy. The MD Anderson has also reported that there are 40 human studies, 55 animal studies, 37 *in vitro* studies, and 11 reviews published concerning *T. versicolor* or its extract PSK (*http://www.mdanderson.org/education-and-research/resources-for-professionals/clinical-tools-and-resources/cimer/therapies/herbal-plant-biologic-therapies/coriolus-versicolor-scientific.html*).

1.3.1.2 Fatigue

The treatment can be physically exhausting for the patient who might already be very tired from cancer-related fatigue. Chemotherapy can cause or potentiate fatigue and may produce mild to severe anemia. Therapeutic options to mitigate anemia include hormones to boost blood production (erythropoietin), iron supplements, and blood transfusions.

1.3.1.3 Tendency to Bleed Easily

Medications that kill rapidly dividing cells or blood cells are likely to reduce the number of platelets in the blood, which can result in bruises and bleeding. Extremely low platelet counts may be temporarily boosted through platelet transfusions. Sometimes, chemotherapy treatments are postponed to allow platelet counts to recover. Extremely low platelet counts can be expected in all dose-intense chemotherapy protocols, mainly for those protocols with hematopoietic stem cell rescue and all induction chemotherapy protocols for malignant hematological disorders, when an aplasia is part of the treatment strategy. Because chemotherapy is not administered routinely in extreme dose intensities in solid tumors, this adverse effect can be well managed.

1.3.1.4 Gastrointestinal Distress

Nausea and vomiting are common side-effects of chemotherapeutic medications that kill fast-dividing cells. This can also produce diarrhea or constipation. Malnutrition and dehydration can result when the patient is unable to eat or drink sufficient amounts, or when the patient vomits frequently because of gastrointestinal damage. This can result in rapid weight loss or occasionally in weight gain, if the patient eats too much in an effort to allay nausea or heartburn. Weight gain can also be caused by some steroid medications. These side-effects can frequently be reduced or eliminated with antiemetic drugs. Self-care measures, such as eating frequent small meals and drinking clear liquids, or ginger tea, are often recommended. This is a temporary effect and frequently resolves within a week of finishing treatment. Chemotherapy-induced nausea and vomiting is common with many treatments and some forms of cancer. Drugs called 5-HT$_3$ antagonists are the most effective antiemetics, and constitute the single greatest advance in the management of nausea and vomiting in patients with cancer. These drugs block one or more of the nerve signals that cause nausea and vomiting. During the first 24 h after chemotherapy, the most effective approach appears to be blocking the 5-HT$_3$ nerve signal. Approved 5-HT$_3$ inhibitors include dolasetron, granisetron, and ondansetron. The newest 5-HT$_3$ inhibitor, palonosetron, also prevents delayed nausea and vomiting, which occurs during 2–5 days after treatment [12]. Since some patients have trouble swallowing pills, these drugs are often available by injection, as orally disintegrating tablets, or as patches. The substance P inhibitor aprepitant (Emend®), which became available in 2005, is also effective in controlling the nausea of cancer chemotherapy [13]. A few studies indicate that the use of cannabinoids derived from marijuana during chemotherapy greatly reduces nausea and vomiting, and enables the patient to eat [13]. Some synthetic derivatives of the active substance in marijuana (tetrahydrocannabinol) such as Marinol® may be practical for this application. Natural marijuana, known as medical cannabis is also used and recommended by some oncologists, although its use is regulated and not legal everywhere [14].

1.3.1.5 Hair Loss

Some medications that kill rapidly dividing cells cause dramatic hair loss; other medications may cause hair to thin out. These are temporary effects – hair growth usually returns a few weeks after the last treatment, sometimes with a tendency to curl (a "chemo perm"). Hair loss seems more a psychological problem because it is immediately visible that a person is under anticancer treatment. It is a kind of stigma that can be very distressing for the patient. All treatments to avoid hair loss are only partly successful. The best results have been seen with cool caps, which limit the circulation of the cytostatic agents, thus preventing damage to the hair follicle in the scalp. Nevertheless, the procedure itself is associated with some pain during the cooling procedure. For all longer infusion protocols with cytostatic agents, this procedure is not effective in avoiding hair loss.

1.3.2
Damage to Specific Organs

Damage to specific organs may occur, with resultant symptoms.

1.3.2.1 Cardiotoxicity

The myocardium consists of cells that have limited regenerative capability, which may render the heart susceptible to permanent adverse effects from chemotherapeutic agents. The effects of antineoplastic agents on the heart can be predictable or

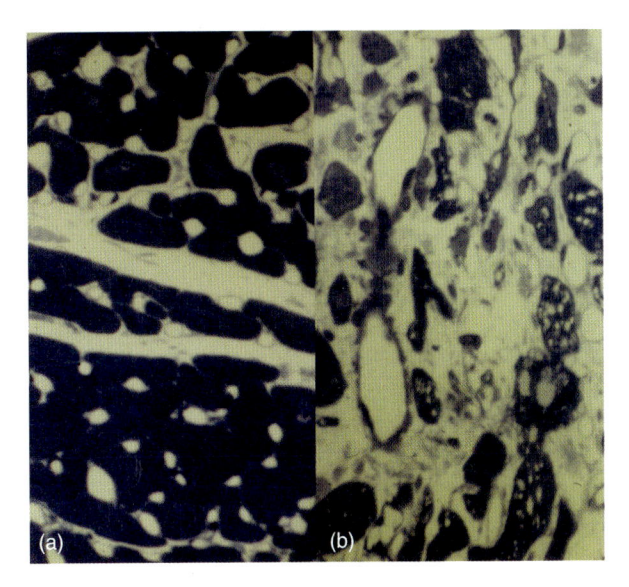

Figure 1.8 Normal (a) and damaged (b) cardiac tissue in mice: destruction of the myocytes and vacuolization. (Reproduced with permission from [17], © Zuckschwerdt Verlag.)

unpredictable, fixed or cumulative [15]. The anthracyclines are feared because acute toxicities include supraclavicular tachycardia, ventricle ectopy, myopericarditis, electrocardiogram changes, cardiomyopathy, and sudden death. Severe irreversible cardiotoxicity is rarely seen at grades 2–4. The most important cardiotoxicity is cumulative late cardiomyopathy, which generally occurs 5 or more years after anthracycline therapy [16]. This kind of toxicity is dose dependent, symptomatic with a progressive decrease in the left ventricular function often resulting in congestive heart failure. Figure 1.8 histologically depicts the damage to the myocytes of the hearts of mice under cumulative treatment with doxorubicin [17].

This is especially a problem in young children because the heart of these patients is much more vulnerable than in older patients. Anthracyclines are an important part of curative therapy for treating most malignant tumors of children [18]. The problem of injury to the heart has probably been underestimated in the past. In the case of anthraquinones such as mitoxantrone, similar but less cardiac damage has been observed. The use of vinca alkaloids has also been associated with heart toxicity related to the vasoconstrictive properties of this group of drugs. Under treatment with 5-FU, myocardial ischemia has been observed. 5-FU has been shown to induce a plethora of cardiac abnormalities. The putative mechanisms of ischemia and other cardiac toxic effects of 5-FU are not known, but there is evidence that coronary vasospasms may play a critical role [19].

1.3.2.2 Hepatotoxicity

Hepatotoxicity is mainly judged by liver function tests because of the ease of determining liver-associated enzyme activities. Apart from hepatic damage by cytostatic agents, other potential causes of abnormal liver function must be considered, such as other medications, alcohol, chemicals, infections, and localized or diffuse infiltrating liver metastases. The spectrum of liver toxicities ranges from the usually incidental elevations of transaminases observed, for example, with nitrosurea to life-threatening massive hepatic necrosis observed with dacarbazine. At doses higher than 16 mg/kg busulfan, veno-occlusive disease develops in a significant number of patients undergoing hematopoietic stem cell transplantation. 6-MP-induced hepatotoxicity occurs in a variety of clinical settings when the dosage exceeds the usual daily dose of 2 mg/kg. The histological pattern includes features of both intrahepatic cholestasis and parenchymal cell necrosis. Bilirubin increases with a moderate increase of transaminases and alkaline phosphates. Since liver function tests do not adequately reflect the degree of hepatic injury, the presence or absence of liver damage is best assessed by serial fine needle biopsies of the liver. Several antineoplastic drugs are metabolized in the liver and excreted via the bile ducts, and are thus relatively nontoxic to the liver. Transient liver enzyme elevations with normalization is the most common reaction profile [20, 21].

1.3.2.3 Nephrotoxicity

The most prominent drugs that are toxic for the kidney are cisplatin, ifosfamide, methotrexate, and mitomycin. Chemotherapeutic agents can produce a variety of acute and chronic kidney toxicities. Awareness of the toxicity potential of each anti-cancer drug in use is important. Either the glomeruli, tubules, or renal vasculature might be at risk, with clinical manifestations ranging from asymptomatic serum creatinine to acute renal failure requiring dialysis. Several factors can potentiate renal dysfunction and contribute to the nephrotoxic potential of antineoplastic drugs: the use of several other drugs, other comorbidities, diabetes mellitus, and heart failure, which might contribute to a decrease of renal function. An acute, mainly proximal tubular impairment occurs with platinum complexes. Proximal tubular damage is marked by a considerable reduction in the reabsorbtive capacities for sodium and water, which is followed by disruption of glomerular filtration and impaired distal tubular function. Forcing diuresis is the method of choice. For the alkylating agents ifosfamide and cyclophosphamide, forced diuresis, and splitting the dose in the case of ifosfamide, is the method of choice for protecting the kidney. For mitomycin, renal failure and microangiopathic hemolytic anemia termed thrombocytopenic purpura/hemolytic uremic syndrome is well known. Ten percent of all patients treated with mitomycin C can develop this severe syndrome. Azacitidine, a pyrimidine analog, has been observed to induce a proximal tubular defect in up to 70% of patients. Methotrexate-induced nephrotoxicity has been managed with high-dose leucovorin, hemodialysis, and with the recombinant enzyme carboxypeptidase G_2, which cleaves methotrexate to produce inactive metabolites [22].

1.3.2.4 Pulmonary Side-Effects

Early-onset chemotherapy-induced lung injury can be classified as inflammatory interstitial pneumonitis, pulmonary edema, bronchospasm, or pleural effusions [23]. In late-onset chemotherapy-induced lung injury, present more than 2 months

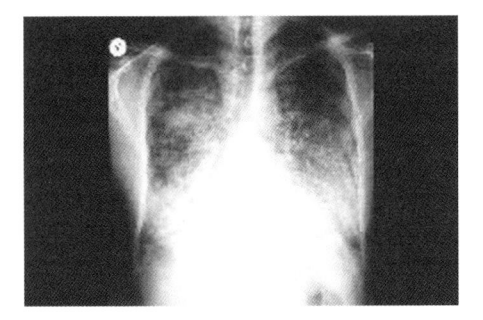

Figure 1.9 Respiratory distress syndrome induced in a patient receiving gemcitabine (strong infiltration in both lungs induced by gemcitabine, 1000 mg/m^2). (Reproduced with permission from [24].)

after the completion of therapy, the most common manifestation is pulmonary fibrosis. The agents with the highest incidence include bleomycin, busulfan, carmustine (bis-chloronitrosourea; BCNU®), and mitomycin. In rare cases even gemcitabine can cause pulmonary damage, as shown in Figure 1.9 [24].

Finally, chemotherapy-induced pulmonary toxicity remains an elusive entity to diagnose. Clinicians should be ever vigilant in watching the clinical signs and symptoms of lung injury, and include this in their differential diagnosis.

1.3.2.5 Vascular Adverse Effects

It has long been recognized that thrombosis and thromboembolic disease may complicate cancer-associated symptoms. There is increasing evidence that vascular toxicity is associated with the administration of chemotherapeutic agents. Such vascular toxicities encompass a heterogeneous group of disorders, including asymptomatic arterial lesions, pulmonary veno-occlusive disease, hepato veno-occlusive disease, Budd–Chiari syndrome, Raynaud's phenomenon, myocardial infarction and ischemia, thrombotic microangiopathy, thrombosis, thromboembolic events, hypotension, hypertension, acral erythema, leukocytoclastic vasculitis, and retinal toxicity. The origin of cytotoxic drug-induced vascular disorders is not clear. One possible mechanism is damage to the endothelial cell by antineoplastic agents or their metabolites. Bleomycin causes a direct toxic effect on endothelial cells in capillaries and small arterioles. Another possible mechanism is drug-induced perturbation of the clotting system or platelet activation. It is apparent that a variety of vascular disorders can be seen after chemotherapies. However, it is not always apparent whether their manifestations are related to the cytotoxic drugs or the malignancy itself and further research in this field is necessary [25].

1.3.2.6 Tissue Damage (Extravasation)

Some of the chemotherapeutic agents are strong tissue-damaging agents, which occurs when the drug is not administered intravenously [26]. The symptoms of extravasation reactions can range from pain, localized tissue inflammation, necrosis to the ulceration of skin and underlying structures (Figure 1.10). Most lesions heal

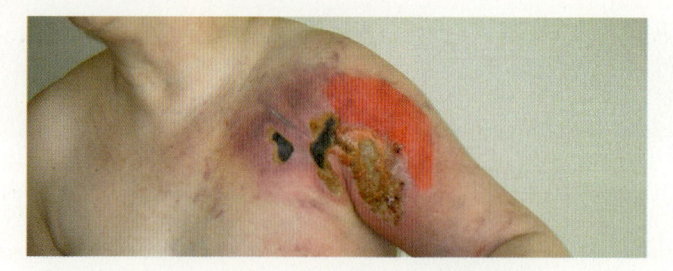

Figure 1.10 Severe tissue ulceration by anthracycline extravasation; epirubicin was administered in the tissue due to a misleading Port-a-Cath needle. (Reproduced with permission from [27].)

poorly and slowly. Vesicant (ulcerogenic) drugs have the capacity to induce the formation of blisters and cause tissue destruction.

Irritant drugs can cause pain with or without inflammation reaction. Nonvesicant drugs rarely produce acute reactions or tissue damage. Chemotherapeutic agents that bind to nucleic acids such as anthracyclines cause direct cell death with necrosis. The drugs that do not bind to nucleic acids may undergo clearance, which limits the degree of tissue injury. A high vesicant potential is known for actinomycin, daunorubicin, doxorubicin, epirubicin, idarubicin, mechlroethamine, vinblastine, vincristine, vindesine, and vinorelbine. The drug amount and the localization of the paravasate determines the amount of tissue damage/irritation. Since extravasation is one of the most serious complications when administering chemotherapeutic agents, oncologists need to take all precautions and care that accidents are avoided. Each location, either in hospitals or outpatients wards or doctor's offices, where intravenous administrations of chemotherapy is carried out should have written guidelines and standard operating procedures for minimizing tissue damage [28].

1.3.2.7 Neurological Side-Effects

Microtubule-stabilizing agents (MTSAs), including the taxanes and epothilones, stabilize microtubules, block mitosis, and induce cell death [29]. A major toxicity associated with this mechanism is peripheral neuropathy. The mechanism of MTSA-induced peripheral neuropathy is not fully understood. As the neurons require that proteins and other components be actively transported along long axons from the neuron's cell body to its distal synapses, MTSA treatment disturbs this active transport. The incidence of peripheral neuropathy depends on the dose of MTSA per treatment cycle. There is a significant difference in the incidence of peripheral neuropathy depending on treatment schedules. Weekly paclitaxel is more neurotoxic than 3-week schedules. The onset of peripheral neuropathy generally depends on the cumulative dose of MTSAs. Other risk factors may include diabetes mellitus, platinum compounds (especially cisplatin), and older patients who are more prone to MTSA-induced peripheral neuropathy. To date, the best strategy is to stop treatment with any potentially neurotoxic drug as soon as neurotoxicity becomes clinically apparent. Administering potentially neuroprotective drugs to prolong treatment with MTSA has failed and unfortunately there are no effective drugs available that reduce this drug-induced toxicity. The reversibility of neurotoxicity is very limited [30].

1.3.2.8 Secondary Neoplasms

The development of secondary neoplasms after successful chemotherapy and or radiotherapy treatment can occur. The most common secondary neoplasm is secondary acute myeloid leukemia (myelodysplastic syndrome), which develops primarily after treatment with alkylating agents or topoisomerase inhibitors. Other studies have shown a 13.5-fold increase from the general population in the incidence of secondary neoplasm occurrence after 30 years from treatment.

1.3.2.9 Infertility

Distinct chemotherapy regimens are gonadotoxic and may cause infertility. Chemotherapies with high risk include procarbazine and alkylating drugs such as cyclophosphamide, ifosfamide, busulfan, melphalan, chlorambucil, and mechloroethamine. Drugs with medium risk include doxorubicin and platinum analogs such as cisplatin and carboplatin [31]. Therapies with a low risk of gonadotoxicity include plant derivatives such as vincristine and vinblastine, antibiotics such as bleomycin and dactinomycin, and antimetabolites such as methotrexate, 6-MP, and 5-FU.

Patients may choose between several methods of fertility preservation prior to chemotherapy, including cryopreservation of semen, ovarian tissue, oocytes, or embryos [32].

1.3.2.10 Other Side-Effects

Patients with particularly large tumors, such as large lymphomas, can develop a tumor lysis syndrome from the rapid breakdown of malignant cells. Although prophylaxis is available and is often initiated in patients with large tumors, this is a dangerous side-effect that can lead to death if left untreated.

Less-common side-effects include pain, red skin (erythema), dry skin, hand and foot syndrome damaged fingernails, a dry mouth (xerostomia), water retention, and sexual impotence. Some medications can trigger allergic or pseudoallergic reactions.

Some patients report fatigue or nonspecific neurocognitive problems, such as an inability to concentrate; this is sometimes called postchemotherapy cognitive impairment (referred to as "chemo brain" by patient groups) [33]. Specific chemotherapeutic agents are associated with organ-specific toxicities, including cardiovascular disease (e.g., doxorubicin), interstitial lung disease (e.g., bleomycin), and occasionally secondary neoplasm (e.g., MOPP therapy for Hodgkin's disease).

1.4 Supportive Care

The development of new drugs to prevent nausea (the prototype of which was ondansetron) was of great practical use as was the design of indwelling intravenous catheters (e.g., Hickman lines and Port-a-Cath systems) that allowed safe administration of chemotherapy as well as supportive therapies via an intravenous line. Supportive care includes treatment of infections, treatment with growth factors, treatment with blood products, and treatment of pain, diarrhea, psychological derangement, depression, and anxiety by oncologists, psycho-oncologists, and specialized nursing staff.

1.5
New Approaches Complementing Current Cancer Chemotherapy

Despite the success of certain anticancer agents in curing certain malignant diseases, mostly hematological cancers or neoplasms with a low prevalence, and the gradual improvement of treating the most common solid tumors with combination therapy in the adjuvant or palliative setting, oncologists appeared to have hit a wall in terms of achieving major breakthroughs with conventional cytostatic agents.

An important asset at this point was the recognition that hormonal therapy was beneficial for several types of cancers derived from hormonally responsive tumors, including breast, prostate, endometrium, adrenal cortex, and endocrine tumors. Effective strategies for starving tumor cells of growth- and survival-promoting hormones was to use drugs that inhibit the production of those hormones (e.g., estrogens or testosterone for breast and prostate cancer, respectively) or to administer hormone receptor antagonists. Both classes are often used prior or after chemotherapy in the subpopulation of patients that have a positive hormone receptor status, and can inhibit tumor growth for many months and are also beneficial in preventing a tumor relapse after successful surgery or chemotherapy. For some tumors, such as endocrine tumors, an analog of the peptide hormone somatostatin, octreotide, is the best option of treating endocrine tumors of different origin and carcinoid tumors.

From the 1980s onwards, advances in molecular biology allowed a progressive elucidation of the mechanisms underlying cancer and a profound understanding of the genetic nature of cancer. The molecular and genetic approaches uncovered entirely new signaling networks of intra- and extracellular kinases, growth factor receptors, and antigens that regulate activities of tumor cells and tumor tissue, such as their proliferation and survival as well as angiogenesis – the formation of tumor blood vessels that are necessary for a solid tumor to grow once it has reached a size of approximately 1 cm^3.

As a result, the pharmaceutical and biotech industry invested heavily into a new drug generation and the expression "targeted therapy" was coined, referring to treating cancer by blocking the growth of cancer cells by interfering with specific cellular targets needed for carcinogenesis and tumor growth.

The two categories of targeted therapy are small molecules and monoclonal antibodies (mAbs). The most successful example of targeted development for small molecules is imatinib mesylate (Gleevec$^®$) – a small molecule that inhibits the signaling molecule kinase Bcr–Abl kinase that causes chronic myelogenous leukemia

(CML). Gleevec® has dramatically improved the treatment of this malignancy. The next generation of drugs (dasatinib and nilotinib) has now been approved and is available, inducing a more effective molecular remission in CML than imatinib.

Subsequent developments for treating solid tumors have resulted in tyrosine kinase inhibitors such as gefitinib (Iressa®) [34], which targets the epidermal growth factor receptor (EGFR) tyrosine kinase and is approved for treating non-small-cell lung cancer (NSCLC), and erlotinib (Tarceva®), which acts by a similar mechanism as gefitinib. Both drugs work best for EGFR receptor kinase mutations in NSCLC [35]. This type of cancer is a distinct type of cancer where personalized medicine can be successfully used when the biomarker EGFR activating mutations is present. Another good example is the treatment of NSCLC with an anaplastic lymphoma kinase (ALK) inhibitor (crizotinib) in the case of (echinoderm microtubule-associated protein-like) EML4-ALK-positive tumors [36]. EML4-ALK is a fusion-type protein tyrosine kinase that is present in only about 5% of NSCLC patients. A crucial factor is the identification of this small subgroup through prospective tumor genotyping as a prerequisite for a successful treatment. Three other multikinase inhibitors (sunitinib, sorafenib, and pazopanib) are approved, but not for major tumor types, such as breast, lung, colon, and prostate cancer. The approvals comprise less-common tumors such as kidney cancer, gastrointestinal stromal tumor, and primary liver cancer, and to date it is unclear if these drugs can be successfully integrated in the treatment strategies of major tumors. Recent results showed that sunitinib failed in phase III studies in colon and breast cancer. Another interesting aspect is the fact that all new drugs failed in pancreatic cancer, and most in prostate cancer, indicating that these tumors cannot currently be treated effectively by targeted therapy.

Bortezomib (Velcade®) is an inhibitor of the proteasome – an intracellular protein complex that degrades unneeded or damaged proteins – and is approved to treat multiple myeloma that no longer responds to chemotherapy.

Another new class of targeted small molecules is represented by the histone deacetylase (HDAC) inhibitors that inhibit the proliferation of tumor cells by inducing cell cycle arrest, differentiation, and/or apoptosis. Histone acetylation and deacetylation play pivotal roles in the regulation of gene transcription. Vorinostat® is the first HDAC inhibitor to be approved for the treatment of cutaneous T cell lymphoma.

The alternative approach to conventional chemotherapy has been the development of mAbs that are directed toward tumor-associated antigens. The advent of chimeric or humanized, or human mAbs in which only the variable, the hypervariable, or none of the regions of the binding domain carry murine sequences, has resolved the initial drawback of provoking a immune reaction in cancer patients. As a consequence, six antibodies, trastuzumab (Herceptin®, used in the treatment of HER2/*neu* breast cancer), alemtuzumab (Campath®, targets the antigen CD52 expressed on in chronic lymphatic leukemia), rituximab (Rituxan®, used in the treatment of CD20$^+$ Hodgkin's lymphoma), bevacizumab (Avastin®, used in the treatment of colon cancer, breast cancer, and NSCLC inhibiting the vascular endothelial growth factor receptor that is important for angiogenesis) [37], and cetuximab (Erbitux®) and panitumumab (Vectibix®), both of which target the EGFR and are used in the treatment of colon cancer, are approved and a large number of other antibodies are in clinical trials [38]. The next mAb that will very likely be approved is ipilimumab, which blocks cytotoxic T-lymphocyte-associated antigen-4 to potentiate an T-cell response for the treatment of metastatic melanoma [39].

Although the new generation of targeted therapies have undoubtedly improved the therapeutic options of treating cancer, four important issues need to be considered: (i) the use of approved targeted drugs have improved the overall survival of cancer patients by 3–12 months; (ii) treatment with these drugs causes side-effects that range from skin toxicity, cardiac toxicity, effusions, diarrhea, fatigue, and hypertension to other side-effects that can be severe, approaching grade 3 and 4 toxicity, which is encumbering for the patient and sometimes requires another treatment to ameliorate these side-effects; (iii) resistance against targeted therapy occurs just like with conventional anticancer agents; and (iv) targeted therapy is generally used in combination with conventional chemotherapy and the best therapeutic results are achieved in such regimens.

1.6
Conclusions and Perspectives

The era of cancer chemotherapy began in the 1940s with the first use of nitrogen mustards and folic acid antagonist drugs. Cancer drug development has developed since then into a multi-billion dollar industry. Conventional cytotoxic chemotherapy has shown the ability to cure some cancers, including testicular cancer, chorioncarcinoma, rhabdosarcoma, Hodgkin's disease, non-Hodgkin's lymphoma, and some leukemias. It has also proved effective in the adjuvant setting, in reducing the risk of recurrence after surgery for high-risk breast, colon, and lung cancers, among others. In the palliative setting, the continuing evaluation of combination therapies has improved the quality of live and over two decades has shown a slow but gradual increase in the overall survival rates of patients with solid tumors.

The overall impact of chemotherapy on cancer survival can be difficult to estimate, since improved cancer screening, prevention (e.g., antismoking campaigns), and detection all influence statistics on cancer incidence and mortality. To date, the World Health Organization predicts that deaths from cancer worldwide are projected to rise continuously, with an estimated 12 million deaths in 2030.

The addition of targeted therapies has significantly improved the treatment of a few malignancies such as CML, lung tumors with adeno cancer, kidney cancer, colon cancer, or multiple myeloma, and has in combination with classic anticancer agents improved the quality of life and the overall survival for patients with many solid tumor by approximately 3–12 months in the palliative setting. However, for some common solid tumors such as metastatic breast cancer the overall survival has remained more or less constant during nearly three decades, albeit several subgroups (e.g., HER2/*neu* receptor-positive) have an significant advantage by additionally using a HER2/*neu* receptor-specific antibody (Herceptin®).

With the better understanding of carcinogenesis, angiogenesis, and signal transduction pathways there were high hopes that therapy with targeted therapies with or without conventional chemotherapy would revolutionize cancer therapy with malignant diseases being treated as a chronic disease with long-term improvement or stabilization of the disease. Unfortunately, we are still far from reaching this goal. With succeeding generations of tumor cells, differentiation is typically lost, growth becomes less regulated, and tumors become less responsive to most chemotherapeutic or targeted agents. Near the center of some solid tumors, cell division has effectively ceased, making them insensitive to chemotherapy. Further challenges for treating solid tumors are due to the fact that the chemotherapeutic agent often does not reach the core of the tumor. Finally, with increasing tumor mass and the formation of metastases, cancer cells become more resistant to chemotherapy treatments.

The three volume compendium gives an overview of the drug delivery systems that have been developed over the past decades with the aim of improving the therapeutic index of anticancer drugs. This is a central goal for treating malignant diseases with conventional anticancer drugs or targeted drugs, with the first drug delivery systems now approved and many others in clinical trials. Such drug delivery systems will be a valuable asset for the oncologist in his/her options of treating cancer patients as effectively as possible, very likely in combination with established clinical protocols. As we move toward a more personalized approach of treating over 100 different tumor indications, we should learn from the mistakes of putting all our eggs in one basket and disregarding long experience with conventional chemotherapy in the hope that new approaches, whether they are called targeted therapies, immunotherapy, gene therapy, or nanomedicine, will find a quick medical solution. It is more likely that all these fields will make advances and it will be a tailor-made combination of different therapeutic strategies that will achieve the best results when faced with such a complex disease as cancer.

References

1. Li, J.J. (2006) *Laughing Gas, Viagar, Liptor; The Human Stories behind the Drugs We Use*, Oxford University Press, Oxford, p. 8.
2. Goodman, L.S., Wintrobe, M.M., Dameshek, D., Goodman, M.J., Gilman, A., and McLennan, M.T. (1946) Nitrogen mustard therapy; use of methyl-bis (β-chloroethyl) amine hydrochloride and tris (β-chloroethyl) amine hydrochloride for Hodgkin's disease, lymphosarcoma, leukemia and certain allied and miscellaneous disorders. *J. Am. Med. Assoc.*, **132**, 126–132.
3. Farber, S. and Diamond, L.K. (1948) Temporary remissions in acute leukemia in children produced by folic acid antagonist, 4-aminopteroyl-glutamic acid. *N. Engl. J. Med.*, **238**, 787–793.
4. Li, M.C., Hertz, R., and Bergenstal, D.M. (1958) Therapy of choriocarcinoma and related trophoblastic tumors with folic acid and purine antagonists. *N. Engl. J. Med.*, **259**, 66–74.
5. Newman, D.J. and Cragg, G.M. (2007) Natural products as sources of new drugs over the last 25 years. *J. Nat. Prod.*, **70**, 461–477.

6. Frei, E., Jaffe, N., Gero, M., Skipper, H., and Watts, H. III (1978) Adjuvant chemotherapy of osteogenic sarcoma: progress and perspectives. *J. Natl. Cancer Inst.*, **60**, 3–10.
7. Bonadonna, G., Valagussa, P., Rossi, A., Tancini, G., Brambilla, C. et al. (1985) Ten-year experience with CMF-based adjuvant chemotherapy in resectable breast cancer. *Breast. Cancer Res. Treat.*, **5**, 95–115.
8. Tkaczuk, K.H. (2009) Review of the contemporary cytotoxic and biologic combinations available for the treatment of metastatic breast cancer. *Clin. Ther.*, **31**, 2273–2289.
9. Skipper, H.E. (1964) Perspectives in cancer chemotherapy: therapeutic design. *Cancer Res.*, **24**, 1295–1302.
10. Higgins, C.F. (2007) Multiple molecular mechanisms for multidrug resistance transporters. *Nature*, **446**, 749–757.
11. Primeau, A.J., Rendon, A., Hedley, D., Lilge, L., and Tannock, I.F. (2005) The distribution of the anticancer drug doxorubicin in relation to blood vessels in solid tumors. *Clin. Cancer Res.*, **11**, 8782–8788.
12. MASCC (2004) Prevention of chemotherapy- and radiotherapy-induced emesis: results of the 2004 Perugia International Antiemetic Consensus Conference. *Ann. Oncol.*, **17**, 20–28.
13. Gralla, R.J., de Wit, R., Herrstedt, J., Carides, A.D., Ianus, J. et al. (2005) Antiemetic efficacy of the neurokinin-1 antagonist, aprepitant, plus a 5HT$_3$ antagonist and a corticosteroid in patients receiving anthracyclines or cyclophosphamide in addition to high-dose cisplatin: analysis of combined data from two phase III randomized clinical trials. *Cancer*, **104**, 864–868.
14. Tramer, M.R., Carroll, D., Campbell, F.A., Reynolds, D.J., Moore, R.A. et al. (2001) Cannabinoids for control of chemotherapy induced nausea and vomiting: quantitative systematic review. *Br. Med. J.*, **323**, 16–21.
15. Hijiya, N., Hudson, M.M., Lensing, S., Zacher, M., Onciu, M. et al. (2007) Cumulative incidence of secondary neoplasms as a first event after childhood acute lymphoblastic leukemia. *J. Am. Med. Assoc.*, **297**, 1207–1115.
16. Elliott, P. (2006) Pathogenesis of cardiotoxicity induced by anthracyclines. *Semin. Oncol.*, **33**, S2–S7.
17. Mross, K. (ed.) (1993) *Klinische und Pharmakologische Untersuchungen zur Pharmakokinetik, Metabolisierung, Pharmakodynamik und Toxizität von Anthranzklinen in Aktuelle Onkologie 76*, Zuckschwerdt Verlag, München.
18. Floyd, J.D., Nguyen, D.T., Lobins, R.L., Bashir, Q.B., Doll, D.C., and Perry, M.C. (2005) Cardiotoxicity of cancer therapy. *J. Clin. Oncol.*, **23**, 7685–7696.
19. Lipshultz, S.E. (2006) Exposure to anthracyclines during childhood causes cardiac injury. *Semin. Oncol.*, **33**, S8–S14.
20. Field, K.M., Dow, C., and Michael, M. (2008) Part I: liver function in oncology: biochemistry and beyond. *Lancet Oncol.*, **9**, 1092–1102.
21. Filed, K.M. and Michael, M. (2008) Part II: liver function in oncology: towards safer chemotherapy use. *Lancet Oncol.*, **9**, 1191–1190.
22. de Jonge, M.J.A. and Verweij, J. (2006) Renal toxicities of chemotherapy. *Semin. Oncol.*, **33**, 68–73.
23. Meadors, M., Floyd, J., and Perry, M.C. (2006) Pulmonary toxicity of chemotherapy. *Semin. Oncol.*, **33**, 98–104.
24. Fuxius, S., Unger, C., and Mross, K. (1999) Pulmonary toxicity resulting from treatment with gemcitabine. *Onkologie*, **22**, 146–149.
25. Doll, D.C. and Yarbo, J.W. (1992) Vascular toxicity associated with antineoplastic agents. *Semin. Oncol.*, **19**, 580–596.
26. Ener, R.A., Meglathery, S.B., and Styler, M. (2004) Extravasation of systemic hemato-oncological therapies. *Ann. Oncol.*, **15**, 858–862.
27. Frost, A., Gmehling, D., Azemar, M., Unger, C., and Mross, K. (2006) Treatment of anthracycline extravasation with dexrazoxane – clinical experience. *Onkologie*, **29**, 314–318.
28. Mader, I., Fürst-Weger, P.R., Mader, R.M., Nogler-Semenitz, E., and Wassertheurer, S. (2006) *Paravasation von Zytostatika*, Springer, Wien.

29. Lee, J.J. and Swain, S.M. (2006) Peripheral neuropathy induced by micotubule-stabilizing agents. *J. Clin. Oncol.*, **24**, 1633–1642.
30. Mielke, S., Mross, K., Gerds, T.A., Schmidt, A., Wäsch, R. et al. (2003) Comparative neurotoxicity of weekly non-break paclitaxel infusions over 1 versus 3 hours. *Anti-Cancer Drugs*, **14**, 785–792.
31. Brydoy, M., Fossa, S.D., Dahl, O., and Bjoro, T. (2007) Gonadal dysfunction and fertility problems in cancer survivors. *Acta. Oncol.*, **46**, 480–489.
32. Gurgan, T., Salman, C., and Demirol, A. (2008) Pregnancy and assisted reproduction techniques in men and women after cancer treatment. *Placenta*, **29** (Suppl. B), 152–159.
33. Tannock, I.F., Ahles, T.A., Ganz, P.A., and Van Dam, F.S. (2004) Cognitive impairment associated with chemotherapy for cancer: report of a workshop. *J. Clin. Oncol.*, **22**, 2233–2239.
34. Kwak, E.L., Bang, Y.-J., Camidge, D.R., Shaw, A.T., Solomon, B. et al. (2010) Anaplastic lymphoma kinase inhibition in non small-cell-lung-cancer. *N. Engl. J. Med.*, **363**, 1693–1703.
35. Maemondo, M., Inoue, A., Kobayyashi, K., and Sugawara, S. (2010) Gefitinib or chemotherapy for non-small cell lung cancer with mutated EGFR. *N. Engl. J. Med.*, **352**, 2380–2388.
36. Paz-Ares, L., Soulieres, D., Melezinek, I., Moecks, J., Keil, L. et al. (2010) Clinical outcomes in non-small-cell lung cancer patients with EGFR mutations: pooled analysis. *J. Cell. Mol. Med.*, **14**, 51–69.
37. Mross, K. (ed.) (2007) *Angiogeneseinhibition in der Onkologie*, Uni-Med Verlag, Bremen.
38. Ferris, R.L., Jaffee, E.M., and Ferrone, S. (2010) Tumor antigen-targeted, monoclonal antibody-based immunotherapy: clinical response, cellular immunity, and immunoescape. *J. Clin. Oncol.*, **28**, 4390–4399.
39. Hodi, F.S., O'Day, S.J., Dermott, D., Weber, R.W., Sosman, J.A. et al. (2010) Improved survival with ipilimumab in patients with metastatic melanoma. *N. Engl. J. Med.*, **363**, 711–723.

2
Pathophysiological and Vascular Characteristics of Solid Tumors in Relation to Drug Delivery

Peter Vaupel

2.1
Introduction

Most, if not all, solid tumors begin as avascular aggregates of malignant cells. "Microscopic tumors" exchange nutrients and breakdown products of metabolism with their surroundings by simple diffusion [1–6]. The growth of an avascular three-dimensional aggregate of tumor cells is therefore self-limiting (up to 1–2 mm in diameter). Small tumors can stay dormant for a very long time period until the so-called angiogenic switch occurs [7]. Rapid tumor growth, tumor progression, invasion, local spread, and distant metastasis to other organs or tissues following the avascular growth period are possible only if convective transport (nutrient supply and waste removal) is initiated through nutritive blood flow (i.e., flow through tumor microvessels that guarantees adequate exchange processes between the microcirculatory bed and the cancer cells). This notion has led to the dogmatic assumption that both tumor growth and tumor spread are dependent on rigorous angiogenesis (for a review, see [8]). This implies that vascularization is a prerequisite for tumor growth, invasion, and metastasis. At the same time the tumor microcirculation – besides diffusion – is the major transport mechanism for the effective delivery of therapeutic molecules. A compromised microcirculation is therefore considered as an obstacle in drug delivery.

In this chapter, the consequences of the irregular structure and function of the tumor microcirculation for drug delivery will be described. Special emphasis will be given to (i) delivery by the heterogeneous microcirculation, (ii) extravasation through the leaky vessel walls, and (iii) traversing of the special interstitial compartment. These different steps are characterized by special barriers to therapy that may not be shared by hemoblastoses. In addition, emphasis is also put on the role of hypoxia and acidosis in the development of acquired drug resistance.

2.2
Basic Principles of Blood Vessel Formation in Solid Tumors

When considering the continuous and indiscriminate formation of a vascular network in rapidly growing tumors, six different mechanisms have been described [4–6, 9, 10]:

1) Angiogenesis by endothelial sprouting from pre-existing venules.
2) Co-option of existing vessels.
3) Vasculogenesis.
4) Intussusception.
5) Vascular mimicry.
6) Microvessel formation by bone marrow-derived myeloid cells.

2.2.1
Angiogenesis

The avascular (= prevascular) growth phase characteristic of a "dormant" tumor and the vascular phase in which "explosive" growth ensues in many solid tumors are separated by the "angiogenic switch" [11]. This switch is "off" when the effect of proangiogenic molecules is balanced by that of antiangiogenic molecular players. It is "on" when the net balance is tipped in favor of angiogenesis [12]. Pro- and antiangiogenic molecules can be released from cancer cells, endothelial cells, stromal and inflammatory cells, or can be mobilized from the extracellular matrix [9, 10]. The "angiogenic switch" – a pivotal and early event in tumor progression – greatly depends on one or more positive regulators, such as growth factors, permeability regulating factors, migration stimulators, proteolytic enzymes (balanced with their inhibitors), extracellular matrix molecules, and adhesion molecules (Table 2.1).

1) Vascular-specific growth factors include vascular endothelial growth factors (VEGFs) and their receptors, the angiopoietin family (Ang) and Tie receptors, and the ephrins.
2) Nonspecific factors comprise platelet-derived growth factor (PDGF), fibroblast growth factors (FGFs), transforming growth factor (TGF)-β, tumor necrosis factor (TNF)-α, epidermal growth factor (EGF), and several others.

A central inducer of growth of new blood vessels is VEGF (originally identified as "vascular permeability factor"). Expression of VEGF is regulated by hypoxia [15, 16], hypoglycemia [17], acidosis [9], activation of oncogenes or deletion of tumor-suppressor genes that control production of angiogenesis regulators [18], cytokines, and hormones (M. Neeman, personal communication).

The process of angiogenesis is extremely complex and requires balanced interactions with biologic redundancy. Major steps in the "angiogenic cascade" include (besides the "angiogenic switch" and upregulation of proangiogenic molecules,

Table 2.1 Angiogenic proteins regulating tumor angiogenesis and major actions of these growth factors (selection) (adapted from [13, 14]).

Factors	Major actions
Specific factors	
VEGF	increases vascular permeability, promotes proliferation, and endothelial cell migration, upregulates proteases for matrix degeneration, inhibits endothelial cell apoptosis, stabilizes vessels
Ang-1	stabilizes endothelium, suppresses endothelial cell apoptosis, promotes vessel maturation and vascular hierarchy, stimulates sprout and lumen formation, inhibits hyperpermeability
Ang-2	antagonizes Ang-1 signaling, destabilizes endothelium, promotes endothelial sprouting
Ephrins	guide vessel branching, determine endothelial cell specialization
Non-specific factors	
PDGF	promotes endothelial cell proliferation and migration, stimulates pericyte and smooth muscle cell recruitment, stimulates DNA synthesis in endothelial cells
FGFs	stimulate proliferation and migration of endothelial cells, promote endothelial cell tube formation, induce and synergize VEGF
TGF-β	regulates proliferation and migration of endothelial cells, regulates vessel maturation, stimulates production of extravascular matrix
TNF-α	stimulates angiogenesis and tube formation
EGF	stimulates endothelial cell proliferation

binding of the latter to specific endothelial cell receptors and ligand–receptor interaction):

- Dilation of existing vessels.
- Endothelial cell activation.
- Hyperpermeability of postcapillary venules and vessel destabilization.
- Localized degradation of basement membrane.
- Matrix remodeling [degradation of extracellular matrix in response to activation of matrix metalloproteinases (MMPs), formation of a new provisional extravascular matrix by leaked plasma proteins].
- Migration of endothelial cells.
- Cell–cell contacts, sprout formation.
- Extension of sprouts by endothelial cell proliferation.
- Tube formation ("canalization"), fusion to form vascular loops.
- (Nonmandatory) recruitment of pericytes and smooth muscle cells.
- (Often improper) vessel maturation.

These different steps are partly concurrent, partly in series and sequential. They occur in different parts of primary tumors and in metastases at the same time.

2.2.2
Vascular Co-option

Tumor cells often appear to co-opt vessels (i.e., they can incorporate pre-existing vessels within a vascularized host tissue to initiate vessel-dependent tumor growth as opposed to classic angiogenesis) [10]. Later, in the co-opted vessels, endothelial cells release Ang-2 (probably by autocrine action), which leads to vascular destabilization and vascular collapse. The resultant hypoxia and nutrient deprivation then yield an upregulation of VEGF and "secondary" angiogenesis [19].

2.2.3
Vasculogenesis

De novo vessel formation through incorporation of circulating endothelial precursor cells (angioblasts) from bone marrow or peripheral blood is mandatory for vasculogenesis.

2.2.4
Intussusception

In intussusception, interstitial tissue columns insert into the lumen of pre-existing vessels and lead to partition of the initial vessel lumen [20].

2.2.5
Vascular Mimicry

De novo generation of pseudovascular channels without the participation of endothelial cells has been described in central areas of melanomas. A contribution of cancer cells to the wall of tumor vessels has also been reported for tumor entities other then melanomas [10, 21]. The concept of vascular mimicry is, however, still controversial [22].

2.2.6
Microvessel Formation by Myeloid Cells

Microvessel formation may also be triggered by a subset of bone marrow-derived myeloid cells infiltrating solid tumors.

The tumor vasculature is characterized by vigorous proliferation leading to immature, structurally, defective and, in terms of perfusion, ineffective microvessels. "Tumor vessels lack the signals to mature" and tumor vasculature is often described as an "aberrant monster" [23]. Consequently, tumor blood flow is chaotic and heterogeneous (Section 2.4).

2.3
Tumor Lymphangiogenesis

Although the metastatic spread of tumor cells to regional lymph nodes is a common feature of many human cancers, it is not clear whether shedding tumor cells utilize existing lymphatic vessels or whether tumor dissemination requires *de novo* formation of lymphatics [10]. The notion that tumor microcirculation may be supported by a newly formed, tumor-induced lymphatic network has so far not been confirmed convincingly. VEGF-C, VEGF-D, and their corresponding receptors have been identified as specific lymphangiogenic factors in several tumors [10, 24]. It has been proposed that functional lymphatics in the tumor margin are sufficient for lymphatic metastasis, because the tumor center was found to contain no functional lymphatics [25]. The intratumoral lymphatic vessels are usually collapsed (compressed) due to the high interstitial pressure caused by the growing tumor mass in a confined space. In the tumor periphery VEGF-C causes lymphatics to enlarge, collecting interstitial fluid and metastatic cancer cells [9].

2.4
Tumor Vascularity and Blood Flow

As already mentioned, the key players in tumor angiogenesis are VEGF, angiopoietins, ephrins, and their corresponding receptors. However, their excessive production causes the formation of structurally and functionally abnormal blood vessels. The tumor vasculature can be described as a system that is maximally stimulated, yet only minimally fulfilling the metabolic demands of the growing tumor that it supplies [26].

Microvessels in solid tumors are often dilated, tortuous, elongated, and saccular (Figure 2.1). There is significant arteriovenous shunt perfusion accompanied by chaotic vascular organization that lacks any regulation matched to the metabolic demands or functional status of the tissue. Excessive branching is a common finding, often coinciding with blind vascular endings. Incomplete or even missing endothelial lining and discontinuous or even absent basement membranes result in an increased vascular permeability with extravasation of blood plasma and of red blood cells expanding the interstitial fluid space and drastically increasing the hydrostatic pressure in the tumor interstitium (Table 2.2). In solid tumors there is a *rise in viscous resistance to flow*, due mainly to hemoconcentration. Aberrant vascular morphology and a decrease in vessel density are responsible for an *increase in geometric resistance to flow*, which can lead to an inadequate perfusion. Substantial spatial heterogeneity in the distribution of tumor vessels and significant temporal heterogeneity in the microcirculation within a tumor [27] may result in a considerably anisotropic distribution of tumor tissue oxygenation and of a number of other factors, which are usually closely linked and which define the so-called metabolic microenvironment. Variations in these relevant parameters between

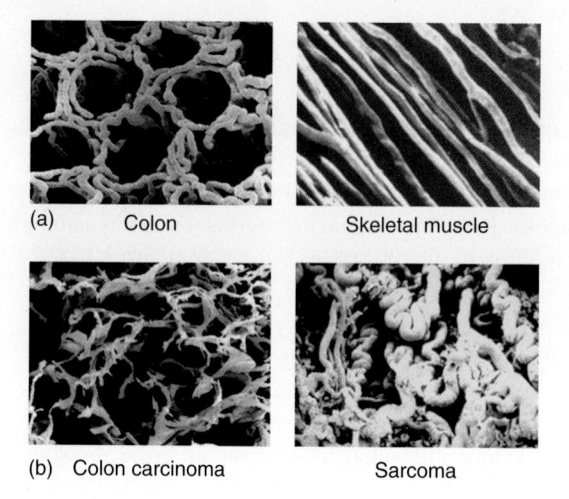

Figure 2.1 Microvasculature of normal tissues (a) and malignant tumors (b). (Modified from [4]).

tumors are often more pronounced than differences occurring between different locations or microareas within a tumor [28–30].

Blood flow in solid tumors can vary considerably, ranging from around 0.01 to 3.0 ml/g/min (Figure 2.2). Tumors can thus have flow rates similar to those measured in tissues with a high metabolic rate or can exhibit perfusion rates comparable to those of tissues with low metabolic turnover. Flow data from multiple sites of measurement show marked heterogeneity within individual tumors. (Delivery of anticancer drugs is similarly compromised.) When measuring the microregional distribution of perfusion within a tumor using the H_2-clearance technique, microflow rates of 0.01–3.0 µl/µl tissue/min (median microflow: 0.5 µl/µl/min) were observed with an accumulation of measured values less than 0.01 µl/µl/min. Considering all flow values assessed by this technique, flow data can vary by a factor of approximately 300 (Figure 2.3). This flow variability in experimental animal tumors is thus significantly larger than that seen in individual tumor entities in the clinical setting (100-fold; see Figure 2.2). This heterogeneous flow distribution clearly mirrors the chaotic microvasculature found in solid tumors [35]. However, tumor-to-tumor variability seems to be more pronounced than intratumor heterogeneity [28].

2.5
Arteriovenous Shunt Perfusion in Tumors

First rough estimations concerning the arteriovenous shunt flow in malignant tumors showed that at least 30% of the arterial blood can pass through experimental tumors without participating in the microcirculatory exchange processes [36–38]. In patients receiving intra-arterial chemotherapy for head and neck cancer, shunt

Table 2.2 Major structural and functional irregularities of tumor microvessels (updated from [5, 6, 30]).

Blood vessels	Lymphatic vessels
Missing differentiation Loss of vessel hierarchy (disorganized vascular network) Increased intervessel distances, existence of a vascular areas Large diameter (sinusoidal) microvessels Elongated, tortuous (convoluted) vessels Contour irregularities Saccular microvessels, blind endings Aberrant branching [31] Haphazard pattern of vessel interconnection Incomplete endothelial lining, fenestrations Interrupted or absent basement membranes Presence of lumen-less endothelial cell cords ("nonproductive angiogenesis") Existence of vessel-like cavities not connected to the blood stream Existence of tumor cell-lined vascular channels ("vascular mimicry") Arteriovenous anastomoses (shunt perfusion) Vessels originating from the venous side Missing innervation Lack of physiological/pharmacological receptors Lack of smooth muscle cells Poor or absent coverage by pericytes Absence of vasomotion and flow regulation Increased vascular permeability, plasma leakage Increased geometric resistance to flow Increase in hematocrit within tumor microvessels by 5–14% Increased viscous resistance to flow Unstable flow velocities (about 85% of all microvessels [32]) Fluctuating red blood cell fluxes [33] Unstable direction of flow Intermittent flow, regurgitation (about 5% of all microvessels [33]) Flow stasis (about 1% of all microvessels [33]) Plasma flow only (about 8% of all microvessels [33]) Formation of platelet/leukocyte clusters [34]) Thrombus formations Formation of red blood cells aggregates Reduced Fahraeus–Lindqvist effect Acidosis-induced rigidity of red blood cells	Commonly infiltrated by tumor cells (periphery) Flattened vessels without lumen (center) VEGF-C- and VEGF-D-induced growth at tumor margin Inadequate lymphatic drainage in the tumor center Interstitial fluid flow Interstitial hypertension

It is not only the quantity of microvessels that counts, but also – or even more so – the quality of vascular function in terms of the tumor tissue supply or drainage!

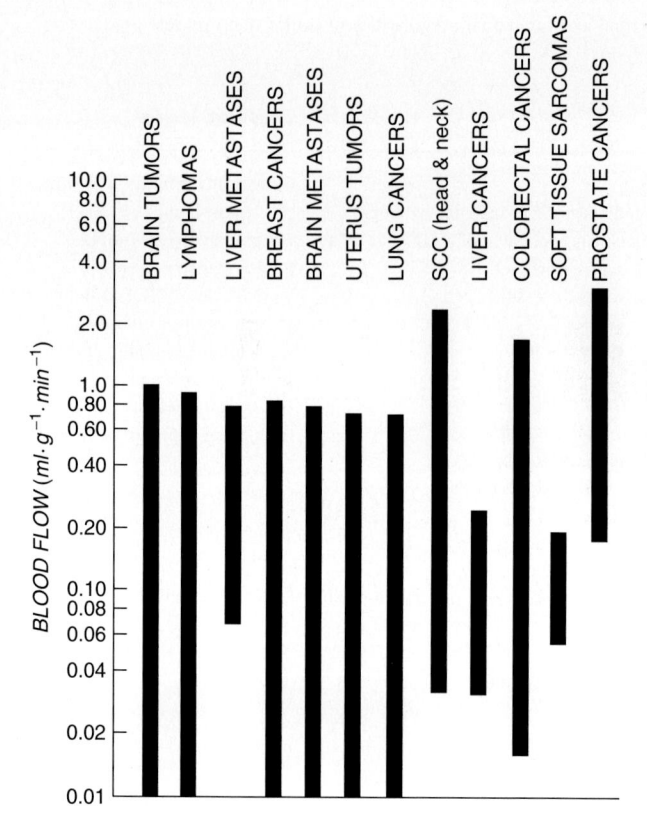

Figure 2.2 Variability of blood flow rates in solid tumors. SCC, squamous cell carcinomas. (Updated from [6]).

flow is reported to be 8–43% of total tumor blood flow – the latter consistently exceeding normal tissue perfusion of the scalp [39]. The mean fractional shunt perfusion of tumors was 23 ± 13% in studies utilizing ^{99m}Tc-labeled macroaggregated albumin (diameter of particles: 15–90 µm). The significance of this shunt flow on local, intratumor drug distribution (pharmacokinetics) and on relevant metabolic phenomena has not yet been systematically studied and remains speculative.

2.6
Volume and Characteristics of the Tumor Interstitial Space

The interstitial compartment of solid tumors is significantly different from that of most normal tissues [40]. In general, the tumor interstitial space is characterized by:

- A distension of its volume, which is 3–5 times larger than in most normal tissues (Figure 2.4).
- A relatively high interstitial diffusivity.

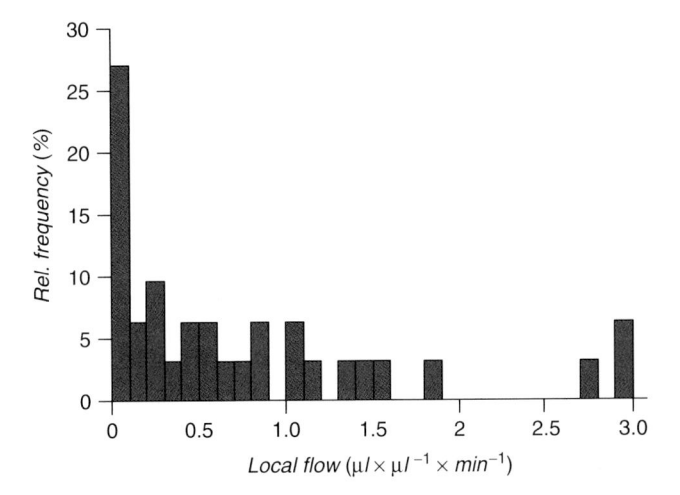

Figure 2.3 Frequency distribution of measured blood flow values in superficial regions of C3H mouse adenocarcinoma using the hydrogen clearance technique for assessment of local perfusion rates ("microflow" rates). (Modified from [35]).

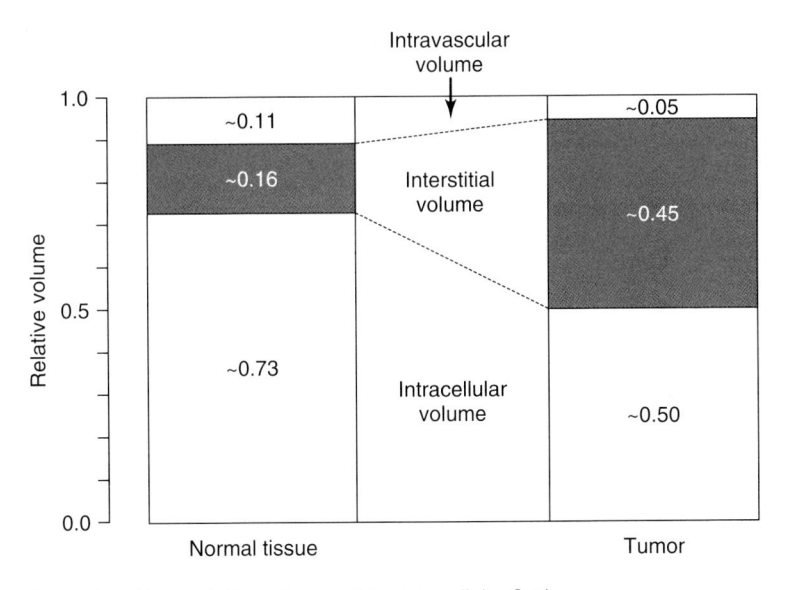

Figure 2.4 Mean relative volumes of the intracellular fluid, the vascular compartment, and the interstitial fluid space in malignant tumors (right panel) and in normal tissue (left panel). (Adapted from [3]).

- A relatively large quantity of free fluid in contrast to normal tissues where almost all of the fluid is in the gel phase.
- A quick diffusion of low-molecular weight, water-soluble agents (e.g., contrast agents, drugs) [41].
- A compromised convective transport of high-molecular-weight substances.

2.7
Interstitial Fluid Pressure in Tumors

As already mentioned, the growing tumor produces new, often abnormally leaky (hyperpermeable) microvessels, but is unable to form its own functional lymphatics [42]. As a result, there is significant bulk flow of free fluid into the interstitial space as long as a relevant pressure difference (both hydrostatic and oncotic) between the intra- and extravascular space exists. Whereas convective currents into the interstitial compartment are estimated to be about 0.5–1% of plasma flow in normal tissue, in human cancers water efflux into the interstitium can reach 15% of the respective plasma flow [3].

After seeping copiously out of the highly permeable tumor microvessels – an equilibrium is reached when the hydrostatic and oncotic pressures within the microvessels and the respective interstitial pressures become equal – fluid accumulates in the tumor extracellular matrix and a high interstitial fluid pressure (IFP) builds up in solid tumors [43–47].

Apart from vessel hyperpermeability and lack of functional lymphatics, interstitial fibrosis, contraction of the interstitial space mediated by stromal fibroblasts, and high oncotic pressures within the interstitium may contribute to the development of interstitial hypertension [48]. Whereas in most normal tissues IFP is slightly subatmospheric ("negative") or just above atmospheric values [49], an interstitial hypertension with values up to 60–70 mmHg [48, 50] (Table 2.3) develops in cancers, which forms a "physiologic" barrier to the delivery (via convection) of therapeutic macromolecules (e.g., monoclonal antibodies), liposomes, nanoparticles, or gene vectors to the cancer cells [51].

The tumor IFP is rather uniform throughout the center of the tumor, but drops steeply in the periphery. Fluid is squeezed out of the high- to the low-pressure regions at the tumor/normal tissue interface, carrying away antitumor drugs and contrast agents.

Despite increased overall leakiness, not all tumor microvessels are leaky. Vascular permeability varies from tumor to tumor and exhibits spatiotemporal heterogeneity ("4D heterogeneity") within the same tumor as well as during tumor growth or regression. Furthermore, IFP in tumors fluctuates with changing microvascular pressures [52].

Transmural coupling between IFP and microvascular pressure due to the high permeability of tumor microvessels can abolish perfusion pressure differences between up- and downstream tumor microvessels, and thus can lead to blood flow stasis in tumors without "physically" occluding (compressing) the vessels [42]. The

Table 2.3 Interstitial fluid pressure in normal tissues and in human tumors (adapted from [6, 30]).

Type of tissue	Mean IFP (mmHg) (range)
Normal tissues	
Breast tissue	0
Skin	−2
	−0.3
	0.4
Subcutis	−3
Fibrous tissue	−3
Submucosa (paravaginal)	1
Tightly encased tissues	
brain	4–6
kidney	6
Malignant tumors	
Renal cell carcinomas	38
Cervix cancers	(6–76)
Liver metastases (colorectal)	21 (4–45)
Head and neck carcinomas	15 (4–33)
Breast carcinomas	17 (4–33)
Breast cancer (invasive, ductal)	29
Melanomas	29 (0–110)
Metastatic melanomas	33 (20–50)
Non-Hodgkin's lymphomas	5 (1–12.5)
Lung carcinomas	10

equilibration of hydrostatic pressures between the interstitial and microvascular compartments is accompanied by a similar equilibration of oncotic pressures in both spaces (20.0 mmHg in plasma versus 20.5 mmHg in solid tumors [53]).

2.8
Role of the Disorganized, Compromised Microcirculation as an Obstacle in Drug Delivery

2.8.1
Blood-Borne Delivery

As already mentioned, there is a disturbed balance of pro- and antiangiogenic molecules (yielding an unregulated angiogenesis), which leads to the development of a disorganized microvasculature and significant arteriovenous shunt perfusion, and thus to an inefficient delivery of therapeutic molecules (e.g., drugs, cytokines, antibodies) and nutrients (e.g., oxygen and glucose) through the vascular system of the tumor (Table 2.4). The situation is further aggravated by flow-dependent

Table 2.4 Chaotic tumor microcirculation as a barrier of drug delivery (selection).

Pathophysiological condition	Leads via	To
Inadequate and heterogeneous perfusion (4D heterogeneity)	inefficient and heterogeneous delivery of cytotoxic agents	impaired pharmacokinetics of drugs, impaired delivery of therapeutic macromolecules and gene therapies
	inefficient and heterogeneous nutrient supply yielding decreasing cell proliferation rates/cell cycle arrest with increasing distance from tumor blood vessels (development of marked gradients in the cell proliferation rate)	protection from cytotoxic therapies whose activity is selective for rapidly dividing cells (cell cycle-active drugs)
Arteriovenous shunt vessels	shunt perfusion (i.e., flow bypassing exchange vessels)	impaired delivery of cytotoxic agents
Enlarged diffusion distances	compromised penetration of cytotoxic agents (development of steep gradients in drug concentration, and drug uptake and retention in (tumor) cells close to blood vessels)	insufficient concentrations of drugs and therapeutic macromolecules in tumor regions distant to patent blood vessels; not all tumor (stem) cells are exposed to a potentially lethal drug concentration

spatiotemporal heterogeneities in the distribution of plasma-borne drugs (and their metabolites). These "4D heterogeneities" are not static, but instead are quite dynamic (and therefore more complex than has been previously assumed).

The considerable impediment of fluctuating (intermittent) perfusion to successful cancer therapy has been comprehensively reviewed by Durand [54] and Durand and Aquino-Parsons [55, 56].

The mean vascular density in most tumor areas is generally lower than that in normal tissues and thus diffusion distances are enlarged. Penetration of drugs from tumor capillaries to tumor cells that are distant from them is therefore compromised. As shown by Primeau et al. [57], the concentration of drugs decreases exponentially with distance from tumor blood vessels, decreasing to half its perivascular concentration at a distance of about 40–50 μm. (Note that intervessel distances in solid tumors can vary between 10 and 1000 μm with a grand median of approximately 100 μm [58].) Thus, many viable tumor cells are not exposed to detectable concentrations of low-molecular-weight drugs following a single injection (Figure 2.5). In these tumor regions distant to patent microvessels some

(d)

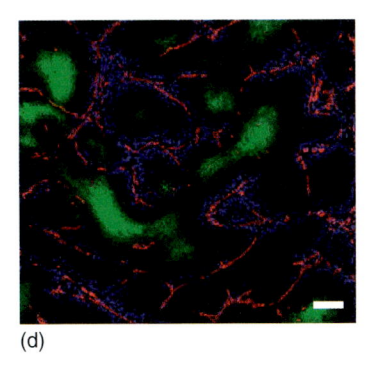

Figure 2.5 Perivascular distribution of doxorubicin (blue) in relation to microvessels (red) and hypoxic regions (green) in a tissue section from experimental mouse tumours; bar: 100 µm. (From [57]).

drugs (i.e., preferentially drugs with a short half-life within the circulation) cannot achieve sufficient concentrations to exert lethal toxicity for all of the viable cells further away from the tumor microvasculature system [57, 59, 60]. In addition, in these tumor regions, the concentrations of the key nutrients are also low, leading to marked gradients with higher cellular turnover rates close to blood vessels and lower cell proliferation rates (and cell cycle arrest) further from the nearest microvessel before treatment, and to repopulation of surviving tumor cells after/between treatments [61–63].

Cells dividing at a reduced rate would be protected from the effects of cytotoxic therapies whose activity is "selective" for rapidly dividing cell populations with a short cell cycle, a large proportion of cells in S phase, and, therefore, a large growth fraction [64, 65]. There is a strong indication that the growth fraction decreases as tumor size increases, at least in experimental tumor systems.

Antiangiogenic therapy for solid tumors using inhibition of VEGF signaling can generate an early phase of "normalization" of tumor vasculature [66]. This occurs via the recruitment of pericytes to the tumor microvasculature – an effect associated with a temporary, short-lived stabilization of the vessels and a (still hypothetic) improvement in blood flow. The latter may be accompanied by improved oxygen and drug delivery, creating a window of opportunity for the delivery of anticancer agents [67]. The postulated increase in pericyte recruitment is thought to be mediated by Ang-1 and MMPs [68].

2.8.2
Extravasation of Anticancer Agents

Therapeutic (and diagnostic) molecules cross the leaky vessel walls by two major mechanisms: diffusion and convection. Diffusion is the prevailing molecular transport of small-size molecules driven by concentration gradients. Convection is driven by hydrostatic pressure gradients, and is the dominant mode of transport for large molecules, liposomes, and other particles [69]. Due to the increased interstitial pressure (interstitial hypertension), significant hindering of the transport of macromolecules into the extravascular space has to be considered.

2.9
Interstitial Barriers to Drug Delivery

As already outlined, the interstitial compartment of tumors is significantly different to that of normal tissues. As a result of (i) vessel leakiness, (ii) lack of functional lymphatics, (iii) interstitial fibrosis, and (iv) contraction of the interstitial matrix mediated by stromal fibroblasts, most solid tumors have an increased IFP [47, 48, 70–72].

Increased IFP within solid tumors decreases extravasation and inhibits the extravascular transport of larger molecules (e.g., monoclonal antibodies, cytokines) by convection (Table 2.5). Macromolecules rely more heavily on convection as

Table 2.5 Interstitial barriers for drug delivery in tumors (selection).

Pathophysiological condition	Leads via	To
Interstitial hypertension	decreased extravasation and compromised interstitial transport of macromolecules	impaired delivery of therapeutic macromolecules (e.g., passive immunotherapy) and gene therapies, disturbed immigration of immune effector cells
Dense network of collagen fibers	compromised interstitial transport of macromolecules	impaired delivery of therapeutic macromolecules (e.g., passive immunotherapy)
IFP drop at the tumor/normal tissue interface	centrifugal interstitial fluid flow	loss of anticancer agents
	diversion of blood from tumor center to periphery	loss of anticancer agents in the tumor periphery
Transmural coupling between IFP and microvascular pressure	critical reduction in perfusion pressure	flow stasis compromising intra-tumor pharmacokinetics
Expansion of the interstitial space	increase in distribution space for anticancer (and diagnostic) agents	time necessary for drug concentration equilibrium between vascular and interstitial space may be prolonged

opposed to simple diffusional transport of low-molecular-weight drugs. Interstitial transport of macromolecules is further impaired by a much denser network of collagen fibers in the extracellular matrix of tumors as compared to normal tissues. Collagen content in tumors is much higher and collagen fibers are much thicker than in normal tissues, leading to an increased mechanical stiffness of the tissue [48, 73]. The interstitium also contains stromal cells and enzymes that can affect the activity and delivery of drugs to the tumor cells [69].

As already mentioned, IFP is almost uniform throughout a tumor and drops precipitously at the tumor/normal tissue interface. For this reason, the interstitial fluid oozes out of the tumor into the surrounding normal tissue, carrying away anticancer agents with it [42]. As another consequence of this drop in IFP, blood may be diverted away from the tumor center toward the periphery where anticancer agents may be lost from larger vessels.

Transmural coupling between IFP and microvascular pressure can critically reduce perfusion pressure between up- and downstream tumor blood vessels, leading to blood flow stasis and, thus, inadequate delivery of anticancer agents, in addition to the mechanisms impairing blood flow already mentioned above.

Interactions between cancer cells and the extracellular matrix can affect their response to chemotherapy. The basic mechanisms involved in so-called "adhesion-mediated drug resistance" are rather complex and still under investigation. Agents that can modulate cell adhesion might enhance the effects of chemotherapy [65].

Since increased IFP in malignant tumors can impair the delivery of therapeutic agents, interventions that can reduce IFP may improve drug delivery. Several types of treatment have been shown to decrease tumor IFP in patients. These compounds include VEGF antagonists, corticosteroids, hyaluronidase, and prostaglandin E_1 [48, 72, 74–77].

2.10
Pathophysiological Tumor Microenvironment as an Obstacle in Tumor Therapy

As mentioned above, the tumor microvasculature and interstitium can limit the delivery of anticancer drugs (and diagnostic agents). In addition, the dysfunctional microcirculation also creates a hostile pathophysiological microenvironment. Unique (and mostly adverse) aspects of this microenvironment are, among others, hypoxia (Figure 2.6) and extracellular acidosis (Figure 2.7), which can markedly alter the activity (and the distribution) of drugs, and thus the response of malignant tumors to cytotoxic drugs, immunotherapy, and hormones. Apart from "direct" effects (i.e., effects of hypoxia or acidosis *per se*), such as reduced generation of reactive oxygen species, increased DNA repair, modulation of the transmembrane transport of agents, drug distribution between the extra- and intracellular space, and so on, "indirect" effects are mostly based on changes in the transcriptome, in differential regulation, of gene expression, and in alterations of

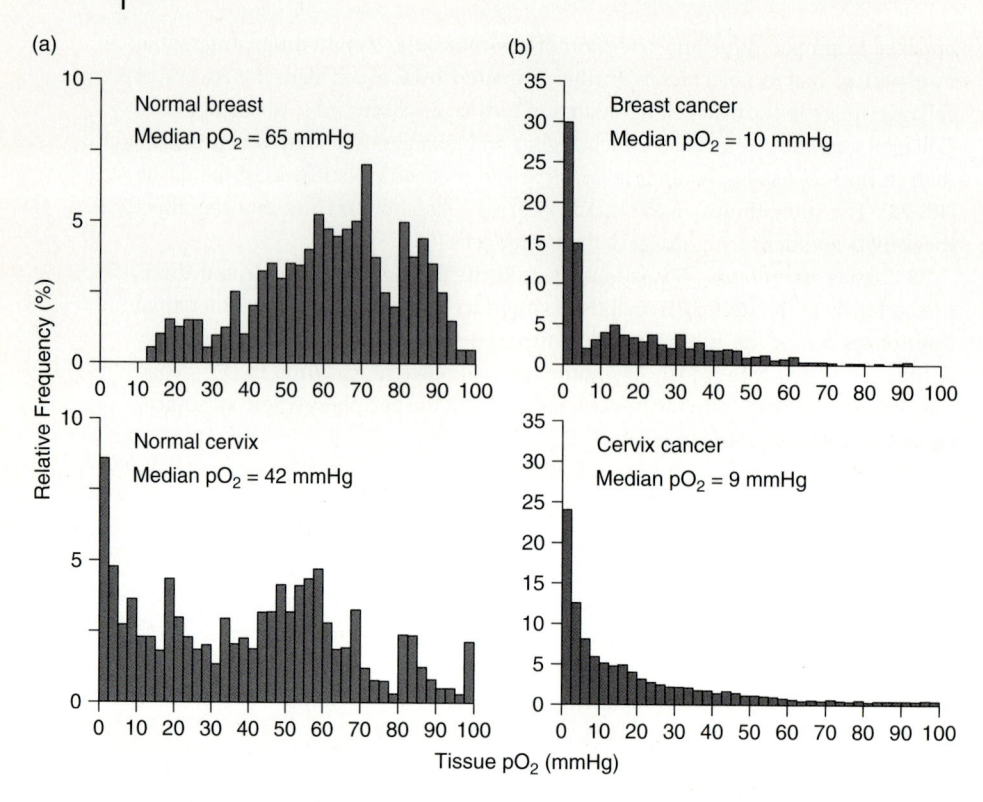

Figure 2.6 Frequency distributions (histograms) of oxygen partial pressures measured in normal tissues (a), and in cancers of the breast and of the uterine cervix (b). (Updated from [6]).

the proteome and/or genome [51]. Many microenvironmental factors with impacts on pharmacodynamics are indirectly influenced by the abnormal microcirculation.

2.10.1
Hypoxia as an Obstacle in Drug Therapy

Hypoxia protects tumor cells from damage by anticancer drug therapies that are directly or indirectly oxygen dependent (or both, see Figure 2.7; for reviews, see [78–88]).

2.10.1.1 Direct Effects
Direct effects (i.e., effects of hypoxia *per se*) are mediated via deprivation of molecular O_2 and thus reduced generation of free radicals that some chemotherapeutic agents (e.g., the antibiotics bleomycin and doxorubicin [89]) and photodynamic therapy require to be maximally cytotoxic.

2.10 Pathophysiological Tumor Microenvironment as an Obstacle in Tumor Therapy

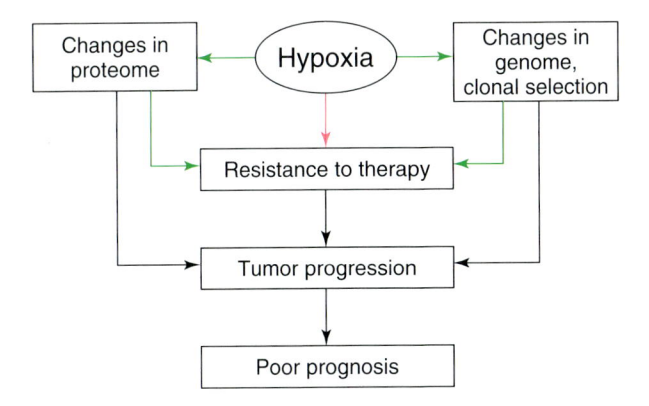

Figure 2.7 Schematic representation of major hypoxia-induced mechanisms causing treatment resistance and malignant progression finally leading to poor long-term prognosis. Red arrow: direct effect; green arrows: indirect effects.

In normoxic conditions, many anticancer drugs form free radicals that can damage DNA. Hence, cytotoxicity of drugs mediated by free radicals will decrease in hypoxia (Table 2.6).

2.10.1.2 Indirect Effects Based on Changes in the Transcriptome, in Differential Regulation of Gene Expression, and in Alterations of the Proteome

Indirect effects, which to a great part are reversible and which may occur upon exposure to oxygen levels below 1% ($pO_2 < 7mmHg$), rely on the hypoxia-mediated modulation (stimulation or inhibition) of gene expression and post-transcriptional or post-translational effects resulting in changes in the proteome and leading, among others, to:

- Modulation of proliferation kinetics, perturbations of the cell cycle distribution, number of tumor cells accumulating in G_1 phase, and reduction in the fraction of active S-phase cells (e.g., the vinca alkaloids and methotrexate exhibit cell cycle phase specificity [90]). As a rule, the portion of proliferating cells decreases with increasing hypoxia and increasing duration of hypoxia. Thus, the fraction of hypoxic and not proliferating – but still viable – tumor cells is of special interest;
- Quantitative changes in cellular metabolism (e.g., intensified glycolysis in hypoxic tumors with tissue acidosis, which in turn can have an impact on cellular activation, intracellular accumulation, and membrane transport of drugs), increased enzyme activities, elevated intracellular concentrations of glutathione (GSH), and associated nucleophilic thiols that can compete with the target DNA for alkylation (Table 2.6).
- Increased transcription of membrane transporters (e.g., glucose transporter-1 (GLUT1) facilitating the efflux of vinblastine [96]), DNA repair enzymes,

Table 2.6 Tumor hypoxia and acquired treatment resistance (selection of mechanisms) (adapted from [51]).

Treatment affected	Mechanisms involved	Examples	References
Directs effects			
Chemotherapy[a]	reduced generation of free radicals	antibiotics (bleomycin, doxorubicin)	Erlichman [89]
Indirect effects			
Chemotherapy[b]	cell cycle effects, modulation of proliferation kinetics	vinca alkaloids, methotrexate, platinum compounds, taxanes, doxorubicin	Chabner et al. [90]
	increased activity of repair enzymes	alkylating agents, platinum compounds, etoposide, anthracyclines	Chabner et al. [90] Zeller [91]
	elevated intracellular levels of glutathione	melphalan	–
	increased telomerase activity	telomerase inhibitors	Nishi et al. [92] Anderson et al. [93]
	development of an aggressive phenotype	–	Lunt et al. [50]
	amplification and increased synthesis of dihydrofolate reductase	methotrexate	Rice et al. [94]
	increased synthesis of growth factors (e.g., TGF-β, basic FGF)	–	Wei and Au [95]
	increased transcription of membrane transporters (e.g., GP-170, GLUT1)	vinca alkaloids, anthracyclines, etoposide, taxanes	Vera et al. [96] Comerford et al. [97]
	increased expression of antiapoptotic proteins, selection of apoptosis-resistant cells	alkylating agents, cisplatin, anthracyclines, etoposide	Cole and Tannock [98]
Endocrine theraphy	modulation of receptor function		Vaupel [51]
Immunotherapy	impaired cytokine production		Vaupel [51]

[a] Anemia acts as a factor worsening tumor hypoxia.
[b] Anemia acts as a factor that intensifies tumor hypoxia and that may impair transport of some cytotoxic drugs by red blood cells.

autocrine and paracrine growth factors (e.g., TGF-β), proteins involved in cell detachment and tumor invasiveness, and resistance-related proteins. Many hypoxia-inducible genes are controlled by several transcription factors such as hypoxia-inducible factor-1, nuclear factor κB, and activator protein-1 [99–101]. Signaling through inhibition of the mammalian target of rapamycin kinase and through activation of the unfolded protein response is also responsive to hypoxia.

In addition to hypoxia, other epigenetic microenvironmental factors (e.g., acidosis, glucose depletion, lactate accumulation) may also be involved in the mechanisms described above. (For more details on hypoxia-mediated proteome changes, see [88, 94, 102–113].)

2.10.1.3 Indirect Effects Based on Enhanced Mutagenesis, Genomic Instability, and Clonal Selection

Therapeutic resistance can also result from (progressive) genome changes and clonal selection at tissue O_2 concentrations below 0.1% ($pO_2 < 0.7$ mmHg; [4, 114]).

Increasing resistance toward nonsurgical therapy concomitant with primary tumor growth can also be driven by transient or persistent genomic changes and clonal selection (often associated with subsequent clonal dominance) due to a hypoxia-related strong selection pressure. Hypoxia promotes genomic instability (through point mutations, gene amplification, and chromosomal rearrangements), thus increasing the number of genetic variants, and thereby promoting clonal and intrinsic tumor cell heterogeneity. Emancipative proliferation of resistant clonal variants in a "survival of the fittest" scenario and malignant progression are the final results (Table 2.6).

Hypoxia-mediated clonal selection of tumor cells with persistent genomic changes can lead, among others, to a loss of differentiation and of apoptosis, which can stabilize or further aggravate tumor hypoxia and which in turn again promotes malignant progression [114, 115]. Thus, hypoxia is involved in a vicious circle that is regarded as a fundamental biologic mechanism of malignant disease (for reviews, see [88, 114, 116]). Other consequences of hypoxia-induced malignant progression are an increased locoregional spread and enhanced metastasis [117, 118].

For more details on hypoxia-mediated genome changes and expansion of aggressive tumor subclones, see [88, 106, 119–127].

2.10.1.4 Tumor Hypoxia: An Adverse Parameter in Chemotherapy

In addition to restricted delivery and uneven distribution (due to poor and heterogeneous blood flow) as well as reduced diffusional flux (due to enlarged diffusion distances), oxygen dependency has been documented for a broad range of cytotoxic drugs (e.g., cyclophosphamide, methotrexate, 5-fluorouracil, etoposide, carboplatin, bleomycin, and doxorubicin) under *in vitro* and *in vivo* conditions [83, 84, 128–130]. However, these investigations have been qualitative and clear hypoxic thresholds for O_2-dependent anticancer agents are still not available, although they presumably exist for each agent [131]. Thus, additional research is necessary to provide quantitative data on hypoxia-induced chemoresistance, although this information may be difficult to obtain under *in vivo* conditions. Multiple (direct and indirect) mechanisms are probably involved in the hypoxia-induced resistance to chemotherapeutic agents, including a reduced generation of free radicals (e.g., bleomycin, anthracyclines), the increased production of nucleophilic substances such as GSH that can compete with the target DNA for alkylation (e.g., in the acquired resistance to alkylating agents), an increased activity of DNA repair enzymes (e.g., alkylating agents, platinum compounds [90]), an inhibition of cell proliferation, and tissue acidosis, which is often observed in hypoxic tumors with a high glycolytic rate [79, 80]. Furthermore, hypoxic stress proteins, the loss of apoptotic potential, and multidrug resistance proteins can impart resistance to certain chemotherapeutic drugs [132–134]. It was recently shown that hypoxia decreased the responsiveness of human hepatoma cell line HepG2 to etoposide at least by two independent pathways involving p53 inhibition and *c-jun* activation [135].

Anemia is an independent risk factor for survival in most cancers treated with chemotherapy (e.g., [136–139]). As with radiotherapy, the presence of anemia and its association with inferior results of chemotherapy may be – at least partially – linked to severe hypoxia and its profound effect on tumor biology (e.g., development of an aggressive phenotype). However, anemia as a result of a reduced red blood cell mass may also have a negative impact on pharmacokinetics of chemotherapeutic agents [140]. Red blood cells have been reported to play an important role in storage, transport, and metabolism of particular cytotoxic drugs. Anthracyclines, ifosfamide and its metabolites, and topoisomerase I/II inhibitors are incorporated in erythrocytes, and may be transported by these cells to the tumor tissue and mobilized by active or passive mechanisms [141–143]. 6-Mercaptopurine, methotrexate, and aminotrexate are reported to accumulate in erythrocytes [144, 145]. As shown for oxaliplatin, platinum-derived cytotoxic agents are also bound to erythrocytes and transported by red blood cells [146]. In an animal model, a significant correlation was found between concentrations of melphalan in erythrocytes and the tumor availability of this drug [147]. Owing to their potential ability to take up, transport, and deliver various antineoplastic drugs, erythrocytes have increasingly become interesting objects to be evaluated as biological carriers in clinical oncology. Pretreatment elevation and/or maintenance of hemoglobin levels are therefore essential, irrespective of the way in which this goal is achieved [147].

The oxygen dependence of a number of anticancer drugs, such as cyclophosphamide, carboplatin, and doxorubicin, has been determined both *in vitro* and *in vivo* [130]. The results were quite conflicting and indicated that very high levels of resistance to anticancer drugs can develop through mechanisms that are expressed only *in vivo*. Matthews *et al.* [148] have reported a significant (almost by a factor of 2.6) enhancement of the cytotoxic effect of cisplatin under hypoxic conditions. In addition, the accumulation of cisplatin in cells was increased by a factor of 1.5 and its binding to DNA was increased by a factor of 1.7 under hypoxia compared to that in normoxia.

The enhancement of the cytotoxic action of mitomycin C on HeLa cells cultivated under hypoxic conditions has been described by Kohnoe et al. [149] – an effect that was abolished by low pH of the culture medium. Weak influences of hypoxia on the cytotoxic effect of chlorambucil, cisplatin, daunorubicin, and docetaxel have been observed by Skarsgard et al. [150] and Thews et al. [151].

2.10.2
Tumor Acidosis and Drug Resistance

As already mentioned, tumors have a lower extracellular pH (pH_e) than normal cells (Figure 2.8). This is an inherent characteristic of the malignant phenotype. Like normal cells, tumor cells have a neutral to slightly alkaline cytosolic ("internal") pH (pH_i), which is considered to be permissive for cell proliferation [152]. The result is a reverse (or negative) pH gradient ($pH_i > pH_e$) across the tumor cell plasma membrane *in vivo* compared with normal tissues where $pH_i < pH_e$ (around 7.2 versus around 7.4, see Figure 2.9; reviewed in [2, 153]).

The extracellular acidosis in tumors is not simply caused by excessive production of lactic acid and CO_2, but may also be the result of other mechanisms yielding H^+ ions that are exported into the extracellular space mainly via the H^+-monocarboxylate cotransporter (MCT1) and the Na^+/H^+ antiporter (NHE1), and – to a lesser extent – by a vacuolar type H^+-pump (H^+-ATPase [154]). Taking the various H^+ sources of tumor metabolism into account, it is not surprising that hypoxia is not always correlated with a decrease in extracellular pH (i.e., acidic tumor regions and hypoxic tumor areas are not necessarily congruent).

pH effects on therapeutic modalities were summarized extensively by Wike-Hooley et al. [155], Tannock and Rotin [156], Durand [79, 80], Song et al. [157, 158], Vaupel [86], Gerweck [159], and Stubbs [160]. More recent reviews include Stubbs et al. [161], Evelhoch [162], and Roepe [163].

The transport of drugs into tumor cells (either by diffusion or carrier-mediated mechanisms) and their intracellular metabolism are pH dependent [156]. Since the cellular uptake of drugs by diffusion is efficient only for the nonionized form of compounds and since the extracellular pH in tumors is acidic with the cytosolic pH being maintained in the neutral/slightly alkaline range, the respective pH gradient acts to exclude weakly basic drugs and thus impairs their cellular uptake by diffusion. Since cell membranes are readily permeable only to uncharged drug molecules, weak bases tend to concentrate on the more acid side of the membrane (i.e., in the extracellular space), while weak acids accumulate on the more alkaline side of the membrane (i.e., in the cytosolic compartment). Weakly basic (alkaline) drugs include doxorubicin, idarubicin, epirubicin, daunarubicin, bleomycin, mitoxantrone, and vinca alkaloids [159, 164–167]; weakly acid drugs include chlorambucil, melphalan, 5-fluorouracil, cisplatin and cyclophosphamide.

Multiple indirect mechanisms may additionally be involved in the acidosis-induced resistance to chemotherapeutic agents, including an increased efflux of drugs [168] and resistance to apoptosis [169] – the latter mechanisms being mediated by overexpression of P-glycoprotein. Furthermore, an increased activity of

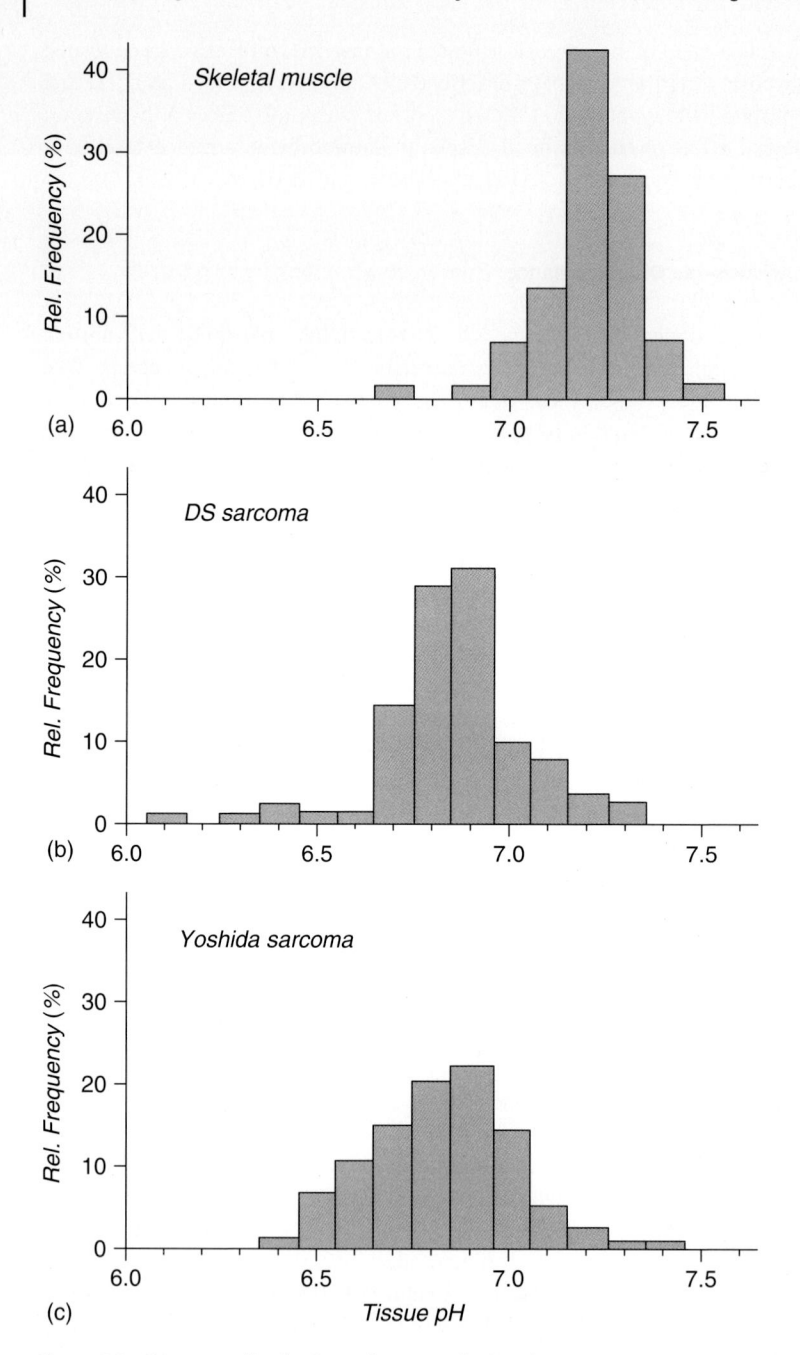

Figure 2.8 Frequency distributions of measured pH values in the extracellular space of skeletal muscle (a), and experimental tumors: DS-sarcoma (b) and Yoshida sarcoma (c). (Modified from [35]).

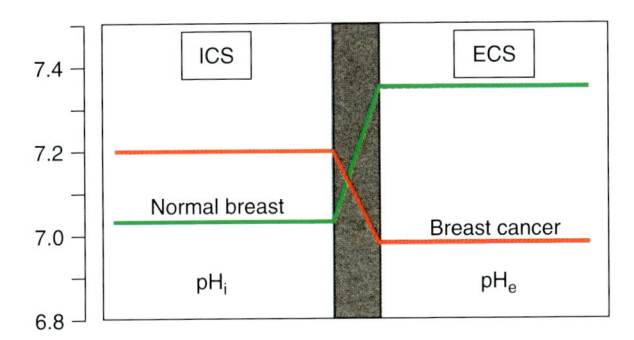

Figure 2.9 Schematic representation of pH gradients between the intracellular space (ICS) and the extracellular space (ECS) of normal breast tissue (green) and in breast cancer (red). (Modified from [6]).

Table 2.7 Tumor acidosis and acquired treatment resistance (selection of mechanisms) (adapted from [51]).

Treatment affected	Mechanisms involved	Examples	References
Chemotherapy	cell cycle effects, reduced cell proliferation rate	–	Wike-Hooley et al. [155] Cole and Tannock [98] Valeriote and van Putten [171]
	reduced active uptake due to ATP depletion	methotrexate	–
	reduced uptake by diffusion	weakly basic drugs	Gerweck and Seetharaman [166]
	increased DNA repair	alkylating agents	Sarkaria et al. [170]
	overexpression of P-glycoprotein, increased drug efflux	anthracyclines vinca alkaloids	Wei and Roepe [168] Lotz et al. [172]
	resistance to apoptosis	overexpression of P-glycoprotein	Robinson et al. [169]
Immunotherapy	inhibition of cell-mediated antitumor immunity		Vaupel [51]

DNA repair enzymes has been convincingly described [170], and an inhibition of cell proliferation and cell cycle effects have extensively been discussed as mechanisms reducing the effectiveness of chemotherapeutic agents in acidic environments (e.g., [171]) (Tables 2.7 and 2.8).

Table 2.8 pH dependence of antitumor drugs (adapted from [173]).

Decreased cytostatic effect at $pH_e < 6.8$	Enhanced cytostatic effect at $pH_e < 6.8$
Doxorubicin[a] (adriamycin)	Chlorambucil[c]
Daunorubicin[a] (daunomycin)	Melphalan[c]
Vinblastin[a]	Cyclophosphamide[c] (in vitro)
Paclitaxel[b] (taxol)	5-Fluorouracil[c]
Methotrexate	Cisplatin
Bleomycin	Tiophosphamide
Mitoxantrone[a]	Mitomycin C
Topotecan (water-soluble camptothecin)	Camptothecin

[a] Weakly alkaline (basic).
[b] Zwitterion.
[c] Weakly acid.

2.11
Conclusions

Apart from "classical" drug resistance (mostly based on the molecular biology of tumor cells, e.g., mutations, alterations of gene expression, and epigenetic changes), which can only partly explain the lack of treatment efficacy, substantial experimental and clinical evidence suggests that the irregular and heterogeneous structure and function of the microcirculation and the self-perpetuating hostile pathophysiological microenvironment of solid tumor may – to a large extent – mediate resistance of solid tumors to anticancer drugs. Therefore, the distribution of tumor blood flow and relevant flow-related factors of the microenvironment (e.g., hypoxia, extracellular acidosis) are increasingly receiving attention in the clinical setting. One of the goals of translational cancer research is to obtain a better understanding of the compromised delivery and distribution of chemotherapeutic drugs in solid tumors (intratumor pharmacokinetics) in order to improve patients' outcomes.

Acknowledgments

The valuable assistance of Mrs. Anne Deutschmann-Fleck and Dr. Debra K. Kelleher in preparing this manuscript is greatly appreciated.

References

1. Brem, S., Brem, H., Folkman, J. et al. (1976) Prolonged tumor dormancy by prevention of neovascularization in the vitreous. *Cancer Res.*, **36**, 2807–2812.

2. Vaupel, P., Kallinowski, F., and Okunieff, P. (1989) Blood flow, oxygen and nutrient supply, and metabolic microenvironment of human tumors: a

review. *Cancer Res.*, **49**, 6449–6465.
3. Vaupel, P.W. (1994) *Blood Flow, Oxygenation, Tissue pH Distribution, and Bioenergetic Status of Tumors*, Lecture, Vol. 23, Ernst Schering Research Foundation, Berlin.
4. Vaupel, P. (2004) Tumor microenvironmental physiology and its implications for radiation oncology. *Semin. Radiat. Oncol.*, **14**, 198–206.
5. Vaupel, P. (2006) Abnormal microvasculature and defective microcirculatory function in solid tumors in *Vascular-targeted Therapies in Oncology* (ed. D.W. Siemann), John Wiley & Sons, Ltd, Chichester, pp. 9–29.
6. Vaupel, P. (2009) Pathophysiology of solid tumors in *The Impact of Tumor Biology on Cancer Treatment and Multidisciplinary Strategies* (eds M. Molls, P. Vaupel, C. Nieder, and M.S. Anscher), Springer, Berlin, pp. 51–92.
7. Schneider, V., Rischke, H.C., and Drevs, J. (2009) Tumor angiogenesis in *The Impact of Tumor Biology on Cancer Treatment and Multidisciplinary Strategies* (eds M. Molls, P. Vaupel, C. Nieder, and M.S. Anscher), Springer, Berlin, pp. 39–50.
8. Sividris, E., Giatromanolaki, A., and Koukourakis, M.I. (2003) The vascular network of tumours – what is it not for? *J. Pathol.*, **201**, 173–180.
9. Carmeliet, P. and Jain, R.K. (2000) Angiogenesis in cancer and other diseases. *Nature*, **407**, 249–257.
10. Ribatti, D., Vacca, A., and Dammacco, F. (2003) New non-angiogenesis dependent pathways for tumour growth. *Eur. J. Cancer*, **39**, 1835–1841.
11. Bergers, G. and Benjamin, L.E. (2003) Tumorigenesis and the angiogenic switch. *Nat. Rev. Cancer*, **3**, 401–410.
12. Hanahan, D. and Weinberg, R.A. (2000) The hallmarks of cancer. *Cell*, **100**, 57–70.
13. Yancopoulos, G.D., Davis, S., Gale, N.W. et al. (2000) Vascular-specific growth factors and blood vessel formation. *Nature*, **407**, 242–248.
14. Papetti, M. and Herman, I.M. (2002) Mechanisms of normal and tumor-derived angiogenesis. *Am. J. Physiol*, **282**, C947–C970.
15. Semenza, G.L. (2000) HIF-1: using two hands to flip the angiogenic switch. *Cancer Metastasis Rev.*, **19**, 59–65.
16. Pugh, C.W. and Ratcliffe, P.J. (2003) Regulation of angiogenesis by hypoxia: role of the HIF system. *Nat. Med.*, **9**, 677–684.
17. Shweiki, D., Neeman, M., Itin, A., and Keshet, E. (1995) Induction of vascular endothelial growth factor expression by hypoxia and by glucose deficiency in multicell spheroids: implications for tumor angiogenesis. *Proc. Natl. Acad. Sci. USA*, **92**, 768–772.
18. Kerbel, R.S. (2000) Tumor angiogenesis: past, present and the near future. *Carcinogenesis*, **21**, 505–515.
19. Ellis, L.M., Liu, W., Ahmad, S.A. et al. (2001) Overview of angiogenesis: biologic implications for antiangiogenic therapy. *Semin. Oncol.*, **28**, 94–104.
20. Patan, S., Munn, L.L., and Jain, R.K. (1996) Intussusceptive microvascular growth in a human colon adenocarcinoma xenograft: a novel mechanism of tumor angiogenesis. *Microvasc. Res.*, **51**, 260–272.
21. Ruoslahti, E. (2002) Specialization of tumour vasculature. *Nat. Rev. Cancer*, **2**, 83–90.
22. McDonald, D.M., Munn, L., and Jain, R.K. (2000) Vasculogenic mimicry: how convincing, how novel, and how significant? *Am. J. Pathol.*, **156**, 383–388.
23. Shchors, K. and Evan, G. (2007) Tumor angiogenesis: cause or consequence of cancer? *Cancer Res.*, **67**, 7059–7061.
24. Jussila, L. and Alitalo, K. (2002) Vascular growth factors and lymphangiogenesis. *Physiol. Rev.*, **82**, 673–700.
25. Padera, T.P., Kadambi, A., di Tomaso, E. et al. (2002) Lymphatic metastasis in the absence of functional intratumor lymphatics. *Science*, **296**, 1883–1886.
26. Hirst, D.G. and Flitney, F.W. (1997) The Physiological importance and therapeutic potential of nitric oxide in the tumour-associated vasculature in *Tumour Angiogenesis* (eds R. Bicknell, C.E. Lewis, and N. Ferrara), Oxford University Press, Oxford, pp. 153–167.

27. Gillies, R.J., Schornack, P.A., Secomb, T.W., and Raghunand, N. (1999) Causes and effects of heterogeneous perfusion in tumors. *Neoplasia*, **1**, 197–207.
28. Vaupel, P. and Höckel, M. (2000) Blood supply, oxygenation status and metabolic micromilieu of breast cancers: characterization and therapeutic relevance. *Int. J. Oncol.*, **17**, 869–879.
29. Vaupel, P., Thews, O., and Hoeckel, M. (2001) Treatment resistance of solid tumors: role of hypoxia and anemia. *Med. Oncol.*, **18**, 243–259.
30. Vaupel, P. (2011) Pathophysiology of human tumours in *Tumour hypoxia in the clinical setting* (eds. S. Osiusky, H. Friess, P. Vaupel), Akadem-periodyka, Kiew, 21–66.
31. Konerding, M.A., Fait, E., and Gaumann, A. (2001) 3D microvascular architecture of pre-cancerous lesions and invasive carcinomas of the colon. *Br. J. Cancer*, **84**, 1354–1362.
32. Reinhold, H.S. and van den Berg-Blok, A.E. (1987) Circulation physiology of tumours in *Rodent Tumor Models in Experimental Cancer Therapy* (eds R.F. Kallman), Pergamon Press, New York, pp. 39–42.
33. Kimura, H., Braun, R.D., Ong, E.T. et al. (1996) Fluctuations in red cell flux in tumor microvessels can lead to transient hypoxia and reoxygenation in tumor parenchyma. *Cancer Res.*, **56**, 5522–5528.
34. Baronzio, G., Freitas, I., and Kwaan, H.C. (2003) Tumor microenvironment and hemorheological abnormalities. *Semin. Thromb. Hemost.*, **29**, 489–497.
35. Vaupel, P., Kelleher, D.K., and Thews, O. (2000) Microtopology of local perfusion, oxygenation, metabolic and energetic status, and interstitial pH in malignant tumors. Techniques and characterization. *Exp. Oncol.*, **22**, 15–25.
36. Vaupel, P., Grunewald, W.A., Manz, R., and Sowa, W. (1978) Intracapillary HbO_2 saturation in tumor tissue of DS-carcinosarcoma during normoxia. *Adv. Exp. Med. Biol.*, **94**, 367–375.
37. Weiss, L., Hultborn, R., and Tveit, E. (1979) Blood flow characteristics in induced rat mammary neoplasia. *Microvasc. Res.*, **17**, S119.
38. Endrich, B., Hammersen, F., Goetz, A., and Messmer, K. (1982) Microcirculatory blood flow, capillary morphology, and local oxygen pressure of the hamster amelanotic melanoma A-Mel-3. *J. Natl. Cancer Inst.*, **68**, 475–485.
39. Wheeler, R.H., Ziessman, H.A., Medvec, B.R. et al. (1986) Tumor blood flow and systemic shunting in patients receiving intraarterial chemotherapy for head and neck cancer. *Cancer Res.*, **46**, 4200–4204.
40. Vaupel, P. and Mueller-Klieser, W. (1983) Interstitieller Raum und Mikromilieu in malignen Tumoren. *Prog. Appl. Microcirc.*, **2**, 78–90.
41. Reinhold, H.S. (1971) Improved microcirculation in irradiated tumours. *Eur. J. Cancer*, **7**, 273–280.
42. Fukumura, D. and Jain, R.K. (2007) Tumor microenvironment abnormalities: causes, consequences, and strategies to normalize. *J. Cell. Biochem.*, **101**, 937–949.
43. Young, J.S., Llumsden, C.E., Stalker, A.L., (1950) The significance of the tissue pressure of normal testicular and of neoplastic (Brown-Pearce carcinoma) tissue in the rabbit. *J. Pathol. Bacteriol.*, **62**, 313–333.
44. Gutmann, R., Leunig, M., Feyh, J. et al. (1992) Interstitial hypertension in head and neck tumors in patients: correlation with tumor size. *Cancer Res.*, **52**, 1993–1995.
45. Less, J.R., Posner, M.C., Boucher, Y. et al. (1992) Interstitial hypertension in human breast and colorectal tumors. *Cancer Res.*, **52**, 6371–6374.
46. Milosevic, M., Fyles, A., Hedley, D. et al. (2001) Interstitial fluid pressure predicts survival in patients with cervix cancer independent of clinical prognostic factors and tumor oxygen measurements. *Cancer Res.*, **61**, 6400–6405.
47. Milosevic, M., Fyles, A., Hedley, D., and Hill, R. (2004) The human tumor microenvironment: invasive (needle) measurement of oxygen and interstitial fluid pressure. *Semin. Radiat. Oncol.*, **14**, 249–258.

48. Heldin, C.-H., Rubin, K., Pietras, K., and Östman, A. (2004) High interstitial fluid pressure – an obstacle in cancer therapy. *Nat. Rev. Cancer*, **4**, 806–813.
49. Guyton, A.C. and Hall, J.E. (2006) *Textbook of Medical Physiology*, 11th edn, Elsevier, Philadelphia, PA.
50. Lunt, S.J., Kalliomaki, T.M.K., Brown, A. et al. (2008) Interstitial fluid pressure, vascularity and metastasis in ectopic, orthotopic and spontaneous tumours. *BMC Cancer*, **8**, 2.
51. Vaupel, P. (2009) Physiological mechanisms of treatment resistance in *The Impact of Tumor Biology on Cancer Treatment and Multidisciplinary Strategies* (eds M. Molls, P. Vaupel, C. Nieder, and M.S. Anscher), Springer, Berlin, pp. 273–290.
52. Netti, P.A., Baxter, L.T., Boucher, Y. et al. (1995) Time-dependent behavior of interstitial fluid pressure in solid tumors: Implication for drug delivery. *Cancer Res.*, **55**, 5451–5458.
53. Stohrer, M., Boucher, Y., Stangassinger, M., and Jain, R.K. (2000) Oncotic pressure in solid tumors is elevated. *Cancer Res.*, **60**, 4251–4255.
54. Durand, R.E. (2001) Intermittent blood flow in solid tumours – an under-appreciated source of drug resistance. *Cancer Metastasis Rev.*, **20**, 57–61.
55. Durand, R.E. and Aquino-Parsons, C. (2001) Non-constant tumour blood flow: iplications for therapy. *Acta Oncol.*, **40**, 862–869.
56. Durand, R.E. and Aquino-Parsons, C. (2001) Clinical relevance of intermittent tumour blood flow. *Acta Oncol.*, **40**, 929–936.
57. Primeau, A.J., Rendon, A., Hedley, D. et al. (2005) The distribution of the anticancer drug doxorubicin in relation to blood vessels in solid tumors. *Clin. Cancer Res.*, **11**, 8782–8788.
58. Folarin, A.A., Konerding, M.A., Timonen, J. et al. (2010) Three-dimensional analysis of tumour vascular corrosion casts using stereoimaging and micro-computed tomography. *Microvasc. Res.*, **80**, 89–98.
59. Minchinton, A.L. and Tannock, I.F. (2006) Drug penetration in solid tumours. *Nat. Rev. Cancer*, **6**, 583–592.
60. Di Paolo, A. and Bocci, G. (2007) Drug distribution in tumors: mechanisms, role in drug resistance, and methods for modification. *Curr. Oncol. Rep.*, **9**, 109–114.
61. Tannock, I.F. (1968) The relation between cell proliferation and the vascular system in a transplanted mouse mammary tumour. *Br. J. Cancer*, **22**, 258–273.
62. Tannock, I.F. (2001) Tumor physiology and drug resistance. *Cancer Metastasis Rev.*, **20**, 123–132.
63. Hirst, D.G. and Denekamp, J. (1979) Tumour cell proliferation in relation to the vasculature. *Cell Tissue Kinet.*, **12**, 31–42.
64. Hall, E.J. and Giaccia, A.J. (2006) *Radiobiology for the Radiologist*, 6th edn, Lippincott Williams & Wilkins, Baltimore, MD.
65. Trédan, O., Galmarini, C.M., Patel, K., and Tannock, I.F. (2007) Drug resistance and the solid tumor microenvironment. *J. Natl. Cancer Inst.*, **99**, 1441–1454.
66. Jain, R.K. (2001) Normalizing tumor vasculature with anti-angiogenic therapy: a new paradigm for combination therapy. *Nat. Med.*, **7**, 987–989.
67. Jain, R.K. (2005) Normalization of tumor vasculature: an emerging concept in antiangiogenic therapy. *Science*, **307**, 58–62.
68. Lin, M.I. and Sessa, W.C. (2004) Antiangiogenic therapy: creating a unique "window" of opportunity. *Cancer Cell*, **6**, 529–531.
69. Kuszyk, B., Corl, F.M., Franano, F.M. et al. (2001) Tumor transport physiology: Implications for imaging and imaging-guided therapy. *Am. J. Radiol.*, **177**, 747–753.
70. Jain, R.K. (1987) Transport of molecules across tumor vasculature. *Cancer Metastasis Rev.*, **6**, 559–593.
71. Jain, R.K. (1990) Physiological barriers to delivery of monoclonal antibodies and other macromolecules in tumors. *Cancer Res.*, **50**, 814s–819s.

72. Cairns, R., Papandreou, I., and Denko, N. (2006) Overcoming physiologic barriers to cancer treatment by molecularly targeting the tumor microenvironment. *Mol. Cancer Res.*, **4**, 61–70.
73. Netti, P.A, Berk, D.A., Swartz, M.A. et al. (2000) Role of extracellular matrix assembly in interstitial transport in solid tumors. *Cancer Res.*, **60**, 2497–2503.
74. Lee, C.G., Heijn, M., di Tomaso, E. et al. (2000) Anti-vascular endothelial growth factor treatment augments tumor radiation response under normoxic or hypoxic conditions. *Cancer Res.*, **60**, 5565–5570.
75. Willett, C.G., Boucher, Y., di Tomaso, E. et al. (2004) Direct evidence that the VEGF-specific antibody bevacizumab has antivascular effects in human rectal cancer. *Nat. Med.*, **10**, 145–147.
76. Batchelor, T.T., Sorensen, A.G., di Tomaso, E. et al. (2007) AZD2171, a pan-VEGF receptor tyrosine kinase inhibitor, normalizes tumor vasculature and alleviates edema in glioblastoma patients. *Cancer Cell*, **11**, 83–95.
77. Willett, C.G., Boucher, Y., di Tomaso, E. et al. (2005) Surrogate markers for antiangiogenic therapy and dose-limiting toxicities for bevacizumab with radiation and chemotherapy: continued experience of a phase I trial in rectal cancer patients. *J. Clin. Oncol.*, **23**, 8136–8139.
78. Moulder, J.E. and Rockwell, S. (1987) Tumor hypoxia: its impact on cancer therapy. *Cancer Metastasis Rev.*, **5**, 313–341.
79. Durand, R.E. (1991) Keynote address: the influence of microenvironmental factors on the activity of radiation and drugs. *Int. J. Radiat. Oncol. Biol. Phys.*, **20**, 253–258.
80. Durand, R.E. (1994) The influence of microenvironmental factors during cancer therapy. *In Vivo*, **8**, 691–702.
81. Tannock, I.F. and Hill, R.P. (eds) (1992) *The Basic Science of Oncology*, 2nd edn, McGraw-Hill, New York.
82. Teicher, B.A. (ed.) (1993) *Drug Resistance in Oncology*, Dekker, New York.
83. Teicher, B.A. (1994) Hypoxia and drug resistance. *Cancer Metastasis*, **13**, 139–168.
84. Teicher, B.A. (1995) Physiologic mechanisms of therapeutic resistance. *Hematol. Oncol. Clin. North Am.*, **9**, 475–506.
85. Hall, E.J. (1994) Molecular biology in radiation therapy: the potential impact of recombinant technology on clinical practice. *Int. J. Radiat. Oncol. Biol. Phys.*, **30**, 1019–1028.
86. Vaupel, P. (1997) The influence of tumor blood flow and microenvironmental factors on the efficacy of radiation, drugs and localized hyperthermia. *Klin. Pädiat.*, **209**, 243–249.
87. Chaplin, D.J., Horsman, M.R., Trotter, M.J., and Siemann, D.W. (2000) Therapeutic significance of Microenvironmental factors in *Blood Perfusion and Microenvironment of Human Tumors: Implications for Clinical Radiooncology* (eds M. Molls and P. Vaupel), Springer, Berlin, pp. 133–143.
88. Höckel, M. and Vaupel, P. (2001) Tumor hypoxia: definitions and current clinical, biological and molecular aspects. *J. Natl. Cancer Inst.*, **93**, 266–276.
89. Erlichman, C. (1992) Pharmacology of anticancer drugs in *The Basic Science of Oncology*, 2nd edn (eds I.F. Tannock and R.P. Hill), McGraw-Hill, New York, pp. 317–337.
90. Chabner, B., Allegra, C.J., Curt, G.A., and Calabresi, P. (1996) *Goodman and Gilman's The Pharmacological Basis of Therapeutics*, 9th edn, McGraw-Hill, New York, pp. 1233–1287.
91. Zeller, W.J. (1995) Bleomycin in *Onkologie: Grundlagen, Diagnostik, Therapie, Entwicklungen* (eds W.J. Zeller and H. zur Hausen), Ecomed, Landsberg, pp. IV-3.12, 1–7.
92. Nishi, H., Nakada, T., Kyo, S. et al. (2004) Hypoxia-inducible factorIV-3. 1 mediates upregulation of telomerase (hTERT). *Mol. Cell Biol.*, **24**, 6076–6083.

93. Anderson, C.J., Hoare, S.F., Ashcroft, M. et al. (2006) Hypoxic regulation of telomerase gene expression by transcriptional and posttranscriptional mechanisms. *Oncogene*, **25**, 61–69.
94. Rice, G.C., Hoy, C., and Schimke, R.T. (1986) Transient hypoxia enhances the frequency of dihydrofolate reductase gene amplification in Chinese hamster ovary cells. *Proc. Natl. Acad. Sci. USA*, **83**, 5978–5982.
95. Wei, Y. and Au, J.L.-S. (2005) Role of tumour microenvironment in chemoresistance in *Integration/Interaction of Oncologic Growth* (ed. G.G. Meadows), Springer, Amsterdam, pp. 285–321.
96. Vera, J.C., Castillo, G.R., and Rosen, O.M. (1991) A possible role for a mammalian facilitative hexose transporter in the development of resistance to drugs. *Mol. Cell Biol.*, **11**, 3407–3418.
97. Comerford, K.M., Wallace, T.J., Karhausen, J. et al. (2002) Hypoxia-inducible factor-1-dependent regulation of the multidrug resistance (MDR1) gene. *Cancer Res.*, **62**, 3387–3394.
98. Cole, S.P.C. and Tannock, I.F. (2005) Drug resistance in *The Basic Science of Oncology*, 4th edn (eds I.F. Tannock, R.P. Hill, R.G. Bristow, and L. Harrington), McGraw-Hill, New York, pp. 376–399.
99. Koong, A.C., Chen, E.Y., and Giaccia, A.J. (1994) Hypoxia causes the activation of nuclear factor κB through the phosphorylation of IκBα on tyrosine residues. *Cancer Res.*, **54**, 1425–1430.
100. Dachs, G.U. and Tozer, G.M. (2000) Hypoxia modulated gene expression: angiogenesis, metastasis and therapeutic exploitation. *Eur. J. Cancer*, **36**, 1649–1660.
101. Laderoute, K.R., Calaogan, J.M., Gustafson-Brown, C. et al. (2002) The response of c-Jun/AP-1 to chronic hypoxia is hypoxia-inducible factor 1α dependent. *Mol. Cell Biol.*, **22**, 2515–2523.
102. Laderoute, K.R., Grant, T.D., Murphy, B.J., and Sutherland, R.M. (1992) Enhanced epidermal growth factor receptor synthesis in human squamous carcinoma cells exposed to low levels of oxygen. *Int. J. Cancer*, **52**, 428–432.
103. Ausserer, W.A., Bourrat-Floeck, B., Green, C.J. et al. (1994) Regulation of c-jun expression during hypoxic and low-glucose stress. *Mol. Cell Biol.*, **14**, 5032–5042.
104. Graeber, T.G., Peterson, J.F., Tsai, M. et al. (1994) Hypoxia induces accumulation of p53 protein, but activation of a G_1-phase checkpoint by low-oxygen conditions is independent of p53 status. *Mol. Cell Biol.*, **14**, 6264–6277.
105. Sanna, K. and Rofstad, E.K. (1994) Hypoxia-induced resistance to doxorubicin and methotrexate in human melanoma cell lines in vitro. *Int. J. Cancer*, **58**, 258–262.
106. Giaccia, A.J. (1996) Hypoxic stress proteins: survival of the fittest. *Semin. Radiat. Oncol.*, **6**, 46–58.
107. Mattern, J., Kallinowski, F., Herfarth, C., and Volm, M. (1996) Association of resistance-related protein expression with poor vascularization and low levels of oxygen in human rectal cancer. *Int. J. Cancer*, **67**, 20–23.
108. Raleigh, J.A. (1996) Hypoxia and its clinical significance. *Semin. Radiat. Oncol.*, **6**, 1–70.
109. Brown, J.M. and Giaccia, A.J. (1998) The unique physiology of solid tumors: opportunities (and problems) for cancer therapy. *Cancer Res.*, **58**, 1408–1416.
110. Sutherland, R.M. (1998) Tumor hypoxia and gene expression. Implications for malignant progression and therapy. *Acta Olicol.*, **37**, 567–574.
111. Semenza, G.L. (2000) Hypoxia, clonal selection, and the role of HIF-1 in tumor progression. *Crit. Rev. Biochem. Mol. Biol.*, **35**, 71–103.
112. Semenza, G.L. (2000) HIF-1: mediator of physiological and pathophysiological response to hypoxia. *J. Appl. Physiol.*, **88**, 1474–1480.
113. Yokoi, K. and Fidler, I.J. (2004) Hypoxia, increases resistance of human pancreatic cancer cells to apoptosis induced by gemcitabine. *Clin. Cancer Res.*, **10**, 2299–2306.
114. Vaupel, P. (2008) Hypoxia and aggressive tumor phenotype: implications for

therapy and prognosis. *Oncologist*, **13** (Suppl. 3), 21–36.

115. Vaupel, P. (2004) The role of hypoxia-induced factors in tumor progression. *Oncologist*, **9**, 10–17.

116. Vaupel, P., Mayer, A., and Höckel, M. (2004) Tumor hypoxia and malignant progression. *Methods Enzymol.*, **381**, 335–354.

117. Höckel, M., Schlenger, K., Aral, B. et al. (1996) Association between tumor hypoxia and malignant progression in advanced cancer of the uterine cervix. *Cancer Res.*, **56**, 4509–4515.

118. Höckel, M., Schlenger, K., Höckel, S. et al. (1998) Tumor hypoxia in pelvic recurrences of cervical cancer. *Int. J. Cancer*, **79**, 365–369.

119. Young, S.D., Marshall, R.S., and Hill, R.P. (1988) Hypoxia induces DNA over-replication and enhances metastatic potential of murine tumour cells. *Proc. Natl. Acad. Sci. USA*, **85**, 9533–9537.

120. Stoler, D.L., Anderson, G.R., Russo, C.A. et al. (1992) Anoxia-inducible endonuclease activity as a potential basis of the genomic instability of cancer cells. *Cancer Res.*, **52**, 4372–4378.

121. Cheng, K.C. and Loeb, L.A. (1993) Genomic instability and tumor progression: mechanistic considerations. *Adv. Cancer Res.*, **60**, 121–156.

122. Stackpole, C.W., Groszek, L., and Kalbag, S.S. (1994) Benign-to-malignant B16 melanoma progression induced in two stages *in vitro* by exposure to hypoxia. *J. Natl. Cancer Inst.*, **86**, 361–367.

123. Russo, C.A., Weber, T.K., Volpe, C.M. et al. (1995) An anoxia inducible endonuclease and enhanced DNA breakage as contributors to genomic instability in cancer. *Cancer Res.*, **55**, 1122–1128.

124. Graeber, T.G., Osmanian, C., Jacks, T. et al. (1996) Hypoxia-mediated selection of cells with diminished apoptotic potential in solid tumours. *Nature*, **379**, 88–91.

125. Reynolds, T.Y., Rockwell, S., and Glazer, P.M. (1996) Genetic instability induced by the tumor microenvironment. *Cancer Res.*, **56**, 5754–5757.

126. Kim, C.Y., Tsai, M.H., Osmanian, C. et al. (1997) Selection of human cervical epithelial cells that possess reduced apoptotic potential to low-oxygen conditions. *Cancer Res.*, **57**, 4200–4204.

127. Höckel, M., Schlenger, K., Höckel, S., and Vaupel, P. (1999) Hypoxic cervical cancers with low apoptotic index are highly aggressive. *Cancer Res.*, **59**, 4525–4528.

128. Teicher, B.A., Lazo, J.S., and Sartorelli, A.C. (1981) Classification of antineoplastic agents by their selective toxicities toward oxygenated and hypoxic tumor cells. *Cancer Res.*, **41**, 73–81.

129. Teicher, B.A., Holden, S.A., Al-Achi, A., and Herman, T.S. (1990) Classification of antineoplastic treatments by their differential toxicity toward putative oxygenated and hypoxic tumor subpopulations *in vivo* in the FSaII murine fibrosarcoma. *Cancer Res.*, **50**, 3339–3344.

130. Teicher, B.A., Herman, T.S., Holden, S.A. et al. (1990) Tumor resistance to alkylating agents conferred by mechanisms operative only *in vivo*. *Science*, **247**, 1457–1461.

131. Woúters, A., Paúwels, B., Lardon, F. Vermorken, J.B. (2007) Implications of in vitro research on the effect of radiotherapy and chemotherapy under hypoxic conditions. *Oncologist*, **12**, 690–712.

132. Sakata, K., Kwok, T.T., Murphy, B.J. et al. (1991) Hypoxia-induced drug resistance: comparison to P-glycoprotein-associated drug resistance. *Br. J. Cancer*, **64**, 809–814.

133. Hickman, J.A., Potten, C.S., Merritt, A.J., and Fisher, T.C. (1994) Apoptosis and cancer chemotherapy. *Philos. Trans. R. Soc. Lond. B*, **345**, 319–325.

134. Shannon, A.M., Bouchier-Hayes, D.J., Condron, C.M., and Toomey, D. (2003) Tumour hypoxia, chemotherapeutic resistance and hypoxia-related therapies. *Cancer Treat. Rev.*, **29**, 297–307.

135. Cosse, J.-P., Ronvaux, M., and Ninane, N. et al. (2009) Hypoxia-induced decrease in p53 protein level and increase in c-*jun* DNA binding activity results in cancer cell

resistance to etoposide. *Neoplasia*, **11**, 976–986.
136. Harrison, L. and Blackwell, K. (2004) Hypoxia and anemia: factors in decreased sensitivity to radiation therapy and chemotherapy? *Oncologist*, **9**, 31–40.
137. Ludwig, H. (2004) rHuEPO and treatment outcomes: the preclinical experience. *Oncologist*, **9**, 48–54.
138. Vaúpel, P., Höckel, M. (2008) Túmor hypoxia and therapeútic resistance in *Recombinant Húman Erythropoietin (rhEPO) in Clinical Oncology*, 2nd edn (ed. M.R. Nowroúsian), Springer, New York, pp. 283–306.
139. Van Belle, S.J.P. and Cocquyt, V. (2003) Impact of hemoglobin levels on the outcome of cancers treated with chemotherapy. *Crit. Rev. Oncol. Hematol.*, **47**, 1–11.
140. Nowrousian, M.R. (2008) Significance of anemia in cancer chemotherapy in *Recombinant Human Erythropoietin (rhEPO) in Clinical Oncology*, 2nd edn (ed. M.R. Nowrousian), Springer, New York, pp. 207–248.
141. Highley, M.S., Schrijvers, D., van Oosterom, A.T. *et al.* (1997) Activated oxazaphosphorines are transported predominantly by erythrocytes. *Ann. Oncol.*, **8**, 1139–1144.
142. Ramanathan-Girish, S. and Boroujerdi, M. (2001) Contradistinction between doxorubicin and epirubicin: *in vitro* interaction with blood components. *J. Pharm. Pharmacol.*, **53**, 815–821.
143. Schrijvers, D. (2003) Role of red blood cells in pharmacokinetics of chemotherapeutic agents. *Clin. Pharmacokinet.*, **42**, 779–791.
144. Cole, P.D., Alcaraz, M.J., and Smith, A.K. (2006) Pharmacodynamic properties of methotrexate and Aminotrexate™ during weekly therapy. *Cancer Chemother. Pharmacol.*, **57**, 826–834.
145. Halonen, P., Mattila, J., Mäkipernaa, A. *et al.* (2006) Erythrocyte concentrations of metabolites or cumulative doses of 6-mercaptopurine and methotrexate do not predict liver changes in children treated for acute lymphoblastic leukemia. *Pediatr. Blood Cancer*, **46**, 762–766.
146. Luo, F.R., Wyrick, S.D., and Chaney, S.G. (1999) Pharmacokinetics and biotransformations of oxaliplatin in comparison with ormaplatin following a single bolus injection in rats. *Cancer Chemother. Pharmacol.*, **44**, 19–28.
147. Wildiers, H., Guetens, G., de Boeck, G. *et al.* (2002) Melphalan availability in hypoxia-inducible factor-1alpha$^{+/+}$ and factor-1alpha$^{-/-}$ tumors is independent of tumor vessel density and correlates with melphalan erythrocyte transport. *Int. J. Cancer*, **99**, 514–519.
148. Matthews, J.B., Adomat, H., and Skov, K.A. (1993) The effect of hypoxia on cytotoxicity, accumulation and DNA binding of cisplatin in Chinese hamster ovary cells. *Anti-Cancer Drugs*, **4**, 463–470.
149. Kohnoe, S., Emi, Y., Takahashi, I. *et al.* (1991) Hypoxia and acidity increase the cytotoxicity of mitomycin C and carboquone to human tumor cells *in vitro*. *AntiCancer Res.*, **11**, 1401–1404.
150. Skarsgard, L.D., Chaplin, D.J., Wilson, D.J. *et al.* (1992) The effect of hypoxia and low pH on the cytotoxicity of chlorambucil. *Int. J. Radiat. Oncol. Biol. Physiol.*, **22**, 737–741.
151. Thews, O., Gassner, B., Kelleher, D.K. *et al.* (2007) Impact of hypoxic and acidic extracellular conditions on cytotoxicity of chemotherapeutic drugs. *Adv. Exp. Med. Biol.*, **599**, 155–161.
152. Gillies, R.J., Martinez-Zaguilán, R., Peterson, E.P., and Perona, R. (1992) Role of intracellular pH in mammalian cell proliferation. *Cell. Physiol. Biochem.*, **2**, 159–179.
153. Griffiths, J.R. (1991) Are cancer cells acidic? *Br. J. Cancer*, **64**, 425–427.
154. Fais, S., De Milito, A., You, H., and Qin, W. (2007) Targeting vacuolar H$^+$-ATPase as a new strategy against cancer. *Cancer Res.*, **67**, 10627–10630.
155. Wike-Hooley, J.L., Haveman, J., and Reinhold, H.S. (1984) The relevance of tumour pH to the treatment of malignant disease. *Radiother. Oncol.*, **2**, 343–366.

156. Tannock, I.F. and Rotin, D. (1989) Acid pH in tumors and its potential for therapeutic exploitation. *Cancer Res.*, **49**, 4373–4384.
157. Song, C.W., Lyons, J.C., and Luo, Y. (1993) Intra- and extracellular pH in solid tumors: Influence on therapeutic response in *Drug Resistance in Oncology* (ed. B.A. Teicher), Dekker, New York, pp. 25–51.
158. Song, C.W., Park, H., and Ross, B.D. (1999) Intra- and extracellular pH in solid tumors in *Antiangiogenic Agents in Cancer Therapy* (ed. B.A. Teicher), Humana Press, Totowa, NJ, pp. 51–64.
159. Gerweck, L.E. (1998) Tumor pH: implications for treatment and novel drug design. *Semin. Radiat. Oncol.*, **8**, 176–182.
160. Stubbs, M. (1998) Tumour pH in *Blood Perfusion and Microenvironment of Human Tumors: Implications for Clinical Radiooncology* (eds M. Molls and P. Vaupel), Springer, Berlin, pp. 113–120.
161. Stubbs, M., McSheehy, P.M.J., Griffiths, J.R., and Bashford, C.L. (2000) Causes and consequences of tumour acidity and implications for treatment. *Mol. Med. Today*, **6**, 15–19.
162. Evelhoch, J.L. (2001) pH and theraphy of human cancer in *The Tumour Microenvironment: Causes and Consequences of Hypoxia and Acidity*, Novartis Foundation Symposium, Vol. 240 (eds J.A. Goode and D.J. Chadwick), John Wiley & Sons, Ltd, Chichester, pp. 68–84.
163. Roepe, P.D. (2001) pH and multidrug resistance in *The Tumour Microenvironment: Causes and Consequences of Hypoxia and Acidity*, Novartis Foundation Symposium, Vol. 240 (eds J.A. Goode and D.J. Chadwick), John Wiley & Sons, Ltd, Chichester, pp. 232–250.
164. Raghunand, N. and Gillies, R.J. (2000) pH and drug resistance in tumours. *Drug Resist. Updat.*, **3**, 39–47.
165. Raghunand, N. and Gillies, R.J. (2001) pH and chemotherapy in *The Tumour Microenvironment: Causes and Consequences of Hypoxia and Acidity*, Novartis Foundation Symposium, Vol. 240 (eds J.A. Goode and D.J. Chadwick), John Wiley & Sons, Ltd, Chichester, pp. 199–211.
166. Gerweck, L.E. and Seetharaman, K. (1996) Cellular pH gradient in tumor versus normal tissue: potential exploitation for the treatment of cancer. *Cancer Res.*, **56**, 1194–1198.
167. Gerweck, L.E., Vijayappa, S., and Kozin, S. (2006) Tumor pH controls the in-vivo efficacy of weak acid and base chemotherapies. *Mol. Cancer Ther.*, **5**, 1275–1279.
168. Wei, L.Y. and Roepe, P.D. (1994) Low external pH and osmotic shock increase the expression of human MDR protein. *Biochemistry*, **33**, 7229–7238.
169. Robinson, L.J., Roberts, W.K., Ling, T.T. et al. (1997) Human MDR1 protein overexpression delays the apoptotic cascade in Chinese hamster ovary fibroblasts. *Biochemistry*, **36**, 11169–11178.
170. Sarkaria, J.N., Kitange, G.J., James, D. et al. (2008) Mechanisms of chemoresistance to alkylating agents in malignant glioma. *Clin. Cancer Res.*, **14**, 2900–2908.
171. Valeriote, F. and van Putten, L. (1975) Proliferation-dependent cytotoxicity of anticancer agents: a review. *Cancer Res.*, **35**, 2619–2630.
172. Lotz, C., Kelleher, D.K., Gassner, B. et al. (2007) Role of the tumor microenvironment in the activity and expression of the p-glycoprotein in human colon carcinoma cells. *Oncol. Rep.*, **17**, 239–244.
173. Osinsky, S. and Vaupel, P. (2009) *Tumor Microphysiology (in Russian)*, Naukova Dumka, Kiev.

3
Enhanced Permeability and Retention Effect in Relation to Tumor Targeting
Hiroshi Maeda

3.1
Background and Status Quo

We first described the enhanced permeability and retention (EPR) effect of macromolecules in solid tumors under the title of "A new concept for macromolecular therapeutics in cancer chemotherapy: mechanism of tumoritropic accumulation of proteins and the antitumor agent SMANCS" in the December 1986 issue of *Cancer Research* [1]. In prior publications we had described the relationship of plasma half-life of small proteins of about 10 kDa to more than 240 kDa as well as the biocompatibility of proteins in relation to the conformational integrity. For instance, the native versus denatured form of α_2-macroglobulin shows a drastic reduction of plasma half-life when this plasma protease inhibitor of 240 kDa complexes with a protease (trypsin) due to rapid uptake by phagocytotic cells or hepatic entrapment [2–4]. Obviously, inadequate chemical modifications of biocompatible plasma or other proteins will reduce plasma half-life, while appropriate modifications will prolong their half-lives. This effect was noted for the modification of many proteins (e.g., superoxide dismutase (30 kDa) and ribonuclease (12.5 kDa) with divema (divinyl ether–maleic acid copolymer or pyran copolymer), neocarzinostatin (NCS) (12 kDa) with styrene–maleic acid copolymer (SMA) or poly(ethylene glycol) (PEG), etc.) [2–5]. In addition to plasma half-life, two crucial points should be emphasized. Namely, all plasma and other proteins of molecular weight above 40 kDa exhibited tumor-selective accumulation. Thus, we envisaged preferential drug targeting to solid tumors by using macromolecular drugs [1, 2]. We also noted that such macromolecular derivatives accumulated preferentially in the lymphatic tissues [6–8]. The latter point has not received enough attention among oncologists or in the field of cancer chemotherapy, regardless of its importance in relation to lymphatic metastases. Namely, many therapeutic failures in cancer chemotherapy can be attributed to the failure of controlling lymphatic metastases. As a matter of fact, there is no effective treatment for lymphatic metastases, and therapy with common anticancer drugs without lymphotropic accumulation does not control the growth and spread of lymphatic metastases [6–10].

Drug Delivery in Oncology: From Basic Research to Cancer Therapy, First Edition.
Edited by Felix Kratz, Peter Senter, and Henning Steinhagen.
© 2012 Wiley-VCH Verlag GmbH & Co. KGaA. Published 2012 by Wiley-VCH Verlag GmbH & Co. KGaA.

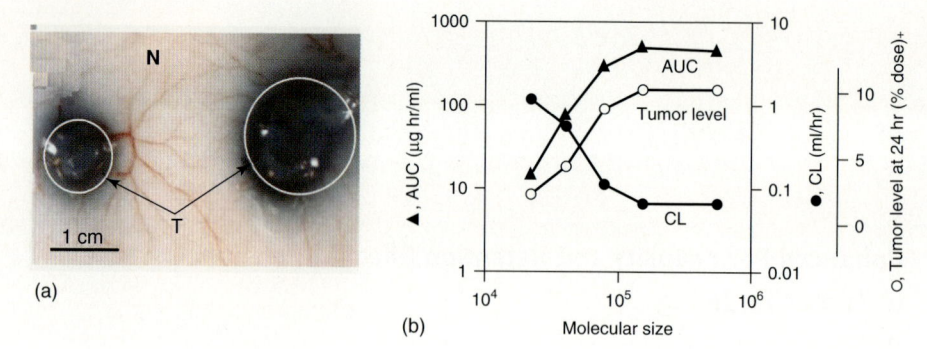

Figure 3.1 (a) EPR effect visualized in experimental mouse tumors where albumin-bound Evans blue (molecular weight 68 kDa) is selectively accumulated only in subcutaneously growing tumor. Arrows 'T' pointing to blue spots are tumors. 'N' is the normal skin that shows no vascular leakage (in contrast to blue-stained tumor). Accumulated Evans blue will remain in the tumor for more than 2–3 weeks. (b) Relation between molecular weight of drugs, plasma level (area under the concentration curve (AUC)), tumor concentration, and renal clearance rate (CL). (Data from [13].)

We have elaborated the EPR effect further by using another biocompatible synthetic polymer, N-(2-hydroxypropyl)methacrylamide (HPMA) copolymers, with discrete molecular size distributions, which were supplied by K. Ulbrich (Prague, Czech Republic) [11–14]. All the data are consistent with the concept of EPR effect, and show that polymers with a molecular weight above 40 kDa exhibited prolonged plasma residence time and preferential accumulation of the polymeric or macromolecular drugs in the tumor tissue [11–16] (Figure 3.1).

Meanwhile, the EPR effect is applicable to a wide range of biocompatible macromolecules, such as proteins/antibodies, liposomes, micelles, DNA or RNA polyplexes, nanocarriers, and lipidic particles for cancer-selective drug delivery [13–16]. The number of papers that cite the EPR effect has increased in a logarithmic manner in recent years, reaching close to 8000 in 2010 (Figure 3.2). In this chapter, I will review the EPR effect briefly, and discuss problems/limitations, solutions, and further augmentation of the EPR effect.

3.2
What is the EPR Effect: Mechanism, Uniqueness, and Factors Involved

The EPR effect is a phenomenon resulting from multiple causes and effects, such as anatomical defects in vascular architecture and higher vascular density as a result of active production of angiogenic factors, especially when tumors are at an early stage and express growth factors such as vascular endothelial growth factors (VEGFs) and nitric oxide (NO). Many vascular permeability factors such as NO (Figure 3.3a–c), bradykinin, prostaglandins, collagenases, matrix metalloproteinases (MMPs), and so on, are overproduced in the tumor tissues (Tables 3.1 and 3.2). They facilitate extravasation of macromolecules in solid tumors [11–21]. As a result, more excessive tumor-selective vascular leakage of

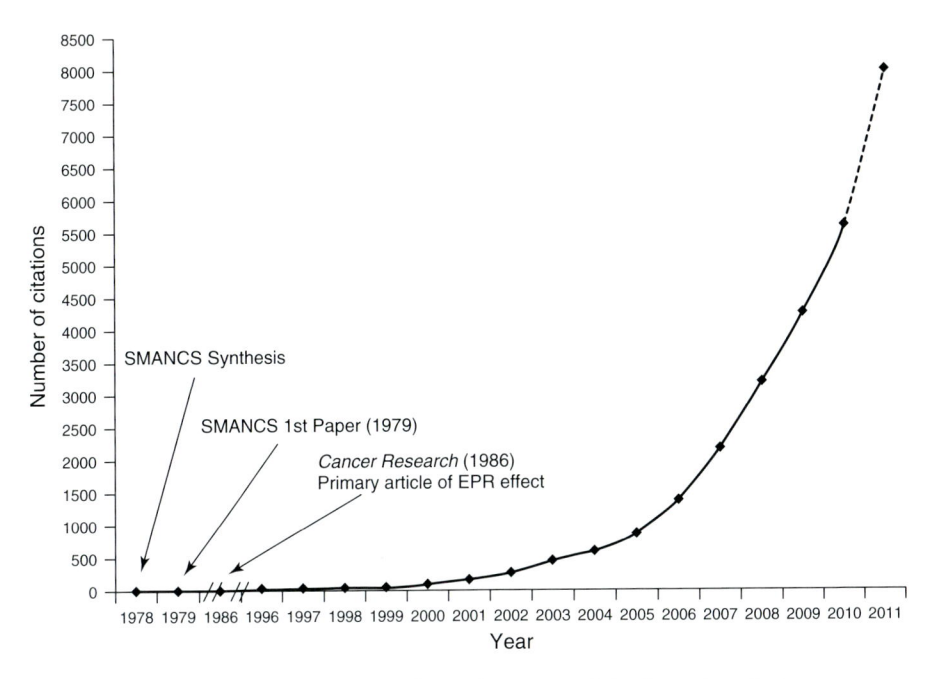

Figure 3.2 Citation numbers of the EPR effect and invention of the first polymeric drug, SMANCS (from *Science Direct* and *SciFinder*). (Adapted from [16].)

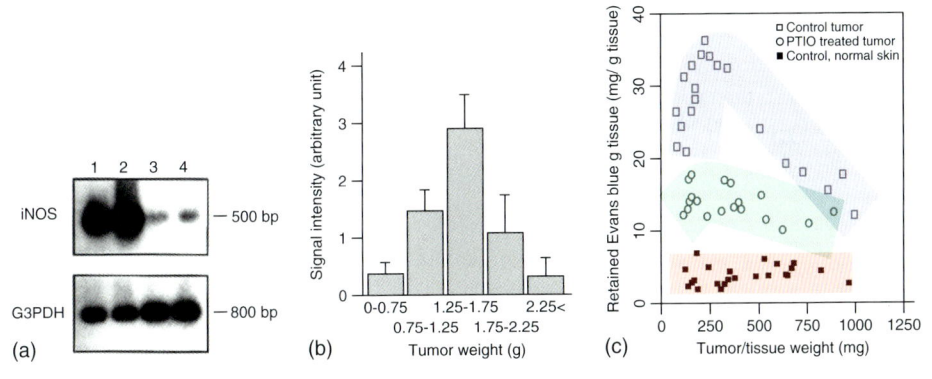

Figure 3.3 (a)–(c) Involvement of NO in the EPR effect: nitric oxide synthase (NOS) induction, relation to tumor size, and effect of NO scavenger by tumor size. (a) Upregulation of the inducible form of NOS (inducible nitric oxide synthase, iNOS) in tumors (lanes 1 and 2) and normal tissues (lanes 3 and 4). (b) Amount of NO generated in solid tumor (S-180) in mice as measured by electron spin resonance spectroscopy with dithiocarbamate–Fe complex and the relation to the size of tumor. (c) Amount of Evans blue–albumin permeation (EPR effect) and effects of NO scavenger (2-phenyl-4,4,5,5-tetramethylimidazolineoxyl-1-oxyl-3-oxide (PTIO), ○) or NOS inhibitor (■) in mouse tumors based on tumor size. Lower zone: control normal tissue; middle zone: treated with PTIO; top zone: control tumor, without NO scavenger. (Adapted from [16, 19].)

Table 3.1 Factors affecting the EPR effect of macromolecular drugs in solid tumors (extensive production of vascular mediators that facilitate extravasation).

Bradykinin
Nitric oxide (NO)
Vascular permeability factor/VEGF
Prostaglandins
Collagenase (MMPs)
Peroxynitrite (ONOO$^-$)
Anticancer agents
Inflammatory cells and H_2O_2
Heme oxygenase-1 (CO)

Table 3.2 Architectural differences and functions.

---

1) Active angiogenesis and high vascular density
2) Defective vascular architecture
    lack of smooth muscle layer
    lack of or fewer receptors for angiotensin II
    large gap in endothelial cell–cell junctions and fenestration
    anomalous conformation of tumor vasculature (e.g., branching or stretching)
3) Defective lymphatic clearance of macromolecules and lipids from interstitial tissue (prolonged retention of these substances)
4) Whimsical and bidirectional blood flow

---

an albumin-bound dye such as Evans blue will occur only at the tumor site, as seen in the examples shown in Figure 3.1a. The uniqueness of this phenomenon is that it will be only seen in tumor tissues, but not in the normal healthy tissue [11, 13–20]. Obviously, normal vasculatures shows no such leakage (Figures 3.1a and 3.3a and c) due to their complete architecture of the blood vasculature as well as little production of vascular mediators as listed in Table 3.1.

Furthermore, macromolecules with a molecular weight more than 40 kDa above the renal threshold such as synthetic polymers, serum proteins, micelles, polymer-based or lipid-based nanoparticles that leak out of the blood vasculature into the interstitial space of tumor tissues remain there for a very long time, even for several weeks, without being cleared (Figures 3.1a,b 3.4, 3.5, and 3.9b) [1, 13, 15]. In contrast to tumors, such micro- or nano- particles, should they leak out of the blood vasculature into normal tissue, will be cleared gradually by the lymphatic system in several days as is usually seen for common inflammations of normal tissue. Neovasculature generated by the tumor is characterized by an irregular shape, dilated, leaky, or defective vessels. The endothelial cells are poorly aligned or disorganized with large fenestrations as illustrated for healthy and tumor vessels in Figure 3.4.

These anatomical features make the vasculature of tumor tissue permeable for macromolecules or even larger nanosized particles such as liposomes or polymeric micelles, whereas in blood vessels of healthy tissue only small molecules can pass

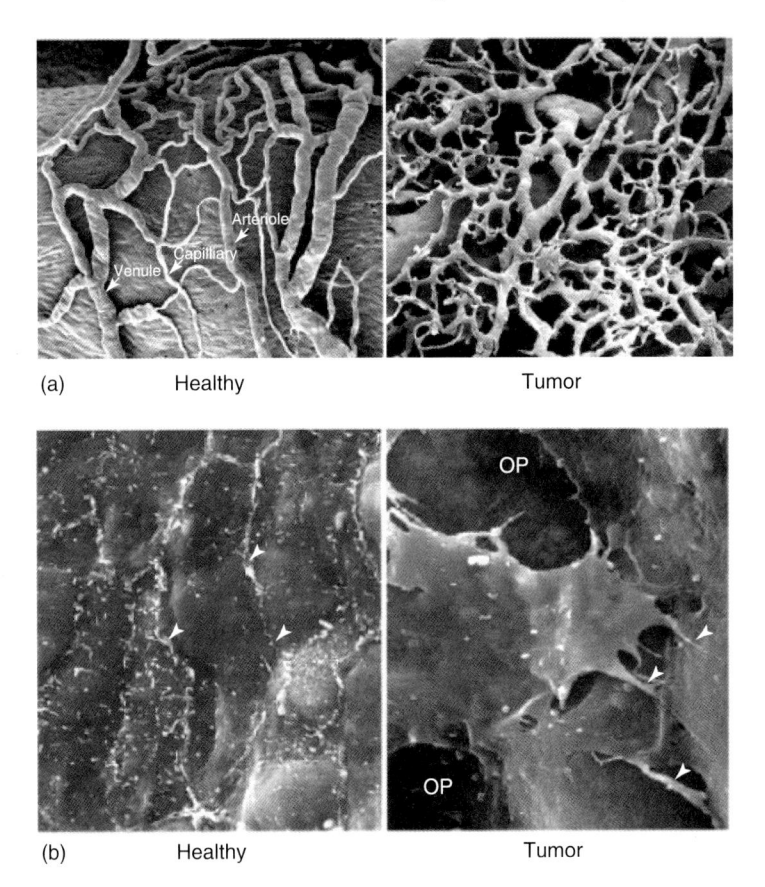

Figure 3.4 (a) Scanning electron microscopy (SEM) imaging of polymer casts of normal (vasa vasorum of rat carotid sinus, left) and tumor (xenograft of human head and neck cancer in nude mouse, right) microvasculature. Marked differences are found in the degree of organization and an apparent lack of conventional hierarchy of blood vessels of the tumor sample. (b) SEM images of the luminal surface of healthy (mouse mammary gland, left) and tumor (MCa-IV mouse mammary carcinoma, right) blood vessels. While the healthy vessel is smooth and has tight endothelial junctions (arrow heads), the tumor vessel shows widened intercellular spaces, overlapping endothelial cells (arrow heads), opening (OP) and other abnormalities. (Reproduced with permission from [22].)

the endothelial barrier. The pore size of tumor microvessels was reported to vary from 100 to 1200 nm in diameter (depending on the anatomic location of the tumor). In contrast, the tight junctions between endothelial cells of microvessels in most normal tissues are less than 2 nm in diameter (noteworthy exceptions are found in postcapillary venules (up to 6 nm), and in the kidneys, liver, and spleen (up to 150 nm)) Figure 3.4b.

The EPR effect is depicted schematically in Figure 3.5.

Figure 3.5 illustrates that blood vessels in most normal tissues have an intact endothelial layer that allows the diffusion of small molecules, but not the entry of

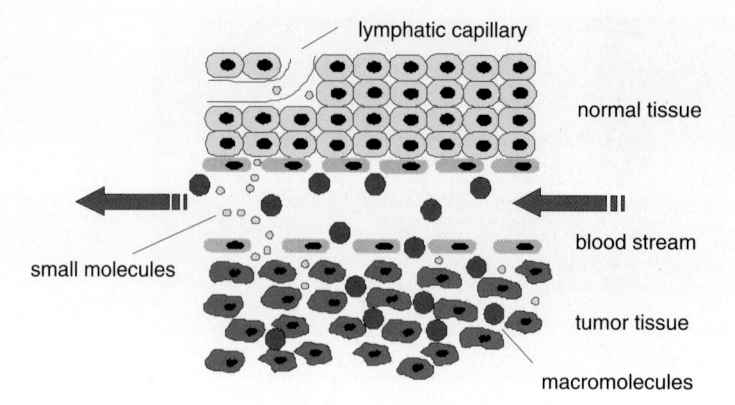

Figure 3.5 Schematic representation of the anatomical and physiological characteristics of normal (upper half) and tumor (lower half) tissues with respect to the vascular permeability and retention of small (lighter circles) and large molecules (darker circles) (see text) [23].

macromolecules into the tissue. In contrast, the endothelial layer of blood vessels in tumor tissue is often leaky so that small as well as large molecules have access to malignant tissue. As tumor tissue does not generally have a lymphatic drainage system, macromolecules are thus retained and can accumulate in solid tumors.

As described above, we can demonstrate this retention effect by injecting Evans blue intravenously, which binds with high affinity and selectivity to the plasma protein albumin (66.5 kDa), and remains in circulation for more than several hours in rodents.

During the long circulation time of Evans blue bound to albumin, the albumin–Evans blue complex will eventually permeate through the porous tumor blood vessels into the interstitial tissue of tumor, thus staining the tumor blue (Figure 3.1a, 3.5). Alternatively, by infusing a lipid contrast agent such as Lipiodol® with/without the polymeric anticancer drug SMANCS (a conjugate of SMA and NCS) via the tumor-feeding arterial route, Lipiodol will be taken up most effectively by the tumor (Figure 3.6a,c and 3.7). In this case, the ratio of the concentration of Lipiodol in the tumor to circulating blood is more than 2000-fold, translating into an extremely tumor pin-pointed targeted delivery [24–26]. When X-ray computed tomography (CT) scans are taken 1 or 2 days after Lipiodol infusion, one can visualize the white Lipiodol-stained tumor areas showing tumor-selective extravasated areas (Figure 3.7a). In this setting, the lipophilic polymeric drug SMANCS dissolved in Lipiodol (thus named SMANCS/Lipiodol) is retained in the tumor tissue selectively. The presence of Lipiodol and SMANCS can be detected as high-election-density areas ("white areas") due to iodine in Lipiodol using X-ray imaging [14, 24–26].

This method allows detection of tumor nodules as small as a few millimeters in diameter [24, 25]. Furthermore, this prolonged retention in tumor tissue is more than just a passive targeting. Namely, when a low-molecular-weight water-soluble contrast agent is infused under identical conditions (known as angiography)

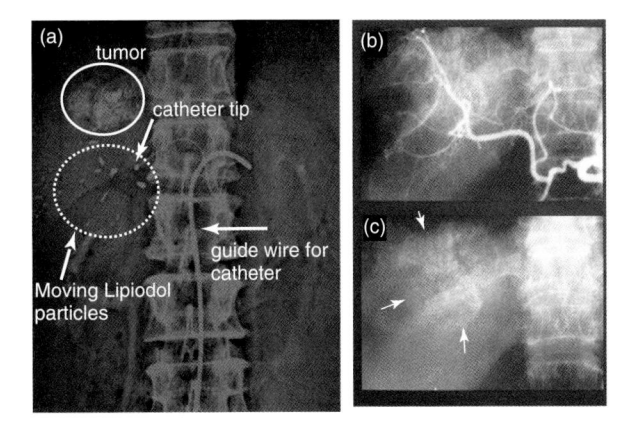

Figure 3.6 (a) Angiographic arterial infusion of SMANCS/Lipiodol using a catheter (Seldinger method) via the hepatic artery (where vascular leakage is seen, but only within 1 min). White Lipiodol particles coming out are captured at the tumor. (b) Arterial phase (blood vessels are visible). (c) Venous phase.

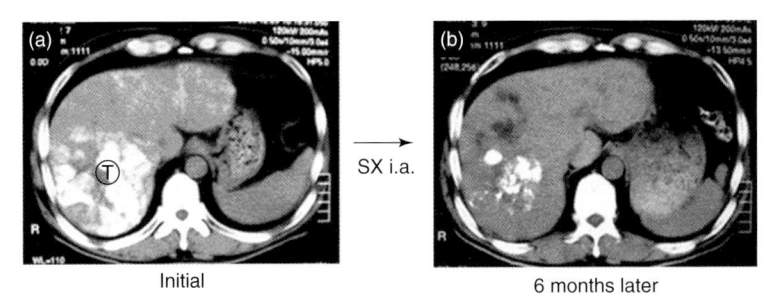

Figure 3.7 X-ray CT scan images of hepatocellular carcinoma (hepatoma) of a patient, where tumor location 'T' and size are visualized by white staining of high-electron-density iodine in the radio contrast agent Lipiodol, which is selectively retained in the tumor. (a) CT image at the first injection. (b) Significant size reduction of the tumor is seen after 6 months of arterial injection of SMANCS 3 times in 6 months via the hepatic artery.

(Figure 3.6a and b) it allows visualization of a solid tumor with the aid of X-ray imaging. However, this tumor staining lasts for only 1–5 min as illustrated by venous-phase staining images (e.g., Figure 3.6c). In contrast to this short time of duration, lipid particles (e.g., Lipiodol) or polymeric drugs, or albumin-bound Evans blue are retained for significantly longer time periods as a result of the EPR effect. The prolonged retention of macromolecules and nanoparticles in the tumor continues for days to weeks, and if they carry a drug this can be released in the vicinity of tumor cells. When an adequate concentration of the active drug in the tumor tissue is attained, it will lead to definite tumor regressions [27]. Thus, the EPR effect is an event observed in *in vivo* settings, but not *in vitro* or cell-free systems, not to mention in normal tissues.

In this context, it may be worth mentioning the enhanced vascular permeability of inflammatory tissues. The enhanced vascular permeability of a tissue is one of the hallmark manifestations of inflammation, which may also involve bradykinin, reactive oxygen species, and other mediators. We had initially observed that bacterial proteases induce activation of a bradykinin-generating cascade [28–32]. Similar events were also discovered in cancer tissues [20, 21, 29–32]. Activation of the kallikrein–kinin cascade leads to the generation of bradykinin that will potentiate the EPR effect instead of suppressing the EPR effect. Another effect is the heterogeneous tumor cell growth with unparalleled angiogenesis resulting in inadequate supply of oxygen (i.e., low pO_2), which will affect induction of p53 or other events that will lead to apoptosis signaling, including the disappearance of vasculature or apoptotic/necrotic tissue death.

If the tumor tissue retained normal or near normal innate immunity such as macrophage functions, it would exert defensive a host response generating NO and superoxide (O_2^-). Both of them react immediately to become peroxynitrite ($ONOO^-$) at confined local vicinities, where $ONOO^-$ is highly toxic and exerts oxidative and nitrating effect, and affects cancer cells [29]. In addition to the cytotoxic effect of $ONOO^-$ (and ClO^-), $ONOO^-$ can activate MMPs (or collagenases) that disrupt tissue matrices and vascular integrity, and facilitate vascular leakage (i.e., the EPR effect) [19, 20, 29, 33]. (The $ONOO^-$ thus generated modifies tyrosine to form nitrotyrosine and guanine to form 8-nitroguanine in nucleic acid as well as 8-nitrocylic GMP [34, 35]. 8-Nitroguanosine becomes a substrate of NADPH-dependent reductase such as cytochrome b_5 reductase and iNOS [36, 37]. As a matter of fact, one can demonstrate the presence of nitrotyrosine and 8-nitroguanosine in tumor cells (by fluorescence immunostaining and high-performance liquid chromatography). The cell-killing potency of $ONOO^-$ is as strong as hypochlorite (ClO^-; i.e., below 10 µM), which is another reactive chemical produced by leukocytes (neutrophils) from H_2O_2 and Cl^- by myeloperoxidase [29].) Tumor tissues under these circumstances are therefore heterogeneous or different from normal pathophysiological tissue.

These vascular effectors that are common among cancer and inflammatory tissues open up the endothelial cell–cell junction, and allow proteins and macromolecules to extravasate into the interstitial tissue. However, they will be gradually recovered via the lymphatic clearance system in a matter of a few to several days. In contrast to this phenomenon of normal tissue, the clearance of drug nanoparticles or drug polymer conjugates from cancer tissue is much slower, and results in sustained access of this type of polymer therapeutics to cancer cells, which is the most desired goal in cancer drug delivery.

3.3
Heterogeneity of the EPR Effect: A Problem in Drug Delivery

The EPR effect is universally observed in rodent, rabbit, and human solid tumors. It is more typical when the tumor size is less than 1 cm. However, as shown in Figure 3.8a–c, when a tumor grows larger than 1 cm, the tumor exhibits more heterogeneity in the EPR effect. Yet it is seen even when tumor nodules are as

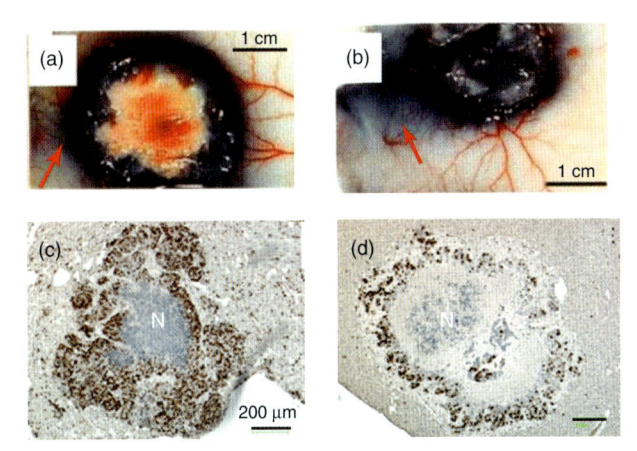

Figure 3.8 Heterogeneity of the EPR effect as seen by extravasation of Evans blue–albumin in tumor. (a) and (b) S-180 tumor in mouse. Macroscopic tumor and the skin, after intravenous Evans blue injection. In both (a) and (b), the tumor tissue shows heterogeneous staining of Evans blue as inhomogeneous extravasation of the blue dye–albumin complex. This type of peripheral uptake of SMANCS/Lipiodol is seen via CT in metastatic human tumors and is classified as B-type staining (26). Arrows in (a) and (b) point to areas in which the EPR effect also occurs in normal tissue as a result of the generation of vascular mediators such as bradykinin. This extravasated blue albumin in normal skin will be cleared via the lymphatics. Ki-67 immunohistochemistry was used to assess tumor proliferation in (c) and (d). Proliferating cells were demarcated by intense brown diaminobenzidine staining in (c). In (d), polymeric drug SMA–pirarubicin reduced tumor proliferation by greater than 75% in 72 h after one intravenous injection. Control tumors of (c) demonstrated a high degree of tumor proliferation. Tumor proliferation was restricted to a thick viable band at the tumor periphery with significant central necrosis (N). (d) Proliferation in SMA–pirarubicin-treated tumors was restricted to the thin viable rim at the tumor periphery. Scale bars = 200 μm [38].

small as 0.5 mm in diameter in metastatic micronodules of the liver (Figure 3.8c,d), although tumor-selective extravasation of a polymeric drug (by the EPR effect) can be observed (Figure 3.9b). In the metastatic liver cancer model of colon cancer, the microheterogeneity of the EPR effect is also observed as viable parts and necrotic parts near the center of the tumor (Figure 3.8c) [38]. However, it should be noted that the tumor-proliferating area is located primarily at the periphery of the solid tumor, which coincides with the area showing an extensive EPR effect, while a hypovascular or avascular appearance is seen in the tumor center (Figures 3.8a and c and 3.10a and b). Despite the heterogeneity of the EPR or the vasculature of the tumor, macromolecular drugs show much more drug accumulation by EPR in the tumor periphery where more proliferating tumor cells exist (see peripheral staining in Figures 3.8a and c and 3.10a,b).

Therefore, the area with a high EPR effect coincides with the tumor growth area. Thus, using cytostatic polymeric drugs is more advantageous from the therapeutic point of view since they act effectively on proliferating cancer cells. In this context, 90–95% suppression of metastatic tumor nodules in the liver by

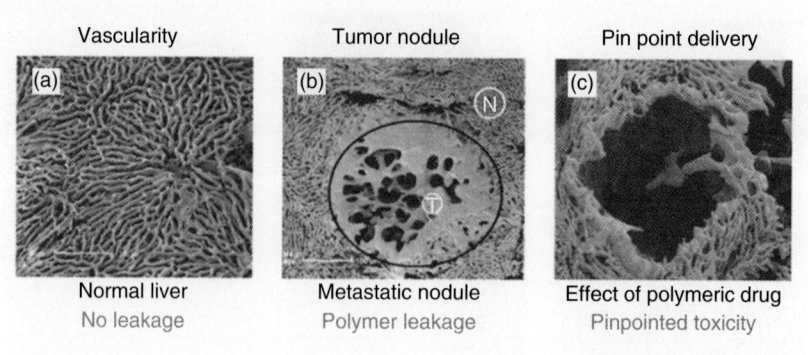

Figure 3.9 SEM images of metastatic colon cancer to the liver. (a) Normal liver vessels. (b) Metastatic micronodule of tumor indicating by 'T' (blood bed) where polymeric resin is extravagated by the EPR effect. (c) After a treatment of tumor-selective polymeric drug (SMA micelles with pirarubicin) by intravenous injection. The nodular blood bed of the metastatic tumor has disintegrated: tumor tissue has undergone apoptosis and necrosis by tumor-selective drug delivery; however, no damage to the normal liver tissue is seen. More than 95% of tumor nodules in the liver are destroyed by this drug given intravenously. The images are courtesy of Dr. J. Daruwalla and Professor C. Christophi of the University of Melbourne, Australia [38].

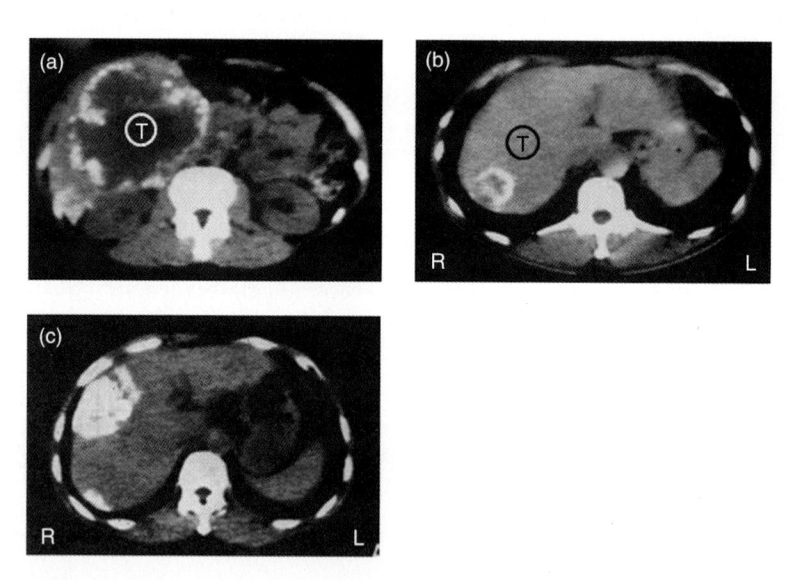

Figure 3.10 X-ray CT scan of the liver cancer after SMANCS/Lipiodol injection via the arterial route under normotensive blood pressure. Heterogeneity of drug uptake in (a) and (b) is remarkable as a ring-like staining. Namely, an avascular or hypovascular area is noted as a dark area in the central part of metastatic liver cancer (a), a massive size metastasized tumor from the gallbladder, and (b) metastatic liver cancer from the colon. In (c), primary liver cancer (hepatocellular carcinoma) seen as a white area at the right side of the liver lobe in the CT image where uptake of SMANCS/Lipiodol is homogeneous.

single intravenous injection of SMA–pirarubicin micelles was significant and a promising result for future drug design in this area of research [38].

In relation to the heterogeneity of the EPR effect, most metastatic tumors in the liver in human patients show hypovascular properties near the tumor center as shown in Figure 3.10. Figure 3.10a is a massive metastatic gallbladder cancer to the liver that shows much less drug (SMANCS/Lipiodol) uptake in the central area when given intra-arterially under normotensive conditions. We have defined these CT images of centrally hypovascular or avascular staining (low density even after Lipiodol infusion) as type B staining [26]. In Figure 3.10b, small-sized metastatic liver cancer originating from the colon in the right lobe also show B-type staining. In contrast, hepatocellular carcinoma (or primary liver cancer) and renal carcinoma usually exhibit complete filling of SMANCS/Lipiodol after arterial infusion under normotensive conditions, and the entire tumor is stained without a central low-density area (Figure 3.10c). This staining was defined type A staining by CT scans, and usually exhibits more homogeneous staining and a good EPR effect [26]. Type A staining is a common feature of tumors with high vascular density such as hepatocellular carcinoma and renal cell carcinoma. Prostate and pancreatic cancers, conversely, show low-density staining, indicating less potential for drug delivery, thus, augmentation of EPR effect is needed as described below.

3.4
Overcoming the Heterogeneity of the EPR Effect for Drug Delivery and How to Enhance the EPR Effect

3.4.1
Angiotensin II-Induced High Blood Pressure

To counteract the heterogeneous EPR effect of hypovascular tumor tissue as described above, which shows reduced drug delivery, we have developed two methods to enhance tumor drug delivery and overcome the problem of EPR-less-dependent tumor tissue. One method is by elevating the blood pressure during the arterial infusion of macromolecular drugs by using angiotensin II (a vasoconstrictor). This can be achieved, for instance, by increasing the systolic blood pressure from 90–120 to 150–160 mmHg and maintaining the hypertensive state for 15–20 min [27, 39, 40]. As shown in Figure 3.11a and b, by angiography of the same experimental rat tumor (window model), the angiotensin-induced hypertension allows the visualization of significantly more blood vessels that are otherwise not visible (Figure 3.11a vs b) [39, 40].

Despite an apparently avascular large tumor mass as shown in Figure 3.11c, e, and g, delivery of SMANCS/Lipiodol was significantly augmented as seen in Figure 3.11 (d, f, and h, respectively). SMANCS/Lipiodol can be delivered effectively to the tumors (see below) and remarkable regression was obtained. It should be noted that when angiotensin II is applied intravenously by slow infusion, blood

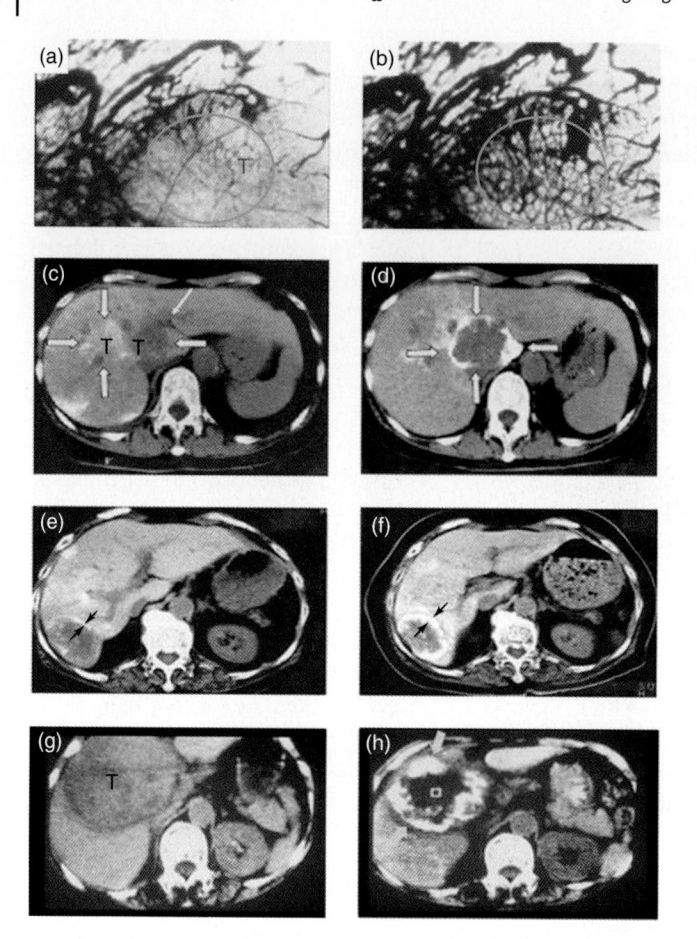

Figure 3.11 Augmentation of the EPR effect by angiotensin II-induced high blood pressure. (a) and (b) Window chamber model of an experimental rat tumor model. Blood vessels are only weekly seen under the normotensive state (circled area) in (a), but the blood vessels became dense as noted in (b) when the systolic blood pressure of 90 mmHg was elevated to 160 mmHg (circled area). (Adapted from [39].) The following examples are results of arterial infusion of SMANCS/Lipiodol of normotensive blood pressure (90–120 mmHg) (c, e, and g) and angiotensin II-infused conditions (to about 150–160 mmHg) (d, f, and h). (c)–(f) Colon cancer → liver metastasis; (g) and (h) a case with massive gallbladder cancer metastasized to the liver. In all these (c, e, and g) difficult-to-treat cases, angiotensin induced a hypertensive state and clearly showed significantly enhanced drug delivery (see arrows, white area).

flow volume increased selectively in the tumor, whereas all normal tissues exhibit a constant blood flow volume regardless of the blood pressure applied [40].

Under this condition, drug delivery to tumor tissue was increased selectively as seen by Evans blue complexed with albumin or radiolabeled albumin. There seems less delivery to normal tissues under this hypertensive condition [41]. Thus, fewer side-effects were seen than in the normotensive state (as revealed by blood cell count, diarrhea, or liver and kidney functions), while this method resulted in a marked increase of drug delivery to the tumor by a factor of 2–3 [41].

In parallel to this increased EPR effect and concomitant drug delivery, we observed an improved therapeutic effect as well as decreased adverse toxicity. This remarkably improved therapeutic effect was observed not only in the rat model, but more importantly also in human patients with difficult-to-treat tumors, such as metastatic liver cancer, pancreatic cancer with liver metastases, massive renal cancer, cancer of the gallbladder with liver metastases, and cholangiocarcinoma [27] (Figure 3.12).

In light of these encouraging results, the next key issue is to optimize the release rate of the drug to attain a drug concentration above the IC_{50} value (inhibitory dose of 50% cell kill) or the minimum inhibitory concentration. SMANCS/Lipiodol of

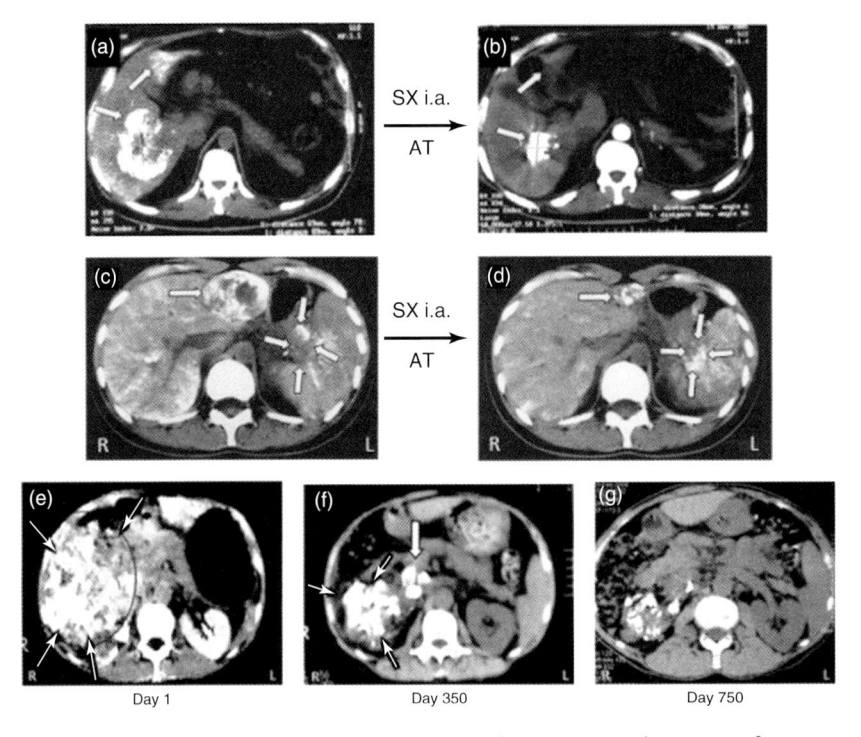

Figure 3.12 Enhanced drug delivery under angiotensin-induced high blood pressure and remarkably improved therapeutic outcome. (a) and (b) A massive metastatic liver cancer originated from stomach cancer regressed considerably in 50 days. It was injected under an angiotensin II-induced hypertensive state. Almost complete filling of the drug (SX) inside the tumor and tumor-selective drug deposition is seen. The white area indicates SMANCS/Lipiodol. (c) and (d) Metastatic liver cancer from a pancreatic cancer. It was similarly treated with SMANCS/Lipiodol given intra-arterially. Both metastatic tumors in the liver and primary tumors in the pancreas regressed considerably within a few months. (e)–(g) Massive renal cell carcinoma treated with SMANCS/Lipiodol similarly regressed remarkably and this patient is still healthy with good a quality of life (longer than 8 years). (From [27].)

1.0–1.5 mg/ml appears ideal in this respect; a higher concentration was recommended for metastatic liver cancer and renal cell carcinoma of 1.3–1.5 mg/ml. For cholangiocarcinoma and pancreatic cancer, a concentration of 1.2–1.3 mg/ml can be recommended [15, 27].

3.4.2
Use of NO-Releasing Agents

The second method we developed recently is the use of nitroglycerin ointment [42]. Nitroglycerin has been used for treating angina pectoris or cardiac infarct in humans for more than 100 years. Both tumor tissue and infarct cardiac tissues show low oxygen tension (pO_2). Nitroglycerin is known to be absorbed from the skin rapidly and enter the general circulation effectively within 5 min. In the hypoxic tissue (where low pO_2 is prevalent) NO_2^- is liberated from nitroglycerin and nitrite (NO_2^-) is further reduced to $NO^\bullet$ (Figure 3.13a).

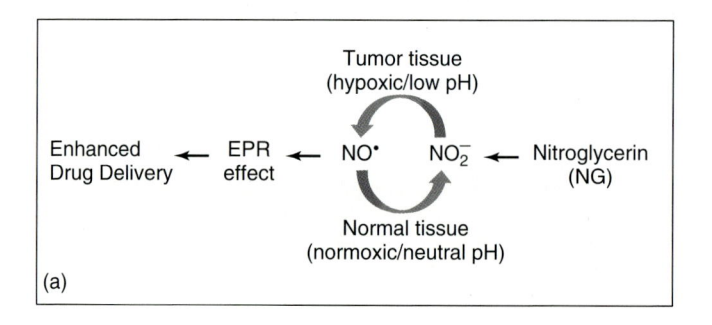

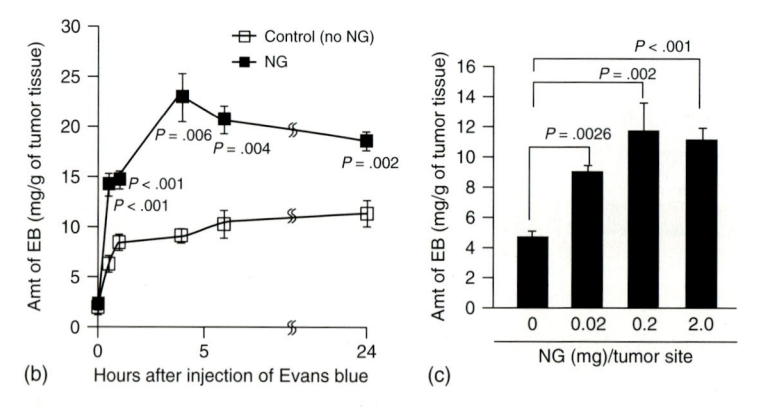

Figure 3.13 Another method to augment the EPR effect in tumor-bearing mice. (a) Conversion of nitroglycerin to nitrite to NO in the tumor. (b) Enhanced drug delivery to the tumor at different timepoints. (c) Effect of the dose of nitroglycerin on the EPR effect measured after 6 h of treatment of glycerin ointment on the skin [42].

It is intriguing that this process occurs more selectively in tumor tissues, such as seen in the infarct cardiac tissue when compared to normal tissues. As stated above, NO is one of the major factors that facilitates the EPR effect [16–20, 29, 42, 43], and hence it will trigger vascular leakage and thus enhance tumor delivery (2- to 3-fold) (Figure 3.13b and c) [42]. Consequently, nitroglycerin application augmented the EPR effect in rodent tumors and hence the therapeutic effect was also augmented in all four experimental tumor models (S-180, colon 38, Meth A, and chemical 7,12-dimethylbenz[a]anthracene-induced rat tumors).

More importantly, this account was validated by Yasuda et al. and Graham et al. even with commonly used anticancer agents in human patients [44–46]. It is also surprising that both mouse and human data showed that nitroglycerin alone has a tumor-suppressive effect that is as good as a single anticancer agent alone without nitroglycerin.

3.4.3
Use of Other Vascular Modulators

In terms of modulation of the EPR effect by use of vascular mediators, we have previously demonstrated enhancement of the EPR effect by angiotensin II-converting enzyme (ACE) inhibitors such as enalapril. As a result of the analogy in the amino acid sequence of angiotensin II and bradykinin, the ACE inhibitor also blocks the degradation of bradykinin. This means that by administrating the ACE inhibitor, the concentration of bradykinin at the tumor site will remain higher because of suppressed degradation of bradykinin. This account is briefly described by Noguchi et al. [47], demonstrating that the increased tumor delivery of even a monoclonal antibody was about 2-fold higher when enalapril and angiotensin II were combined.

We also examined the prostaglandin I_2 agonist, sodium beraprost, in order to enhance the EPR effect. Namely, sodium beraprost given orally has a much longer plasma half-life than parental prostaglandin I_2 and can induce tumor-selective enhanced drug delivery [48].

Very recently, we found CO (gas) is a mediator of EPR effect. CO (carbon mono oxide), together with biliverden and Fe^+, are generated by heme oxygenase using heme and oxygen as substrates. Therefore, induction of heme oxygenase by such as hemin (49), UV irradiation, reactive oxygen species as well as NO (50) can be used as enhancer of EPR effect (49).

3.5
PEG Dilemma: Stealth Effect and Anti-PEG IgM Antibody

As more PEGylated macromolecular drugs are explored, it has been realized in recent years that cellular uptake of PEGylated nanoparticles is not as efficient as one wished for, although PEGylated particles can reach the tumor site selectively by the EPR effect (e.g., [51, 52]). The reason is that the hydrated barrier of the surface of PEGylated particles impedes contact of the PEGylated particle to the cell surface receptors, which can result in less-efficient cellular uptake of the

PEGylated nanoparticles. This is now referred to as the "PEG dilemma" [53, 54]. To overcome this problem, Harashima and others recently [53, 54] proposed to select a shorter chain of PEG or proteolytically cleavable type of bonds between PEG chains and effector molecules for drug delivery. We also reported that PEG linked via an ester bond was more preferred over PEG chains bound through an amide bond [55–57]. Alternatively, different types of polymers (e.g., SMA) have been proposed that exhibit improved cellular uptake [57].

Another problem related to PEGylated drugs as pointed out by Ishida *et al.* [57] is a rapid clearance from the circulating blood, which becomes apparent when a PEGylated drug is injected, not at the first time, but at subsequent injections after 3–7 days of the first injection. They identified PEG-specific IgM antibodies being formed, which is a cause for the rapid elimination from plasma where the IgM antibody complexed with PEGylated drug is cleared by the liver or macrophages [57].

3.6
Concluding Remarks

It is now well known that solid tumor tissue has extensive angiogenesis with pronounced vascular permeability enhancement (EPR effect), albeit some part of the tumor mass may exhibit hypovascular properties or necrotic mass. Thus, tumors may exhibit an inconsistent EPR effect when tumors become larger in size and exhibit a diminished vascular permeability effect. The biological importance of the enhanced vascular permeability is primarily to support the nutritional and oxygen supply to rapidly growing tumor cells.

Heterogeneity of the EPR effect, however, poses a problem in drug delivery that exploits the EPR effect. In this chapter, I have described basic aspects of the EPR effect and its heterogeneity, followed by methods of augmenting drug delivery in tumors with a decreased EPR effect in order to overcome this drawback in relation to passive targeting. Namely, one method to enhance the EPR effect is to utilize angiotensin II-induced hypertension. Some clinical successes using this method were described. Another method is to use the NO generator, nitroglycerin. It was found that nitroglycerin can affect hypoxic tumor tissue more selectively than normal tissues or organs, similar to the cardiac tissue of pectoris angina. Both these methods exhibit significantly improved drug delivery and therapeutic effects.

Our earlier finding regarding the EPR effect of macromolecular drugs in combination with lipid particles could archieve by far the most tumor-selective delivery using arterial infusion into the tumor-feeding artery. Namely, the drug level of tumor to blood ratio is greater than 2000 [24], and no other method is more universally and selectively unique to tumor tissue. Therefore, there is no reason not to utilize further strategies of augmenting the EPR effect in order to achieve an improved tumor-selective drug delivery. Methods such as the use of ACE inhibitors, nitroglycerin, or sodium beraprost, and HO-1 inducer (hemin) or even angiotensin II-induced hypertension are simple. Another important aspect of the EPR effect is its sustained drug retention and release in the tumor tissue. Thus, the use of macromolecular drugs and enhancers of the EPR effect undoubtedly warrants further clinical study. Considering the potential benefit and the great numbers of suffering patients, negligence or unwillingness to adapt such safe and inexpensive therapeutic options is a frustrating reality.

Acknowledgments

The author is indebted to Dr. J. Daruwalla and Professor C. Christophi of the University of Melbourne, Australia and Professor M.A. Konerding *et al.* of the University of Mainz, Germany for SEM images, Dr. K. Hori and Professor M. Suzuki of Tohoku University for vascular images at normotension and hypertension in the rat tumor model (Figure 3.9a and b), and Professor F. Kratz for Figure 3.5; Dr. A. Nagamitsu of Fukuoka for patients data used in this chapter; and also Professor F. Kratz for reviewing and suggestions.

References

1. Matsumura, Y. and Maeda, H. (1986) A new concept for macromolecular therapeutics in cancer chemotherapy: mechanism of tumoritropic accumulation of proteins and the antitumor agent SMANCS. *Cancer Res.*, **46**, 6387–6392.
2. Maeda, H., Matsumoto, T., Konno, T., Iwai, K., and Ueda, M. (1984) Tailor-making of protein drugs by polymer conjugation for tumor targeting: a brief review on SMANCS. *J. Protein Chem.*, **3**, 181–193.
3. Maeda, H., Matsumura, Y., Oda, T., and Sasamoto, K. (1986) Calicheamicin antibody–drug conjugates and beyond in *Protein Tailoring for Food and Medical Uses* (eds R.E. Feeney and J.R. Whitaker), Dekker, New York, pp. 353–382.
4. Oda, T., Akaike, T., Hamamoto, T., and Maeda, H. (1989) Oxygen radicals in influenza-induced pathogenesis and treatment with pyran polymer-conjugated SOD. *Science*, **244**, 974–976.
5. Ogino, T., Inoue, M., Ando, Y., Awai, M., Maeda, H., and Morino, Y. (1988) Chemical modification of superoxide dismutase. *Int. J. Pept. Protein Res.*, **32**, 153–159.
6. Maeda, H., Takeshita, J., and Yamashita, A. (1980) Lymphotropic accumulation of an antitumor antibiotic protein, neocarzinostatin. *Eur. J. Cancer*, **16**, 723–731.
7. Maeda, H. and Matsumura, Y. (1989) Tumoritropic and lymphotropic principles of macromolecular drugs. *Crit. Rev. Ther. Drug Carrier Syst.*, **6**, 193–210.
8. Maeda, H., Takeshita, J., Kanamaru, R., Sato, H., Khatoh, J., and Sato, H. (1979) Antimetastatic and antitumor activity of a derivative of neocarzinostatin: an organic solvent- and water-soluble polymer-conjugated protein. *Gann*, **70**, 601–606.
9. Takeshita, J., Maeda, H., and Kanamaru, R. (1982) *In vitro* mode of action, pharmacokinetics, and organ specificity of poly(maleic acid–styrene)-conjugated neocarzinostatin, SMANCS. *Gann*, **73**, 278–284.
10. Maeda, H., Takeshita, J., and Kanamaru, R. (1979) A lipophilic derivative of neocarzinostatin: a polymer conjugation of an antitumor protein antibiotic. *Int. J. Pept. Protein Res.*, **14**, 81–87.
11. Noguchi, Y., Wu, J., Duncan, R., Strohalm, J., Ulbrich, K., Akaike, T., and Maeda, H. (1998) Early phase tumor accumulation of macromolecules: a great difference in clearance rate

between tumor and normal tissues. *Jpn. J. Cancer Res.*, **89**, 307–314.
12. Seymour, L.W., Miyamoto, Y., Maeda, H., Brereton, M., Strohalm, J., Ulbrich, K., and Duncan, R. (1995) Influence of molecular weight on passive tumour accumulation of a soluble macromolecular durg carrier. *Eur. J. Cancer*, **31**, 766–770.
13. Maeda, H., Wu, J., Sawa, T., Matsumura, Y., and Hori, K. (2000) Tumor vascular permeability and the EPR effect in macromolecular therapeutics. *J. Control. Release*, **65**, 271–284.
14. Maeda, H. (1991) SMANCS and polymer-conjugated macromolecular drugs: advantages in cancer chemotherapy. *Adv. Drug Deliv. Rev.*, **6**, 181–202.
15. Maeda, H., Sawa, T., and Konno, T. (2001) Mechanism of tumor-targeted delivery of macromolecular drugs, including the EPR effect in solid tumor and clinical overview of the prototype polymeric drug SMANCS. *J. Control. Release*, **74**, 47–61.
16. Fang, J., Nakamura, H., and Maeda, H. (2010) EPR effect: unique features of tumor blood vessels for drug delivery, factors involved, and limitation and augmentation of the effect. *Adv. Drug Deliv. Rev.*, **63**, 136–151.
17. Maeda, H. (2001) The enhanced permeability and retention (EPR) effect in tumor vasculature: the key role of tumor-selective macromolecular drug targeting, *Adv. Enzyme Regul.*, **41**, 189–207.
18. Maeda, H. (2010) Tumor-selective delivery of macromolecular drugs via the EPR effect: background and future prospects. *Bioconjug. Chem.*, **21**, 797–802.
19. Maeda, H., Noguchi, Y., Sato, K., and Akaike, T. (1994) Enhanced vascular permeability in solid tumor is mediated by nitric oxide and inhibited by both new nitric oxide scavenger and nitric oxide synthase inhibitor. *Jpn. J. Cancer Res.*, **85**, 331–334.
20. Wu, J., Akaike, T., and Maeda, H. (1998) Modulation of enhanced vascular permeability in tumors by a bradykinin antagonist, a cyclooxygenase inhibitor, and a nitric oxide scavenger. *Cancer Res.*, **58**, 159–165.
21. Maeda, H., Matsumura, Y., and Kato, H. (1988) Purification and identification of [hydroxyprolyl^3]bradykinin in ascitic fluid from a patient with gastric cancer. *J. Biol. Chem.*, **263**, 16051–16054.
22. Konerding, M.A., Miodonski, A.J., and Lametschwandtner, A. (1995) Microvascular corrosion casting in the study of tumor vascularity: a review. *Scanning Microsc.*, **9**, 1233–1244.
23. Kratz, F., Müller, I.A., Ryppa, C., and Warnecke, A. (2008) Prodrug strategies in anticancer chemotherapy. *Chem. Med. Chem.*, **3**, 20–53.
24. Iwai, K., Maeda, H., and Konno, T. (1984) Use of oily contrast medium for selective drug targeting to tumor: enhanced therapeutic effect and X-ray image. *Cancer Res.*, **44**, 2115–2121.
25. Konno, T., Maeda, H., Iwai, K., Maki, S., Tashiro, S., Uchida, M., and Miyauchi, Y. (1984) Selective targeting of anticancer drug and simultaneous image enhancement in solid tumors by arterially administered lipid contrast medium. *Cancer*, **54**, 2367–2374.
26. Maki, S., Konno, T., and Maeda, H. (1985) Image enhancement in computerized tomography for sensitive diagnosis of liver cancer and semiquantitation of tumor selective drug targeting with oily contrast medium. *Cancer*, **56**, 751–757.
27. Nagamitsu, A., Greish, K., and Maeda, H. (2009) Elevating blood pressure as a strategy to increase tumor targeted delivery of macromolecular drug SMANCS: cases of advanced solid tumors. *Jpn. J. Clin. Oncol.*, **39**, 756–766.
28. Matsumoto, K., Yamamoto, T., Kamata, R., and Maeda, H. (1984) Pathogenesis of serratial infection: activation of the Hageman factor–prekallikrein cascade by serratial protease. *J. Biochem.*, **96**, 739–749.
29. Maeda, H., Wu, J., Okamoto, T., Maruo, K., and Akaike, T. (1999) Kallikrein–kinin in infection and cancer. *Immunopharmacology*, **43**, 115–128.
30. Maeda, H. (2002) in *The Encyclopedia of Molecular Medicine*, vol. 4 (ed. T.E. Creighton), John Wiley & Sons, Inc., New York, pp. 2663–2668.

31. Maruo, K., Akaike, T., Inada, Y., Ohkubo, I., Ono, T., and Maeda, H. (1993) EPR effect of microbial and mita protease on low and high molecular weight kininogen. *J. Biol. Chem.*, **268**, 17711–17715.
32. Matsumura, Y., Kimura, M., Yamamoto, T., and Maeda, H. (1988) Involvement of the kinin-generating cascade and enhanced vascular permeability in tumor tissue. *Jpn. J. Cancer Res.*, **79**, 1327–1334.
33. Wu, J., Akaike, T., Hayashida, K., Okamoto, T., Okuyama, A., and Maeda, H. (2001) Enhanced vascular permeability in solid tumor involving peroxynitrite and matrix metalloproteinase. *Jpn. J. Cancer Res.*, **92**, 439–451.
34. Sawa, T., Akaike, T., and Maeda, H. (2000) Tyrosine nitration by peroxynitrite formed from nitric oxide and superoxide generated by xanthine oxidase. *J. Biol. Chem.*, **275**, 32467–32474.
35. Akaike, T., Okamoto, S., Sawa, T., Yoshitake, J., Tamura, F., Ichimori, K., Miyazaki, K., Sasamoto, K., and Maeda, H. (2003) 8-Nitroguanosine formation in viral pneumonia and its implication for pathogenesis. *Proc. Natl. Acad. Sci. USA*, **100**, 685–690.
36. Maeda, H., Sawa, T., Yubisui, T., and Akaike, T. (1999) Free radical generation from heterocyclic amines by cytochrome b_5 reductase in the presence of NADH. *Cancer Lett.*, **143**, 117–121.
37. Sawa, T., Akaike, T., Ichimori, K., Akuta, T., Kaneko, K., Nakamura, H., Stuehr, D.J., and Maeda, H. (2003) Superoxide generation mediate by 8-nitroguanosine, a highly redox active nucleic acid derivative. *Biochem. Biophys. Res. Commun.*, **311**, 300–306.
38. Daruwalla, J., Nikfarjam, M., Greish, K., Malcontenti-WilsonI, C., Muralidharan, V., Christophe, C., and Maeda, H. (2010) *In vitro* and *in vivo* evaluation of tumor targeting SMA–pirarubicin micelles: survival improvement and inhibition of liver metastases. *Cancer Sci.*, **101**, 1866–1874.
39. Suzuki, M., Hori, H., Abe, I., Saito, S., and Sato, H. (1984) Functional characterization of the microcirculation in tumors. *Cancer Metastasis Rev.*, **3**, 115–126.
40. Suzuki, M., Hori, K., Abe, I., Saito, S., and Sato, H. (1981) A new approach to cancer chemotherapy: selective enhancement of tumor blood flow with angiotensin II. *J. Natl. Cancer Inst.*, **67**, 663–669.
41. Li, C.J., Miyamoto, Y., Kojima, Y., and Maeda, H. (1993) Augmentation of tumour delivery of macromolecular drugs with reduced bone marrow delivery by elevating blood pressure. *Br. J. Cancer*, **67**, 975–980.
42. Seki, T., Fang, J., and Maeda, H. (2009) Enhanced delivery of macromolecular antitumor drugs to tumors by nitroglycerin application. *Cancer Sci.*, **100**, 2426–2430.
43. Maeda, H. (2010) Nitroglycerin enhances vascular blood flow and drug delivery in hypoxic tumor tissues: analogy between angina pectoris and solid tumors and enhancement of the EPR effect. *J. Control. Release*, **142**, 296–298.
44. Yasuda, H., Nakayama, K., Watanabe, M., Suzuki, S., Fuji, H., Okinaga, S., Kanda, A., Zayasu, K., Sasaki, T., Asada, M., Suzuki, T., Yoshida, M., Yamada, S., Inoue, D., Kaneta, T., Kondo, T., Takai, Y., Sasaki, H., Yanagihara, K., and Yamaya M. (2006) Nitroglycerin treatment may enhance chemosensitivity to docetaxel and carboplatin in patients with lung adenocarcinoma. *Clin. Cancer Res.*, **12**, 6748–6757.
45. Yasuda, H., Yanagihara, K., Nakayama, Mio, T., Sasaki, T., Asada, M., Yamaya, M., and Fukushima, M. (2010) in *Nitric Oxide and Cancer* (ed. B. Bonavida), Springer, New York, pp. 419–442.
46. Siemens, D.R., Heaton, J., Adams, M., Kawakami, J., and Graham, C. (2009) Phase II study of nitric oxide donor for men with increasing prostate-specific antigen level after surgery or radiotherapy for prostate cancer. *Urology*, **74**, 878–883.
47. Noguchi, A., Takahashi, T., Yamaguchi, T., Kitamura, K., Noguchi, A., Tsurumi, H., Takashina, K., and

Maeda H. (1992) Enhanced tumor localization of monoclonal antibody by treatment with kininase II inhibitor and angiotensin II. *Jpn. J. Cancer Res.*, **83**, 240–243.

48. Tanaka, S., Akaike, T., Wu, J., Fang, J., Sawa, T., Ogawa, M., Beppu, T., and Maeda, H. (2003) Modulation of tumor-selective vascular blood flow and extravasation by the stable prostaglandin I_2 analogue beraprost sodium. *J. Drug Target.*, **11**, 45–52.

49. Fang, J., Qin, H., Nakamura, H., Tsukigawa, K., and Maeda, H. (2011) Carbon monoxide, generated by heme oxygenase-1, mediates the enhanced permeability and retention (EPR) effect of solid tumor. (Submitted)

50. Doi, K., Akaike, T., Fujii, S., Horie, H., Noguchi, Y., Fujii, S., Beppu, T., Ogawa, M., and Maeda, H. (1999) Induction of haem oxygenase-1 by nitric oxide and ischaemia in experimental solid tumours and implications for tumour growth. *Br. J. Cancer*, **80**, 1945–1954.

51. Fang, J., Sawa, T., Akaike, T., and Maeda, H. (2002) Tumor-targeted delivery of polyethylene glycol-conjugated D-amino acid oxidase for antitumor therapy via enzymatic generation of hydrogen peroxide. *Cancer Res.*, **62**, 3138–3143.

52. Fang, J., Sawa, T., Akaike, T., Akuta, T., Greish, K., Hamada, A., and Maeda, H. (2003) *In vivo*, antitumor activity of pegylated zinc protoporphyrin: targeted inhibition of heme oxygenase in solid tumor. *Cancer Res.*, **63**, 3567–3574.

53. Hatakeyama, H., Akita, H., and Harashima, H. (2011) A multifunctional envelope type nano device (MEND) for drug and gene delivery to tumors based on the EPR effect: a strategy for overcoming the PEG dilemma. *Adv. Drug. Deliv. Rev.*, **63**, 152–160.

54. Law, B. and Tung, C.H. (2009) Proteolysis: a biological process adapted in drug delivery, therapy, and imaging. *Bioconjug. Chem.*, **20**, 1683–1695.

55. Tsukigawa, K., Nakamura, H., Fang, J., and Maeda, H. (2010) Annual Meeting of Controlled Release Society, Portland, OR, abstract 24.

56. Nakamura, H., Fang, J., Bharate, G., Tsukigawa, K., and Maeda, H. (2011) Intracellular uptake and behaviour of two types zinc protoporphyrin (ZnPP) micelles, SMA-ZnPP and PEG-ZnPP as anticancer agents; Unique intracellular disintegration of SMA micelles. *J. Control. Release*, in press.

57. Ishida, T., Ichihara, M., Wang, X.Y., Yamamoto, K., Kimura, J., Majima, E., and Kiwada, H. (2006) Injection of PEGylated liposomes in rats elicits PEG-specific IgM, which is responsible for rapid elimination of a second dose of PEGylated liposomes. *J. Control. Release*, **112**, 15–25.

4
Pharmacokinetics of Immunoglobulin G and Serum Albumin: Impact of the Neonatal Fc Receptor on Drug Design

Jan Terje Andersen and Inger Sandlie

4.1
Introduction

The neonatal Fc receptor (FcRn) rescues antibodies of the immunoglobulin G (IgG) class as well as serum albumin (SA) from intracellular degradation via an efficient cellular recycling pathway. The unique mechanism has evolved to secure both ligands a long half-life of approximately 3 weeks and a broad biodistribution. IgG and SA are the two most abundant proteins in blood. FcRn also directs the transport of IgG across mucosal epithelial barriers as well as the placenta, and plays a pivotal role in the biodistribution of IgG and albumin at several other body sites. In light of the expanding use of IgG, IgG Fc (fragment crystallizable), and SA fusions in therapy, the impact of FcRn in the regulation of their pharmacokinetics represents an area of intense interest.

The blood contains a plethora of soluble proteins that are distributed with the bloodstream throughout the body. In this bulk of proteins, IgG and SA dominate; they constitute impressively 80–90% of the total protein pool, and the concentrations are 12 and 40 mg/ml, respectively, in both mouse and man. SA is produced exclusively by the hepatocytes of the liver. It is crucial in maintaining the osmotic blood pressure, and it serves as a multitransporter for several insoluble and hydrophobic endogenous molecules, such as ions, bilirubin, fatty acids, and amino acids [1]. In addition, SA has been found to bind a range of pharmacological drugs such as warfarin and acetylsalicylic acid [1]. SA binds these ligands in distinct binding pockets localized to three structurally related domains, denoted DI, DII, and DIII, which form a heart-shaped structure as revealed by X-ray crystallography [2–4]. The structure of human SA (HSA) is shown in Figure 4.1a. Each domain is stabilized by a complex network of 12 cysteine residues that form six disulfide bridges. DI has one additional free cysteine residue (C34), partially exposed on the surface.

Five classes of antibodies exist: IgA, IgD, IgE, IgG, and IgM. They all have a similar basic structure built up of two identical heavy chains and two identical light chains, each of which are folded into globular Ig domains. The heavy chains are connected via disulfide bridges in the so-called hinge region, while each light chain

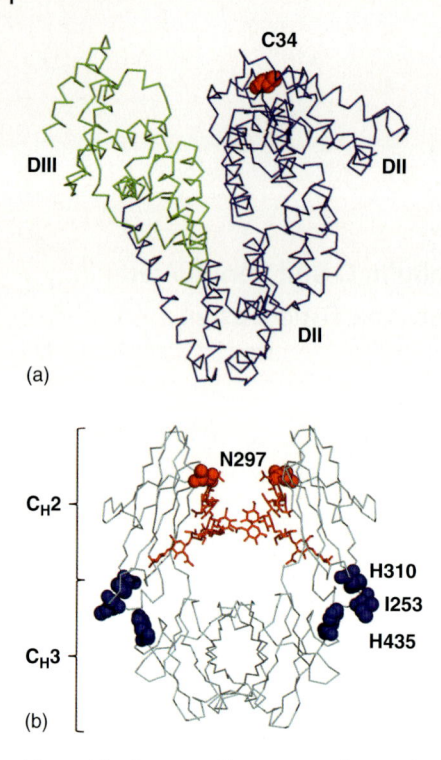

Figure 4.1 Structure illustrations of SA and IgG Fc. (a) Crystal structure of HSA with three subdomains highlighted: DI and DII in dark blue, and DIII in green. The free unpaired C34 in DI is highlighted using red spheres. (b) Crystal structure of human IgG1 Fc. The structures of the two Fc heavy chains are shown in cyan, while the biantennary glycan attached to N297 localized within the C_H2 domain is highlighted in red. The key residues involved in binding to FcRn, I253, H310, and H435, are highlighted using dark blue spheres. The figures were designed using PyMOL (www.pymol.org) with the crystallographic data of HSA and human IgG1 Fc [5, 6].

is covalently coupled to a heavy chain. These four chains are arranged to form two Fab (fragment of antigen binding) arms that are linked to the Fc region. Although they share an overall structural similarity, each antibody class has distinct binding properties toward both soluble molecules and cell-bound receptors, and thus they possess different effector functions in the body at different body sites [7, 8].

IgG is the main antibody class found in the blood. It protects against invading bacteria and viruses. Elimination of such harmful substances depends on its ability to act as an adaptor molecule that links recognition of the foreign substance with appropriate effector functions. Specific recognition of the antigen target is mediated through the variable regions of the two Fab arms while the constant Ig domains of the Fc bind various effector molecules such as Fcγ receptors and complement [7–10]. IgG exists as four subclasses in both humans (IgG1, IgG2, IgG3, and IgG4) and mice (IgG1, IgG2a, IgG2b, and IgG3), in which the heavy chain of each subclass is the product of a unique constant region with differences in amino acid composition that for the most part are just a few amino acids. However, the small variations in sequences create a spectrum of selective and specific binding to the classical Fcγ receptors as recently described by Bruhns et al. [9]. The structural architecture of human IgG1 Fc is shown in Figure 4.1b.

SA and IgG share an unusually long serum half-life of 19–23 days compared to only hours to a few days for other circulating proteins [1, 11, 12]. This unique feature is dependent on their molecular sizes, which are above the renal clearance threshold, as well as their binding specificity for FcRn. In this chapter, we describe our understanding of FcRn biology and the advantages of considering FcRn for drug delivery. We discuss how advanced IgG Fc engineering may improve IgG-based drugs for treatment of various diseases. In light of the finding that FcRn also rescues SA from degradation, we discuss recent developments of SA fused and targeted drugs.

4.2 Discovery of FcRn

FcRn was originally identified as a cell-bound receptor found in the intestinal epithelia of neonatal rats where it was shown to mediate transcellular transport of IgG taken up from mother's milk during the suckling period [13–15]. Thus, the neonatal rodents acquire circulating IgG from their mother via FcRn. The receptor-specific transport mechanism was initially postulated by F.W. Rogers Brambell (1901–1970) long before the receptor was actually identified and cloned [16, 17]. He first discovered that IgG was actively transported from mother to fetus in rabbits via the yolk sac and that the transfer was solely dependent on the Fc part of IgG. Based on this, Brambell described a model with a yet unidentified receptor that could bind specifically to the IgG Fc part in the acidic milieu on the apical side of the small intestine that would subsequently transcytose IgG across the cells for release at the basolateral side at neutral pH. Early cellular assays showed that the receptor binds IgG in a strictly pH-dependent fashion – binding at acidic pH and release or negligible binding at physiological pH [14, 15, 18, 19].

The high concentration of IgG in blood is more or less constant at 12 mg/ml. In 1963, Fahey and Robinson published a study that conclusively showed that the catabolism of IgG increased dramatically when high doses of endogenous IgG or the IgG-derived Fc was injected into mice [20]. Importantly, excess amounts of IgA, IgM, or SA did not affect the clearance of IgG. Based on these findings, Brambell extended his model to include both maternofetal transport and regulation of systemic IgG levels [21]. He postulated a single receptor found within cells that binds the Fc part of IgG and rescues it from intracellular degradation by recycling of bound IgG to the cell surface for release back into the bloodstream.

Cellular studies reported during the 1980s identified such a receptor in the intestinal epithelium of the neonatal rat as a heterodimeric molecule consisting of two chains of 12 and 40–45 kDa, respectively [22, 23]. In 1989, the genes encoding rat FcRn were cloned and surprisingly it shown that the one of the subunits was related to the family of major histocompatibility complex (MHC) class I heavy chains, while the small 12-kDa chain was identical to the common β_2-microglobulin (β_2m) [13]. This discovery inspired its name – the "FcRn."

While the uptake of IgG from the gut of neonatal rats quickly ceases 18–21 days postbirth as a function of downregulation of FcRn, the expression of the receptor has been found to be expressed throughout adult life in the vascular endothelium [14, 24, 25] – a finding that explains its role in prolongation of IgG half-life [24, 26, 27]. Furthermore, the expression of FcRn is remarkably wide, as it has been identified in multiple species [28–33], as well as in several organs and tissues, including cells of the blood–brain barrier (BBB) [34], placenta [35, 36], liver [37, 38], kidneys [39–41], and ocular tissues [42, 43]. An understanding of the roles of FcRn at the different tissue sites is beginning to emerge, as discussed below.

In contrast to the well-characterized interaction between FcRn and IgG, the relationship between FcRn and SA was not discovered until Anderson et al. showed that FcRn binds SA in a pH-dependent manner similar to the IgG–FcRn interaction [44, 45]. Until then, the prolonged half-life of SA had lacked a biological explanation. The interaction was discovered by chance when bovine SA was eluted together with a soluble recombinant form of human FcRn from an IgG-coupled affinity column [44]. This important finding revived a hypothesis postulated by Shultze and Heremans during the 1960s where they proposed that a single cell-bound receptor regulates the half-life of SA [46], similar to the receptor–IgG model proposed by Brambell [21].

4.3
FcRn Structure

The identification and cloning of the rat FcRn heavy chain revealed that it shares a sequence similarity of approximately 20–40% with the family of MHC class I molecules, and both MHC class I and FcRn consist of a transmembrane heavy chain with a short cytoplasmic signaling region [13, 23]. This was followed by reports of the high-resolution X-ray crystallographic structures of soluble recombinant rat FcRn with and without bound rat IgG2a Fc and later the crystal structure of human FcRn [47–49]. The structures show the characteristic MHC class I fold comprising a unique FcRn heavy chain in noncovalent association with the common β_2m. The extracellular part of the heavy chain consists of the N-terminal $\alpha 1 - \alpha 2$ subdomains, which form eight antiparallel β-pleated strands topped by two long α-helices, followed by the membrane proximal $\alpha 3$ domain. The β_2m chain is tightly bound via residues located under the $\alpha 1 - \alpha 2$ platform in addition to the $\alpha 3$ domain.

A hallmark of the FcRn structure is that the peptide-binding groove that is fundamental for MHC class I presentation of antigenic peptides is occluded in the FcRn fold due to a nonconserved proline residue introducing a kink in the structure. Thus, while MHC class I molecules present peptide antigens to CD8$^+$ T-cells, FcRn does not, and instead has evolved to bind both IgG and SA. Illustrations of the cocrystal structure of rat FcRn in complex with rat Fc as well as the structure of human FcRn are shown in Figure 4.2a and b.

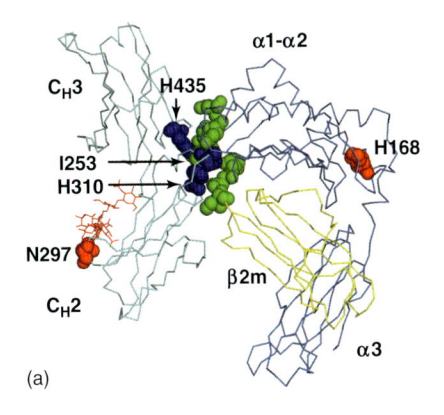

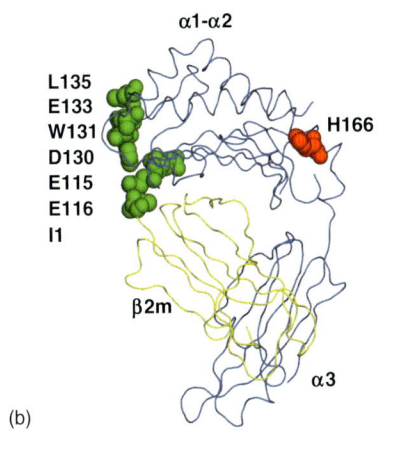

Figure 4.2 Structural illustrations of FcRn in complex with Fc. (a) Structure of rat FcRn in complex with rat IgG2a Fc. The three domains of the heavy chain (α1, α2, and α3) are shown in blue while β$_2$m is shown in yellow. Half of the IgG Fc region (C$_H$2–C$_H$3) is shown in cyan and Fc amino acid residues involved in binding (I253, H310, and H435) with arrows and dark blue spheres, while the corresponding residues on the FcRn heavy chain (E117, E118, E132, W133, E135, and D137) and β$_2$m (I1) are highlighted with green spheres. The biantennary glycan attached to N297 localized within the C$_H$2 domain is highlighted in red. H168 is indicated using red spheres. (b) Structure of human FcRn with the heavy chain in blue and β$_2$m in yellow. The amino acids essential for IgG binding (E115, E116, D130, W131, E133, and L135) and β$_2$m (I1) are shown in green spheres, while H166 is indicated using red spheres. A loop within the α1 domain, near H166, is disordered in the human FcRn structure while it is ordered in the rat FcRn structure. The figures were designed using PyMOL (www.pymol.org) with the crystallographic data of the cocrystal and human FcRn [47, 49].

4.4
FcRn–Ligand Interactions

Our molecular understanding of the FcRn–IgG interaction has been learned from studies using site-directed mutagenesis of monoclonal IgG and IgG Fc derived fragments. Initially, Ward et al. demonstrated that the residues I253, H310, and H435 affected pH-dependent binding to FcRn using human and mouse IgGs [50–52]. Single point mutations at each of these residues reduced the half-life extensively in wild-type mice, exemplified by an almost 9-fold drop in half-life (217.8 versus 26.4 h) when H435 of human IgG1 was mutated to alanine [53]. The cocrystal structure of rat FcRn with rat IgG2a Fc reveals that I253, H310, and H435 are situated at the center of the interaction interface [47]. These residues are highly conserved across species and localized to the Fc elbow region (highlighted in Figure 4.1b). The involvement of conserved histidine residues gives an explanation for the strict pH dependence of the interaction since the isoelectric point of histidine is 6.0. The amino acid is positively charge at pH 6.0 and can interact with negatively charged amino acids on the FcRn heavy chain, as illustrated in Figure 4.2a and b.

The relatively newly discovered FcRn–SA interaction is less well characterized at the molecular level [44, 45], but we have shown that a histidine residue partially exposed on the surface of the heavy chain is involved in binding to SA since mutation of H166 (human) and H168 (mouse) in FcRn to alanines eliminated binding to HSA and mouse SA (MSA) [54, 55]. The histidine is situated within the α2-domain of the heavy chain opposite the major IgG-binding site (Figure 4.2a and b). Thus, IgG and SA may bind simultaneously to FcRn at two distinct and separate binding sites.

Regarding the binding site on SA, no amino acid residues have so far been pointed out, but truncation of the C-terminal DIII of SA has been demonstrated to eliminate binding while DIII alone was capable of binding FcRn in a pH-dependent manner [45, 56]. These data are in agreement with the low serum levels and absence of FcRn binding of a naturally existing HSA polymorphic variant (named Bartin) that lacks almost the entire DIII [56, 57].

4.5
FcRn as a Multiplayer with Therapeutic Utilities

4.5.1
Directional Placental Transport

In parallel with the fact that FcRn was found in the yolk sac in rabbits and mice [17, 58, 59], the human form of FcRn was first cloned from the syncytiotrophoblasts of the placenta where it directs transport of IgG from the maternal circulation to the fetal capillaries of the placental villi [35, 36, 60]. Thus, placentally expressed FcRn acts as an prenatal transporter of IgG that provides the fetus with large amounts of IgG derived from the mother and which serve as a first line of humoral immune defense. Due to ethical considerations, study of FcRn in placental transport has been restricted to *ex vivo* transplacental models [61, 62]. Here, human IgG1 is transported efficiently across placental cotyledones, while a mutant variant (H435A) is not.

This receptor-specific route of transport may have therapeutic benefits in *in utero* therapy. In this regard, IgG molecules that show improved transplacental transport efficiencies are attractive candidates, such as an engineered mutant human IgG1 (H433K/N434F) with considerably increased affinity for FcRn that shows improved transport from the maternal to the fetal compartment relative to wild-type IgG1 [62]. Furthermore, the transport route has been utilized and shown to be valid for Fc fusion molecule delivery. Using a mouse model for a lysosomal storage disease (mucopolysaccharidosis), an Fc fusion protein consisting of the enzyme β-glucuronidase showed efficient prenatal transfer [63]. The pathway may furthermore be blocked in treatment of fetal neonatal immune thrombocytopenia (FNIT) – a severe bleeding disorder in which pathogenic IgGs from the mother cross the placenta for subsequent destruction of fetal/neonatal platelets. In a recent mouse model, development of FNIT depends on FcRn-mediated transplacental transport of pathogenic IgGs [64]. Consequently, FNIT may be treated using FcRn blockers that inhibit IgG transplacental transport. Here, a recently developed synthetic 26-amino-acid peptide (SYN1436) agonist that targets the IgG-binding site on FcRn may be useful [65].

Whether SA is cotransported with IgG across placenta is not fully understood. Brambell reported that SA was transported to the fetus in his rabbit model [66], while Gitlin et al. showed in a human study that IgG was more rapidly transported to the fetus than SA, as no more than 5% of a given SA was found in the infant child [67]. However, conflicting evidence exists on the contribution from other Fcγ receptors found to be expressed in the different placenta cell layers [68–70]. Since Fcγ receptors do not bind SA, it may indicate that SA is prevented from efficient transplacental passage. Two recent reports conclude that Fcγ receptor IIb expressed by the mouse yolk sac does not contribute to IgG transfer [71], while FcRn is required [59].

4.5.2
FcRn at Mucosal Surfaces

In contrast to the restricted expression of FcRn in the neonatal intestine of rats, the human ortholog of FcRn is expressed in the mucosal intestine throughout life and shown to mediate bidirectional transport of IgG [72–75]. Blumberg et al. have shown that FcRn acts in mucosal immunity by binding immune complexes consisting of IgG that are efficiently taken up from the lumen of the intestine and delivered to the lamina propria for induction of T-cell responses [75]. This transport route may be utilized to deliver therapeutic IgGs (Section 4.6).

An interesting question is whether SA is cotransported together with IgG. To our knowledge this has not been addressed. However, there is evidence that SA is present in the small intestine, feces, and saliva in mice [76], and increased secretion of both IgG and SA is demonstrated in polymeric Ig receptor (pIgR)-deficient mice. The authors speculate that it may be due to a significant bulk leakage of serum proteins, but another possibility is that the lack of an IgA/IgM–pIgR pathway leads to upregulation of FcRn expression, and thereby increased selective transport of IgG and SA. This also fits well with the finding that pIgR-deficient mice have increased total systemic IgG and SA levels [76]. Whether SA-based drugs can be administered via the mucosal delivery route is still to be explored.

4.5.3
Systemic FcRn-Mediated Recycling

Although Brambell proposed that the cellular pathways involved in the transfer of IgG from mother to fetus and regulating IgG serum levels might be related, evidence to support this assumption was lacking until Ward *et al.* and others demonstrated that mice deficient in β_2m showed a dramatic increase in clearance of IgG and Fc fragments [24, 26, 27]. This phenomenon was again dependent on I253, H310, and H435. These findings were followed by a pioneering study from the Ward lab where an engineered Fc fragment (T252L/T254S/T256F) that bound FcRn with increased affinity at pH 6.0, and with retained low affinity at physiological pH, showed increased *in vivo* half-life in mice [77]. This proof of concept has inspired the design of a new class of engineered IgG molecules with altered pharmacokinetics, as discussed in Section 4.6.

Using mice lacking expression of the FcRn heavy chain, Anderson *et al.* pinpointed the fundamental role of FcRn in regulation of both IgG and SA half-life [44, 78]. The impact of the receptor is astonishing as the serum levels of IgG and SA are 70–80 and 60% lower, respectively, in deficient mice compared with wild-type mice [44, 78]. In this context, it is of interest to define the major body sites involved in FcRn-mediated protection. Using an engineered mouse strain in which FcRn can be conditionally deleted in endothelial and hematopoietic cells, it was conclusively shown that these cells are primary sites for FcRn-mediated rescue, as the serum levels of IgG and SA were approximately 4- and 2-fold lower, respectively, while the half-life of human IgG1 decreased 21-fold [53]. In line with this are studies that show the involvement of bone marrow-derived cells in the regulation of IgG serum levels [79, 80].

A human example that demonstrates the importance of FcRn is a group of patients with a deficiency in β_2m expression that have abnormally low levels of IgG and SA [81]. The underlying cellular model of how FcRn mediates recycling of IgG and SA is schematically illustrated in Figure 4.3. Within endothelial and hematopoietic cells, FcRn is predominantly localized to intracellular acidic compartments. The cells are bathed in fluid that contains large amounts of IgG and SA that are continuously taken up by fluid-phase endocytosis. The ligands bind FcRn in intracellular vesicles as a function of the low pH that triggers protonation of the histidine residues. Subsequently, the ternary IgG–FcRn–SA complex is recycled to the cell surface membrane where exposure to the physiological pH of the bloodstream triggers release of IgG and SA back into the circulation in a so-called "kiss-and-run" exocytic manner. Ligands that escape binding to the receptor will end up in lysosomal compartments and are destined for proteolytic degradation. The intracellular trafficking of FcRn is under intense investigation using live-cell fluorescence imaging and electron tomography on tissue sections (recently reviewed by Ward and Ober [82]), and is not further discussed here.

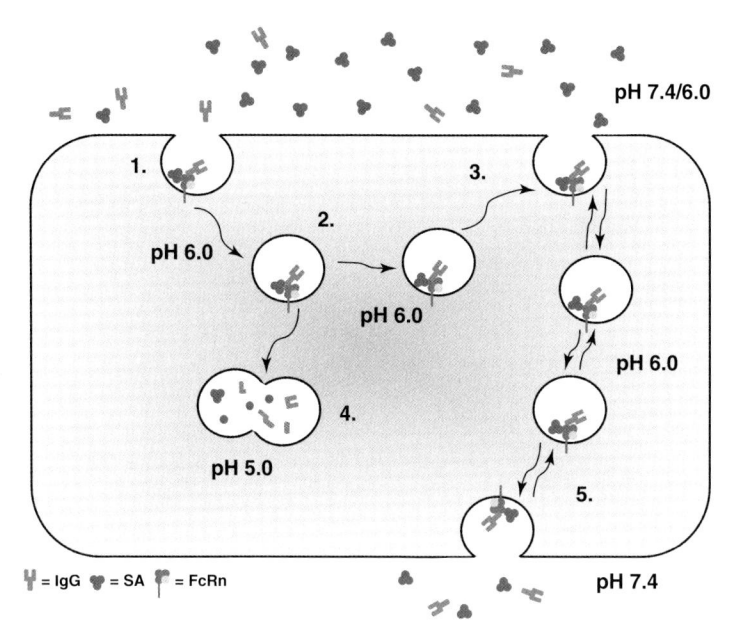

Figure 4.3 Schematic illustration of the FcRn-mediated transport pathways [1]. Large amounts of circulating IgG and SA are continuously taken up by fluid-phase pinocytosis and enter early endosomal compartments where FcRn predominantly resides [2]. The acidified milieu therein facilitates binding of IgG and SA to FcRn [3]. The complex is then recycled to the cell surface where progressive exposure to weaker pH triggers release of IgG and SA out of the cell [4]. IgG and SA that do not bind FcRn are destined for lysosomal compartments and subsequent degradation [7]. FcRn may also transport the ligands bidirectionally across the cellular layer.

4.5.4
Role of FcRn in Antigen Presentation

Hematopoietic cells, including monocytes, macrophages, and dendritic cells, express FcRn and contribute significantly to the increased half-life of IgG by recycling of monomeric IgG. IgG-containing immune complexes, on the other hand, are degraded [79, 83]. Furthermore, recent data demonstrate that FcRn increases antigen presentation by directing IgG-containing immune complexes to lysosomal degradation for loading of antigenic peptides onto MHC class II molecules and subsequent induction of T-cell proliferation [79]. Similarly, FcRn in antigen-presenting cells has been shown to contribute to IgG-mediated pathogenesis of colitis in mice [84] and FcRn expressed by neutrophils has a role in enhancement of IgG-mediated phagocytosis of bacteria [85]. Whether or not FcRn is expressed in B cells has been controversial, although new data point to restricted expression in splenic B cells [53, 86]; however, so far, no function of the receptor has been described at this particular site. One possibility could be that FcRn in these cells contributes to secretion of IgG as a function of pH-dependent binding of newly synthesized IgG.

4.5.5
FcRn at Immune-Privileged Sites

In the central nervous system, FcRn is expressed in cells found at the BBB where it might be involved in removal of IgG, as supported by several studies that show transport of IgG from the brain to the blood via FcRn [34, 87–89]. The pathway may be relevant in diseases where the brain is affected by inflammatory IgGs, as demonstrated in a mouse model of Alzheimer's disease where clearance of amyloid β peptide from the brain by IgG specific for amyloid plaque resulted in reduction of pathogenic symptoms [87]. In stark contrast is one report that claims the transport of IgG over BBB to be the same in both wild-type and FcRn-deficient mice [90]. Nevertheless, the presence of FcRn at this site should be further explored as it may guide the design of novel immunotherapeutic strategies to fight Alzheimer's disease or other diseases that affect the brain, such as multiple sclerosis.

Another immune-privileged site with FcRn expression is the eye, including the ocular tissues such as the cornea and retina [42, 43]. Here, evidence supports a role for FcRn in transport of intravitreally administered IgG over the blood–retina barrier for release of IgG into the bloodstream.

4.5.6
FcRn in the Kidneys

The kidneys filtrate an impressive 50 plasma volumes daily and waste products end up in the urine. Renal secretion is highly dependent on the molecular weight, as proteins smaller than approximately 60 kDa are secreted, while proteins larger than 60 kDa are retained. This so-called renal clearance threshold is a size-selective barrier that prevents secretion of IgG (150–170 kDa) and SA (66.7 kDa). However, FcRn expressed in kidney cells such as podocytes has been demonstrated to play a key role in removal of IgG from the glomerular basement membrane. Large amounts of IgG accumulate at this site in mice lacking FcRn, which leads to serum-induced nephritis [40]. Furthermore, a normal level of SA was restored in FcRn-deficient mice after FcRn-expressing kidney transplantation. On the other hand, transplanting an FcRn-deficient kidney into wild-type mice led to the development of hypoalbuminemia [41]. This again supports that the level of SA is controlled by FcRn and not only the selective barrier *per se*. In contrast, renal loss of IgG was minimal in FcRn-deficient mice, but increased in wild-type mice and FcRn-deficient mice transplanted with an FcRn-expressing kidney [41]. The results suggest that FcRn within kidneys handles SA and IgG differently. The issue is important as abnormal receptor function may contribute to kidney damage as observed in several diseases, such as systemic lupus erythematosus. Lastly, it is important in relation to biodistribution/tissue deposition of IgG- and SA-based drugs.

4.5.7
FcRn Expressed by the Liver

SA is synthesized by the liver to a remarkable of concentration 40–45 mg/ml. The SA level is maintained by the FcRn-mediated recycling mechanism that rescues as much SA from degradation as the liver produces [91]. Furthermore, FcRn is expressed by several types of liver cells, including rodent hepatocytes and hepatic sinusoidal cells [37, 38, 80]. One study suggests that FcRn in rat liver mediates serum-to-bile transport, while another study rejects this as serum-to-bile transport was unaffected by the presence of FcRn [37, 38]. Therefore, it is likely that FcRn in liver may be involved in the recycling of IgG. This is supported by several tumor studies using IgG-modified variants, since decreased FcRn binding affinity has been shown to correlate with increased rates of liver accumulation [92, 93].

The handling of SA by FcRn in liver cells has, to our knowledge, not been addressed. An interesting question is whether FcRn expressed by the hepatocytes contributes to the secretion of SA. *In vivo*, hypoalbuminemia, as observed in FcRn-deficient mice, induces increased liver synthesis of SA [91]. Thus, secretion is not dependent on FcRn.

4.6
Engineering IgG for Altered FcRn Binding and Pharmacokinetics

A number of very important scientific and technical breakthroughs have allowed the manufacture of large amounts of monoclonal IgGs. Much of the IgG engineering that followed focused on antigen specificity and affinity to manipulate targeting and blocking properties [94, 95]. However, a lot of interest has also been given the role of the constant Fc region and, in particular, the possibility to fine-tune binding to Fc-binding molecules such as the classical Fcγ receptors and complement [96, 97]. In light of the successful and increasing use of monoclonal IgGs in the clinic, the fundamental role of FcRn in half-life regulation has attracted interest, both in academia and biotech companies, with the aim to develop novel IgG molecules with altered FcRn binding properties to tailor their pharmacokinetic properties. Here, we first describe the impact of Fc fusions followed by how site-directed mutagenesis can be used to module the FcRn–IgG interaction and we then discuss how FcRn may be targeted for improved therapy.

4.6.1
IgG Fc Fusions

The Fc fusion technology has been used successfully to generate several products routinely used in treatment of disease [98, 99]. It is based on the fact that the Fc part of IgG comprises the unit necessary for prolongation of half-life. A major drawback attributed to several classes of promising drug candidates, including small bioactive peptides and proteins such as cytokines or modified protein scaffolds selected from combinatorial libraries, is that they all suffer from a very short *in vivo* half-life, ranging from minutes to hours [100–102]. This is due both to their small size below the renal clearance threshold (Section 4.5.6) and to their susceptibility to proteolytic degradation. An attractive approach to overcome the short half-life is to genetically fuse protein drugs to an IgG-derived Fc moiety.

The Fc fusions are a growing family of therapeutics of which several are approved by the US Food and Drug Administration (FDA). The first product was launched in 1998 when etanercept (Enbrel™), composed of the extracellular part of the tumor necrosis factor (TNF)-α receptor II fused to the Fc of human IgG1, was approved for treatment of rheumatoid arthritis [103]. Enbrel acts as an antagonist by preventing binding of TNF-α to cell-bound TNF receptors and thus inhibits proinflammatory activity. In addition, small bioactive peptides may be fused to Fc and such an Fc fusion of a small phage-display-selected thrombopoietin agonistic peptide, romiplostim (Nplate™), is FDA-approved for the treatment of thrombocytopenia [104]. Other Fc fusions approved are alefacept (Amevive™) and abatacept (Orenica™), while several others are in clinical trials [98, 105, 106].

Enhanced pharmacological efficacy of such drugs has been demonstrated to require FcRn [78]. However, Fc fragments have a shorter half-life than full-length IgG in mice [107] and Fc fusions show overall shorter half-life (4–13 days) compared with monoclonal IgGs (10–27 days) in humans, as reviewed [108]. One reason may be that the fusion causes steric hindrance. In addition, the design of the fusion as well as the nature of the fused drug may influence the FcRn binding capacity. For instance, monomeric erythropoietin fused to only one of the Fc arms binds more strongly to FcRn than a dimeric variant [109, 110]. This technology has recently been extended to treatment of hemophilia where a fusion consisting of a single molecule of Factor IX fused to Fc showed improved pharmacokinetics compared with nonfused Factor IX and the enhanced efficiency was dependent on FcRn [111]. Thus, fusion to Fc extends half-life and increases bioavailability, which allows for less-frequent administrations that may have a great impact on the cost of treatment.

4.6.2
Engineered IgG Variants

The knowledge that FcRn regulates IgG half-life together with structural and interaction analyses have guided the design of a rapidly growing class of modified IgGs with altered FcRn binding properties and pharmacokinetics. Both decreased and increased half-lives have obvious relevance for both diagnostics and therapeutic derived from IgG molecules, and such variants may be generated by introducing single-amino-acid substitutions in the constant Fc region.

To minimize tissue exposure, shortening the half-life of IgG molecules may be desirable when antibodies are conjugated to radionucleotides or toxins – so-called immunoconjugates, used to treat tumor metastasis or to visualize solid tumors by imaging technologies. A range of modified antibody fragments have been developed during the last decade with a spectrum of distinct clearance profiles, by mutating the residues I252, H310, and H435. This generates a hierarchy of FcRn binding affinities, as exemplified by Fc variants with binding affinities ranging from strongest to weakest: wild-type > H435R > H435Q > I253A > H310A > H310A/H435Q. They have corresponding long, intermediate, and short half-lifes when evaluated in wild-type mice [92, 112]. The impact on biodistribution and tumor targeting of such mutations has been demonstrated by Wu *et al.* using Fc variants fused to a scFv (single-chain variable fragment) with specificity for the tumor marker carcinoembryonic antigen (CEA). All show distinct clearance and tumor-targeting profiles [92, 93, 112], as shown in Figures 4.4 and 4.5. When conjugated to a radiometal, the fastest clearing double mutant (H301A/H435Q) was shown to exhibit the highest liver uptake, followed by H310A and I253A. Thus, hepatic accumulation of radiometal correlates with their rates of blood clearance, as I253A had lower liver activity, followed by H310A and H310A/H435Q [92]. As FcRn is expressed in hepatic cells and tissues (Section 4.5.7), the data support the notion that the receptor protects endogenous IgG and radioconjugated Fc fragments with FcRn binding activity while ignoring mutants with no or low binding activity.

During engineering to improve half-life, the binding kinetics should be fine-tuned in such a fashion that increased affinity is obtained at acidic pH only and not at

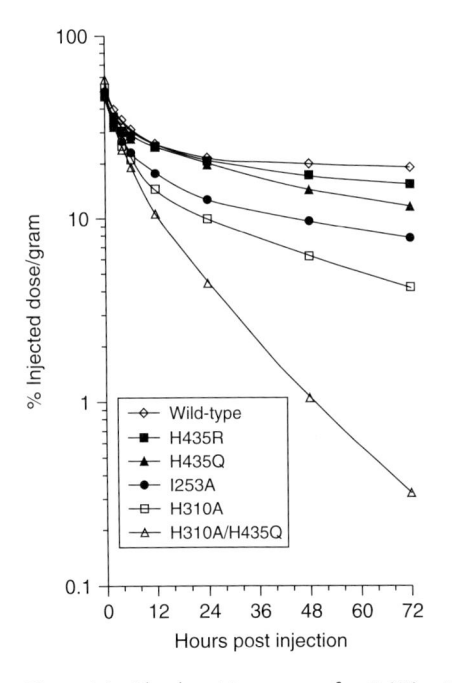

Figure 4.4 Blood activity curves of anti-CEA scFv–Fc variants in mice. Blood activity curves of radiolabeled scFv–Fc variants in BALB/c mice showing order of serum clearance from the slowest to the fastest clearing fragment: wild-type > H435R > H435Q > I253A > H310A > H310A/H435Q [112].

| 4 hours | 18 hours | 48 hours |

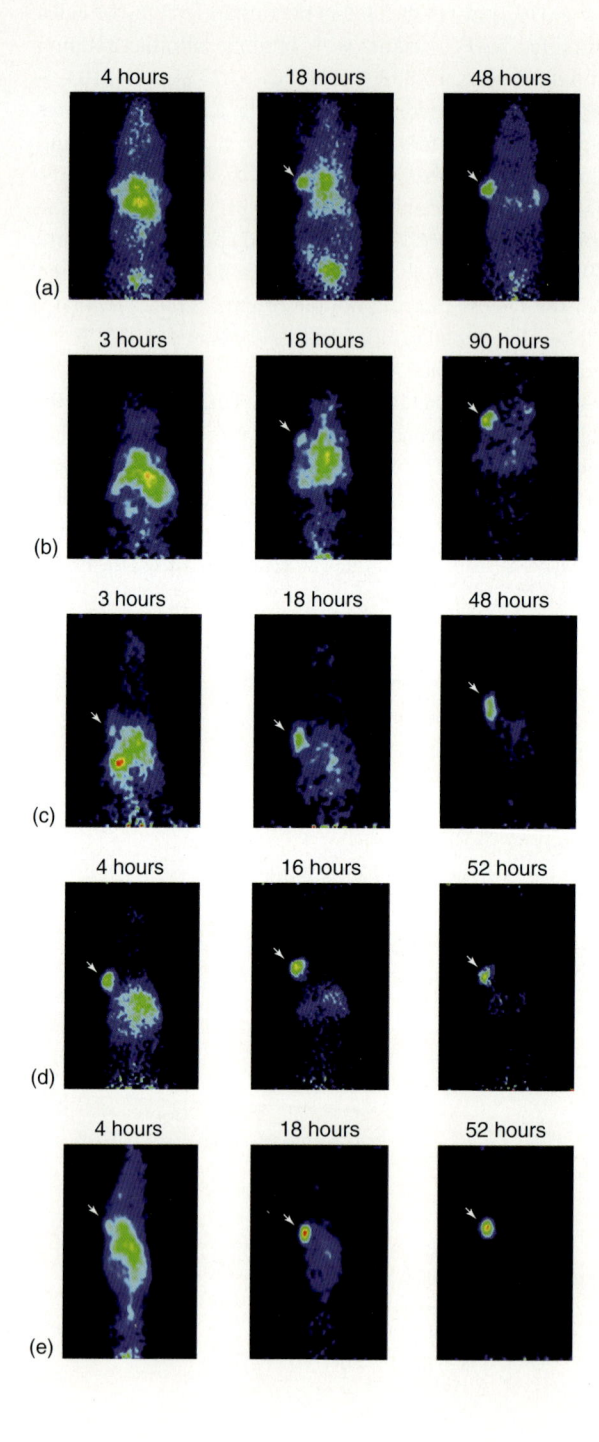

(a)

| 3 hours | 18 hours | 90 hours |

(b)

| 3 hours | 18 hours | 48 hours |

(c)

| 4 hours | 16 hours | 52 hours |

(d)

| 4 hours | 18 hours | 52 hours |

(e)

neutral pH. This was first shown for a phage-display-selected mouse-derived IgG Fc fragment (T252L/T254S/T256F) with increased affinity for FcRn at pH 6 and with retained low affinity at near neutral pH that gave an increased half-life in mice [77]. Recently, a number of engineered IgG molecules with an improved half-life in mice as well as primates have been described. One such variant with 10-fold increased binding at pH 6.0 and maintained pH-dependent binding to cynomolgus monkey and human FcRn is a humanized antirespiratory syncytial virus IgG1 (MEDI-524) containing three point mutations (M252Y/S254T/T256E) [113]. This mutant exhibited an almost 4-fold increase in half-life in cynomolgus monkeys compared with parental MEDI-524 [113]. Another example, a human IgG2 variant with specificity for hepatitis B virus (OST577) and two point mutations (T250Q/M428L) in the Fc region, decreased blood clearance by 2-fold in rhesus monkeys [114]. The same substitutions were also transferable to human IgG1 with a similar improvement in half-life [115]. In stark contrast is an anti-TNF-α human IgG1 variant with the same double mutation. This did not show an extended half-life in cynomolgus monkeys, even though it showed a 40-fold increase in binding to cynomolgus FcRn [116]. Neither have other anti-TNF-α human IgG1 mutants with improved FcRn affinity shown extended half-lifes [116, 117]. Such discrepancies between FcRn binding kinetics and *in vivo* half-lives could be attributed to target-mediated clearance ("antigen sink effect"), differences in techniques used to evaluate IgG–FcRn binding kinetics, or be related to the different species used. This latter issue is clearly illustrated for two engineered IgG1 mutants (N434A and T307A/E380A/N434A) with specificity for human epidermal growth factor receptor-2 (HER2) [118]. While both variants exhibited enhanced binding to human FcRn at pH 6.0, but not at pH 7.4, T307A/E380A/N434A showed binding at both pHs to mouse FcRn while N434A bound mouse FcRn in a pH-dependent manner [118]. In human FcRn transgenic mice they showed 2- to 3-fold improved half-lifes, while in mice they yielded minor half-life differences compared with wild-type IgG [118]. Similarly, a human IgG1 double mutant (H433K/N434F) with increased binding to human FcRn at pH 6.0, but not at pH 7.4, showed increased binding at both pHs to mouse FcRn [62]. These examples demonstrate that half-life data obtained in wild-type mice may not be conclusively transferred to a human setting. Such cross-species limitations will be further discussed in Section 4.8.

Figure 4.5 Coronal micro positron emission tomography (PET) images using anti-CEA scFv–Fc variants in athymic mice bearing LS174T xenografts. MicroPET imaging employed to evaluate the *in vivo* tumor-targeting ability of the anti-CEA scFv–Fc variants. Athymic mice carrying CEA-positive (LS174T colorectal carcinoma) and CEA-negative control (C6 glioma) tumors were injected with radiolabeled scFv–Fc variants. Whole-body microPET scans were obtained at 4, 18, and 48 h postinjection (wild-type); 3, 18, and 90 h (H435Q); 3, 18, and 48 h (I253A); 4, 16, and 52 h (H310A); and 4, 18, and 52 h (H310A/H435Q). Following the imaging studies, tumors were dissected, weighed, and counted in a γ-counter. (a) Wild-type 42.5% ID/g, 185 mg LS174T tumor weight at 48 h postinjection; (b) H435Q 10.6% ID/g, 64 mg at 123 h; (c) I253A 13.7% ID/g, 216 mg at 50 h; (d) H310A 10.6% ID/g, 174 mg at 53 h; and (e) H310A/H435Q 7.3% ID/g, 80 mg at 55 h. (Reproduced with permission from [112].)

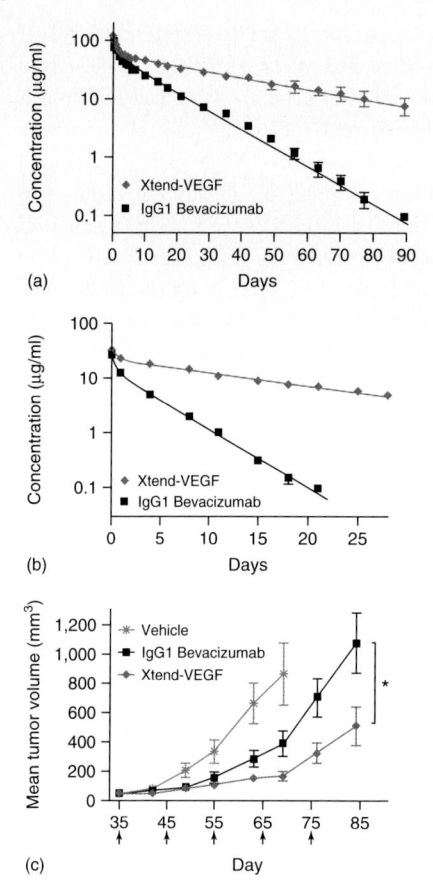

Figure 4.6 Increasing antibody affinity to FcRn extends half-life and improves *in vivo* tumor-killing activity. Blood activity curves expressed as changes in serum concentrations of the anti-VEGF IgG1 bevacizumab and the Xtend double mutant (M428L/ N434S) in (a) cynomolgus monkeys and (b) human FcRn transgenic mice. (c) Xenograft study in hFcRn/Rag1$^{-/-}$ mice comparing activity of anti-VEGF IgG1 bevacizumab and the Xtend variant of bevacizumab against established SKOV-3 tumors. Tumor volume is plotted against day after tumor cell injection. antibodies were dosed at 5 mg/kg every 10 days starting on day 35 (indicated by the arrows). n = 8 mice/group. *$P = 0.028$ at 84 days. (Reproduced with permission from [119].)

Recently, five engineered human IgG1 mutant variants with specificity for either the tumor marker vascular endothelial growth factor (VEGF) or epidermal growth factor receptor (EGFR) were shown to bind FcRn at pH 6.0 with improved affinity (3- to 20-fold) that was almost exclusively due to a slower dissociation rate [119]. When evaluated for their pharmacokinetics in human FcRn transgenic mice as well as cynomolgus monkeys, they all showed extended an half-life compare to their parental counterparts [119]. The lead variant, containing the double substitutions M428L and N434S (Xtend™), with 11-fold improvement in FcRn affinity at pH 6.0, showed a superior enhancement in half-life of 3.2-fold in cynomolgus monkeys, from 9.7 days to impressively 31.3 days – the largest improvement so far achieved by IgG–FcRn interaction engineering. Estimates suggest that this can be translated into a human half-life of more than 50 days. The blood clearance curves for an anti-VEGF human IgG1 antibody (bevacizumab) and the Xtend variant of bevacizumab in cynomolgus monkeys and human FcRn transgenic mice are shown in Figure 4.6a and b. Importantly, the improved half-life of the Xtend variants was shown to translate into a greater antitumor activity in tumor-baring mice xenografted with VEGF- or EGFR-positive tumors [119], as illustrated in Figure 4.6c. The mutations may be translated into the Fc fusion technology described above (Section 4.6.1). The impact of mutant-associated immunogenicity remains to be addressed, however. An overview of selected engineered IgG variants with altered half-lives is given in Table 4.1.

Table 4.1 Engineering IgG half-life.

Fab specificity	IgG subclass	IgG Fc mutations	Host species	$t_{1/2}$(h) mutant versus wild-type	Fold mutant versus wild-type	References
HULys10	human IgG1	H435A	wild-type mice	26.4 versus 169.8	0.2	[53]
	mouse Fc	T252L/T254S/T256F	wild-type mice	152.8 versus 92.8	1.6	[77]
MEDI-524	human IgG1	M252Y/S254T/T256E	cynomolgus monkeys	506.4 versus 146.4	3.5	[113]
OST577	human IgG2	T250Q/M428L	rhesus monkeys	652 versus 351	2.0	[114]
OST577	human IgG1	T250Q/M428L	rhesus monkeys	836 versus 336	2.5	[115]
TNF-α	human IgG1	T250Q/M428L	cynomolgus monkeys	112 versus 121	0.9	[116]
Hu4D5	human IgG1	N434A	wild-type mice	192.0 versus 242.4	0.8	[118]
Hu4D5	human IgG1	N434A	mFcRn$^{-/-}$ hFcRn Tg/Tg mice	230.4 versus 139.2	1.7	[118]
Hu4D5	human IgG1	T307A/E380A/N434A	wild-type mice	202.0 versus 242.2	0.8	[118]
Hu4D5	human IgG1	T307A/E380A/N434A	mFcRn$^{-/-}$ hFcRn Tg/Tg mice	211.2 versus 139.2	1.5	[118]
VEGF	human IgG1	M428L/N434S	cynomolgus monkeys	746.4 versus 232.8	3.2	[119]

HULys10, humanized IgG specific for hen egg lysozyme; MEDI-524, humanized IgG specific for respiratory syncytial virus; OST577, humanized IgG specific for hepatitis B virus; anti-TNF-α, humanized IgG specific for TNF-α; Hu4D5, humanized IgG specific for HER2; Anti-VEGF, humanized IgG specific for VEGF; $t_{1/2}$, serum half-life determined from the β-phase.

4.6.3
Blocking FcRn Recycling

Several autoimmune diseases are characterized by high titers of pathogenic IgGs that destroy cells or tissues [120]. Thus, FcRn recycles autoimmune IgGs and extends their half-lives [121, 122]. Therefore, situations exist where it may be favorable to accelerate the turnover of endogenous IgG. This has extensively been done in the clinic by so-called intravenous Ig (IVIG) therapy where high doses of exogenous IgG are injected. Consequently, the FcRn recycling mechanism is saturated and the half-life of circulating IgG dramatically shortened as demonstrated in several autoimmune mouse models [121–123].

Furthermore, IVIG-induced clearance is a favorable approach to increase the turnover of radiolabeled IgG, and thus reduce the background activity and normal tissue toxicity, as exemplified in both preclinical mouse studies as well as in imaging of tumors in humans [124]. Attractive alternatives to IVIG are IgG mutants designed to bind FcRn strongly with reduced pH dependence that will consequently act as FcRn blockers and hence modulate the levels of endogenous IgG. Such IgG molecules have been named Abdegs ("antibodies that enhance IgG degradation") and have been demonstrated to induce elimination of IgG in mouse model systems [125]. Another approach is to use a phage-display-selected peptide (SYN1436) that binds FcRn and blocks IgG binding [65]. Injection of SYN1436 into cynomolgus monkeys reduced the levels of endogenous IgG by an impressive 80% [65].

4.7
Targeting FcRn by SA

SA had been recognized and utilized for its long half-life before its relationship with FcRn was discovered. In tumor therapy, SA may be an ideal fusion partner of drugs targeted to malignant tissues since tumors are known to have increased fluid-phase uptake of SA (that is used as a major an energy source) compared to healthy tissue [126, 127]. Here, we review several approaches where SA is utilized to improve the pharmacokinetics of drugs. First, molecules chemically or genetically fused to SA are described, followed by examples on how half-life can be extended by targeting SA.

4.7.1
SA Fusions

The presence of high amounts of SA at the site of tumors and inflamed tissues has been utilized in treatments by chemical conjugation of small drugs to the surface of SA. One such therapeutic is the antimetabolite substance methotrexate (SA–MTX) for the treatment of renal carcinomas and autoimmune diseases such as rheumatoid arthritis [128–130]. Another example is the SA-based nanoparticles built up of lipophilic drugs encapsulated with SA under high pressure, which have been extensively evaluated as tumor-targeting vesicles for the mitotic inhibitor paclitaxel (Abraxane™), which has been approved by the FDA for the treatment of metastatic breast cancer [131, 132]. None of these strategies has yet been evaluated regarding their FcRn binding and transport.

A more specific way to chemically target SA is a technology that was recently developed and named Drug Affinity Complex (DAC™) that takes advantage of a free unpaired cysteine residue (C34) exposed on the DI of SA (highlighted in Figure 4.1a). Here, C34 of either exogenous or endogenous SA is bound to the drug in a way which allows rapid, specific and stable binding to SA. One such DAC-based drug is exendin-4 – a glucagon-like peptide-1 homolog (CJC-1131) for treatment of type 2 diabetes that has entered clinical trials [133]. The power of chemical targeting of SA to improve pharmacokinetics is mirrored by the fact that glucagon-like peptide-1 analogs have half-lives of hours only, while C34-bound drugs show a half-life of 9–15 days in human trials [133]. Another example is fusion of a short peptide derived from the HIV envelope protein gp41 to C34 that showed improved half-life in both rats and monkeys, and improved the inhibitory activity of the peptide toward HIV-1 [134]. Presumably, targeting of C34 will not interfere with FcRn recycling since C34 is located to D1, while the FcRn binding site lies within DIII.

Protein-based drugs can be genetically fused to either the N- or C-terminal ends of SA (Figure 4.7a). This strategy is independent of chemical cross-linking and has been broadly applied to small protein drugs with a molecular weight below the renal clearance threshold. A prerequisite is that they are designed in such a fashion that fusion to SA does not affect the bioactivity of the drug. Proteins that have been successfully fused to SA are coagulation Factors IX and VIIa [135–137], thymosin-α_1 [138], CD4 [139], hirudin [140], granulocyte colony-stimulating factor (Albugranin™) [141], growth hormone (Albutropin™) [142], insulin (Albulin™) [143], and interferon (IFN)-α and -β (Albuferon™) [144–146]. Using SA as a carrier, these proteins show improved pharmacokinetics *in vivo* compared to their nonfused counterparts, although their extended half-lifes do not necessarily reach the half-life of endogenous SA in the animal models used (Section 4.8).

One such example is fusion of coagulation factors to SA that aim to improve replacement therapy of individuals with hemophilia. Recombinant Factor VIIa approved for treatment is cleared very fast from the circulation with a half-life of a few hours [136]. Consequently, there is a great need for improved therapeutics to replace recombinant Factor VIIa. A preclinical study in rats shows that fusion of Factor VIIa to HSA improved the half-life by almost 6-fold, although the fusion had an approximately 2-fold lower half-life than HSA [136]. Similarly, fusion of Factor IX to HSA via a cleavable linker showed decreased *in vivo* clearance compared with nonfused Factor IX in mice, rat, and rabbits [135]. Again, the half-life values were far from that of endogenous SA in these animals. The reasons for these aberrations may be that the design of the fusions has an impact on the pharmacokinetics and/or that the model used for preclinical evaluation is not suitable for evaluation of HSA-based fusions, as discussed in Section 4.8.

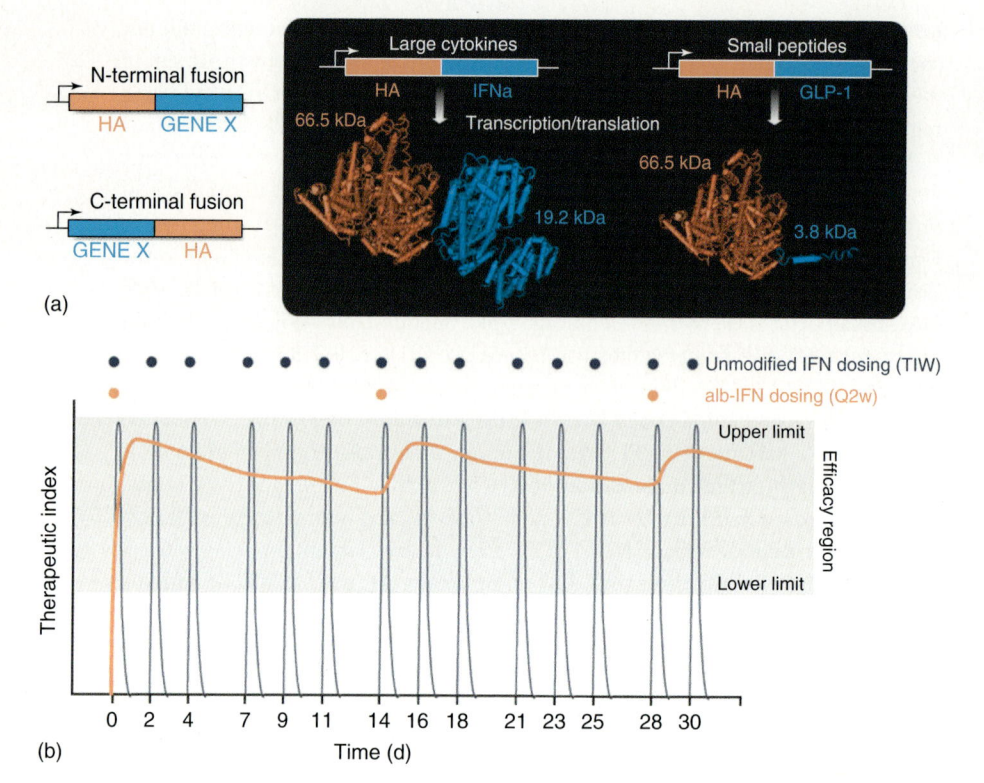

Figure 4.7 SA fusion technology. (a) SA fusion technology permits the design of recombinant, long-acting protein-based drugs by fusing the cDNA (gene X) encoding HSA to cDNAs encoding therapeutically active proteins. Genetic fusion can to done at either the N- or C-terminal of SA. Molecular models depicting SA fusion to a large cytokine (IFNα-2b) or a small peptide (glucagon-like peptide-1 (GLP-1)) illustrate the adaptability of the SA fusion platform. (b) Reduced dosing frequency and sustained exposure. The observed therapeutic index of SA fused to IFN versus unmodified IFN illustrates the sustained exposure and reduced dosing frequency associated with the SA fusion. Unmodified IFN reaches peak levels shortly after administration, followed by a rapid decline to undetectable levels at the end of each dosing interval (TIW = 3 times) dosing, on Monday, Wednesday, and Friday). By contrast, SA-fused IFN administered Q2w (every 2 weeks) provides sustained drug exposure that lies within the range of therapeutic efficacy throughout each dosing interval. Sustained drug exposure accompanied by infrequent dosing might improve tolerability. (Reproduced with permission from [145].)

The lead candidate among the SA fusions is SA fused to IFN-α2b (Albuferon-α2b) that is currently being evaluated in human trials for treatment of chronic hepatitis C [145]. While recombinant IFN-α2b (19 kDa) has a short half-life of only about 4 h in humans, Albuferon-α2b (85.7 kDa) has a 35-fold increased half-life of 141 h [144, 145]. The massive improvement in half-life is far beyond that achieved by conjugation to poly(ethylene glycol) (PEG), which only increased the half-life by 10-fold (40 h) [147]. Such improvement in half-life will likely result in the need of fewer doses required, which will ultimately make treatment more convenient and cost-effective (Figure 4.7b).

While full-length IgG has found broad applications in therapy due to its long half-life, the use of a range of small recombinant antibody molecules such as scFv or bispecific single-chain diabodies (scDbs) has become limiting due to their small size below the renal clearance threshold. For instance, the half-life of Fab and F(ab')$_2$ fragments is only about 1–5% of that of IgG [148, 149]. As an alternative, they may be fused to long-lived SA. The concept was first proven when Fab was chemically cross-linked to rat SA that increased the half-life to that measured for nonconjugated rat SA [150]. In line with this, scFv fragment genetically fused to HSA showed a comparable half-life with HSA in rats [150], although the half-life was again below that of rat SA. Furthermore, bispecific scDbs (scDbCEACD3) with specificity for CEA and the T-cell receptor complex molecule CD3 have been demonstrated to efficiently direct T-cells to tumors for subsequent induction of cell destruction [151]. When scDbCEACD3 was genetically fused to SA it showed an increased half-life in mice compared with naked scDbCEACD3, although its ability to bind target cells was to some extent reduced [152]. Similarly, an anti-CEA scFv fused to SA (immunobumin) showed an improved half-life and enhanced tumor-targeting potential compared with nonfused anti-CEA scFv in a colorectal carcinoma xenografted mouse model [153]. Biodistribution and tumor targeting of anti-CEA immunobumin in athymic mice bearing xenografts of CEA-expressing tumor cells are shown in Figure 4.8. Taken together, these examples show that fusion of antibody fragments to SA is an attractive approach that provides the fragments with beneficial pharmacokinetic properties that enhanced their effectiveness. Examples of half-lives of selected SA variants are listed in Table 4.2.

4.7.2
Targeting SA

SA may also be utilized by reversible noncovalent association. This strategy excludes the need for *in vitro* conjugation or recombinant production of SA fusions. Instead, endogenous SA is targeted *in vivo* postinjection. Since SA acts naturally as a carrier of fatty acids, this property has been utilized using small SA fatty acid affinity tags where affinity for SA correlates with half-life [154–156]. One example is the insulin analog detemir (Levemir™; Novo Nordisk), approved for treatment of diabetes types 1 and 2, which has been engineered to include a myristate tag that efficiently associates with endogenous SA postadministration subcutaneously [157, 158]. Slow reversible dissociation from SA prolongs its bioavailability and therapeutic effect.

Furthermore, a minimal organic SA-binding molecule (2-(3-maleimidopropanamido)-6-(4-(4-iodophenyl)butanamido)hexanoate) chemically conjugated to an engineered free cysteine residue in the C-terminal end of a scFv fragment (scFv-F8(14aa)-Albu) (25 kDa) increased the half-life dramatically (16.6 h) compared with unmodified scFv-F8(14aa)-Cys (0.5 h) in mice [159]. In tumor-bearing

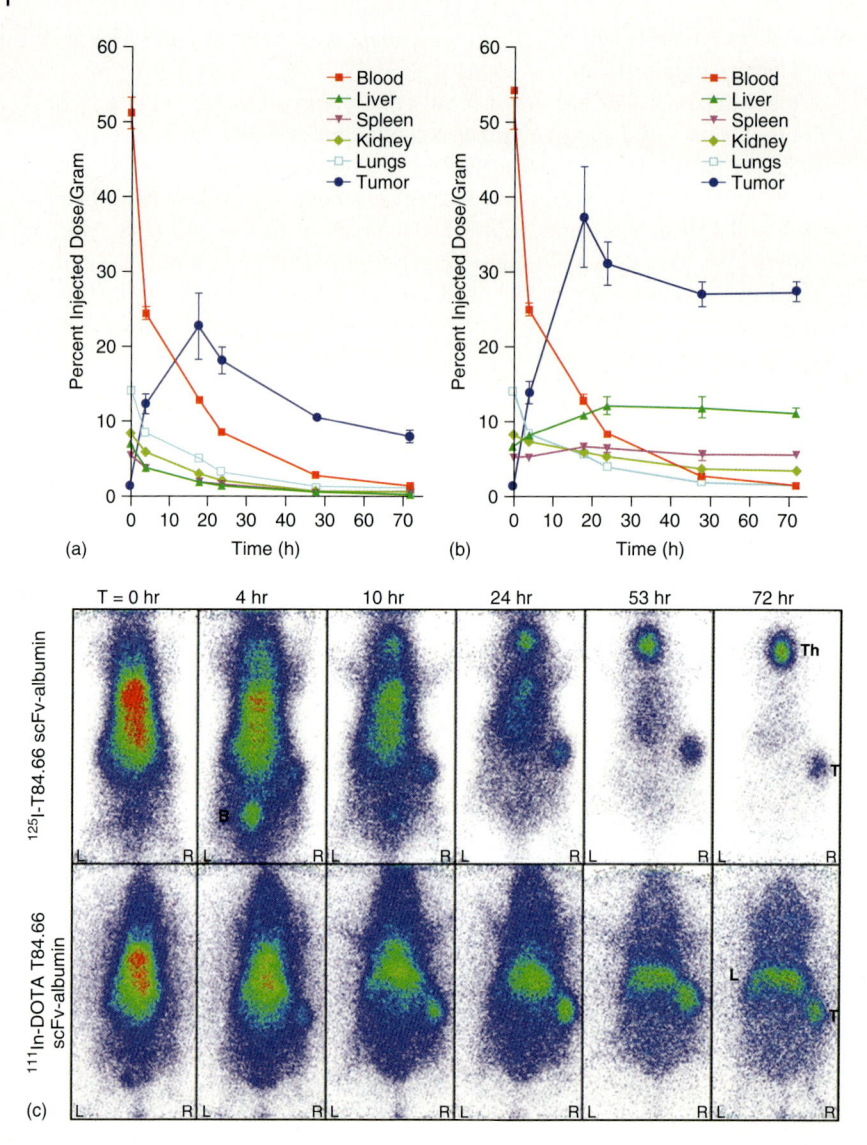

Figure 4.8 Biodistribution and tumor imaging using radiolabeled anti-CEA scFv fused to SA. (a) Tissue distribution of scFv-fused SA in athymic mice bearing LS-174T xenografts. The ^{125}I-labeled immunobumin (a) and ^{111}In-DOTA-labeled immunobumin (b) were intravenously coinjected into xenograft-bearing mice, and tumor-targeting and biodistribution studies performed. Tumor and normal tissue uptake are expressed as percent ID/g and plotted with the standard error of the mean (c) γ-Camera imaging was performed by intravenously injecting ^{125}I-labeled immunobumin and ^{111}In-DOTA-labeled immunobumin. Imaging was performed at 0, 4, 10, 24, 53, and 72 h; all images were half-life-corrected. Tumor (T), bladder (B), thyroid (Th), and liver (L) are noted. DOTA = 1,4,7,10-tetraazacyclododecane-1,4,7,10-tetraacetic acid. (Reproduced with permission from [153].)

Table 4.2 Half-life of SA variants.

Fusion partner	SA species	Host species	$t_{1/2}$(h) nonfused partner	$t_{1/2}$(h) fused	$t_{1/2}$(h) nonfused SA	References
Factor VIIa	human	rat	0.6	4.4	10.3	[136]
IFN-α	human	human	4.0	141.0	~450–500	[144, 145]
Fab	rat	rat	15.9	39.6	49.1	[150]
scFv	human	rat	–	15.2–16.6	14.8	[150]

$t_{1/2}$, serum half-life determined from the β-phase.

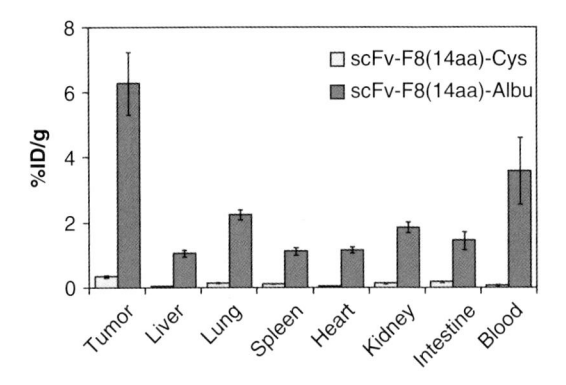

Figure 4.9 Biodistribution profiles of scFv-F8-Cys and scFv-F8-Albu in tumor-bearing mice. Mean targeting results are expressed as %ID/g ± standard error. (Reproduced with permission from [159].)

mice, improved bioavailability as a result of the minimal tag resulted in superior tumor accumulation compared with naked scFv [159]. Biodistribution profiles for radioiodinated scFv-F8-Cys and scFv-F8-Albu in tumor-bearing mice are shown in Figure 4.9.

SA may also be targeted by antibody fragments. Using a bispecific F(ab')$_2$ fragment with one-arm targeted SA, the half-life increased 5-fold compared with monospecific anti-TNF F(ab')$_2$ and reached almost the same half-life of that measured for rat SA (42.5 versus 49.1 h, respectively) [150]. The similarity in half-life strongly supports that the anti-SA Fab arm used in this study does not interfere with FcRn binding to SA. The same trend was seen for small albumin-binding domain (ABD) antibodies (11–13 kDa; AlbudAb™) selected to bind rat SA with low (1 μM) and high (13 nM) affinity that showed half-lives in rats of 43 and 53 h, respectively. Rat SA has a half-life of 53 h, similar to the high-affinity AlbudAb [160]. Notably, AlbudAb binds to DII of SA [161].

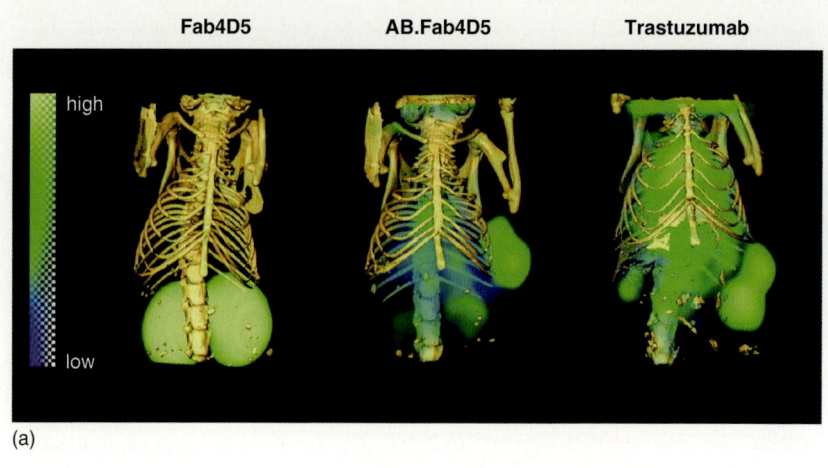

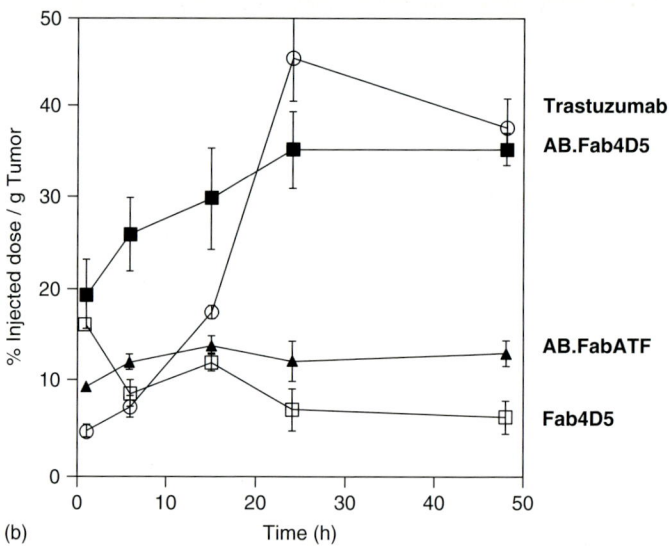

Figure 4.10 Biodistribution of Fab4D5, AB.Fab4D5, and trastuzumab in mice as a function of time determined using single photon emission computed tomography/computed tomography (SPECT/CT) imaging. (a) SPECT/CT fusion images depicting biodistribution of Fab4D5, AB.Fab4D5, and trastuzumab at 18 h. Fab4D5 (left) shows classic kidney clearance. Trastuzumab (right) shows pronounced tumor uptake and substantial remaining blood pool. AB.Fab4D5 (middle) shows distribution more like trastuzumab than Fab4D5, with pronounced tumor uptake, some residual blood pool, and only low-level kidney uptake. (b) Concentration (percent injected dose per gram of tumor) of Fab4D5, AB.Fab4D5, and trastuzumab over time was compared using SPECT/CT imaging. Tumor SPECT intensities of Fab4D5 (□), AB.Fab4D5 (■), trastuzumab (○), and AB.FabATF (negative control) (▲) were converted to percent injected dose per gram by reference to a standard of known activity included in each image. (Reproduced with permission from [164].)

A range of peptides selected by phage display for binding reversibly to SA with the core sequence DICLPRWGCLW has been by described by Dennis *et al.* [162]. One such peptide (SA21) had an impressive 19-fold increase in half-life compared with an unrelated peptide [162]. Moreover, when a range of peptides where fused to a Fab fragment derived from the clinically approved trastuzumab (Herceptin™) with specificity for the tumor marker HER2, a clear correlation between SA affinity and *in vivo* clearance was observed, since AB.Fab fragments (25 kDa) with strong affinity showed longer half-life than those with low-affinity peptides in both mice and rabbits [163].

The AB.Fab concept has also been explored in tumor-targeting approaches [164]. While full-length IgG is known to diffuse slowly into solid tumors, small antibody fragments show superior tumor penetration, but their therapeutic efficiency is hampered by a short *in vivo* half-life and unfavorable accumulation in normal tissues, such as liver and kidneys [165]. In this regard, increasing half-life without affecting the size of small antibody fragments may have great value in tumor-targeting regimes. Furthermore, when AB.Fab4D5 was compared with trastuzumab for their ability to target HER2-positive tumors in a mouse model, AB.Fab4D5 was shown to rapidly target tumor as well as being eliminated much faster from circulation than trastuzumab [164]. Consequently, tumor/normal tissue ratios were significantly improved as high accumulation of AB.Fab4D5 at tumor sites was reached within 2 h postadministration in contrast to 24 h that had passed before the same levels were reached for trastuzumab [164]. Noteworthy is the fact that whereas Fab4D5 accumulated in the kidneys, AB.Fab4D5 did not. This redistribution as a function of SA targeting may be explained by the role of FcRn in rescue of SA in the kidneys (Section 4.5.6), but a prerequisite for such a route is that the AB.Fab fragments in association with SA are able to bind FcRn in a similar manner as SA itself. The SA peptide-targeting strategy may be transferable to any protein of interest to tailor *in vivo* pharmacokinetics. Biodistribution profiles and tumor-targeting properties of Fab4D5 and AB.Fab4D5 compared with trastuzumab are shown in Figures 4.10 and 4.11, respectively.

Finally, minimal SA-binding domains derived from bacterial proteins may be used as SA-targeting modules, such as an ABD derived from *Streptococcus* strain G148 (5 kDa). The strategy has been used to extend the half-life of antibody-derived fragments [166–168]. Fusion of ABD to anti-HER2 Fab4D5 (25 kDa) increased the half-life by 10-fold compared with naked Fab4D5 in mice (21 versus 2 h) [166] and, notably, this is within the same range as that obtained when Fab4D5 was fused to SA-targeting peptides [164]. Similar to the SA-binding peptides, the ABD fusion also accumulated to a lesser extend in the kidneys that nonfused Fab4D5.

Furthermore, fusion of ABD to divalent anti-HER2 affibody (($Z_{HER\ 2:342}$)$_2$) molecules (19 kDa) has demonstrated excellent tumor-targeting properties in preclinical imaging experiments compared with nonfused ($Z_{HER\ 2:342}$)$_2$ [169]. Such affibody molecules consist of a very small domain (around 7 kDa) derived from the IgG-binding domain of staphylococcal protein A that is used as a scaffold in combinatorial phage-display libraries in selection of target binders [170]. Again, targeting of radiolabeled ABD–($Z_{HER\ 2:342}$)$_2$ was shown to give rise to high tumor

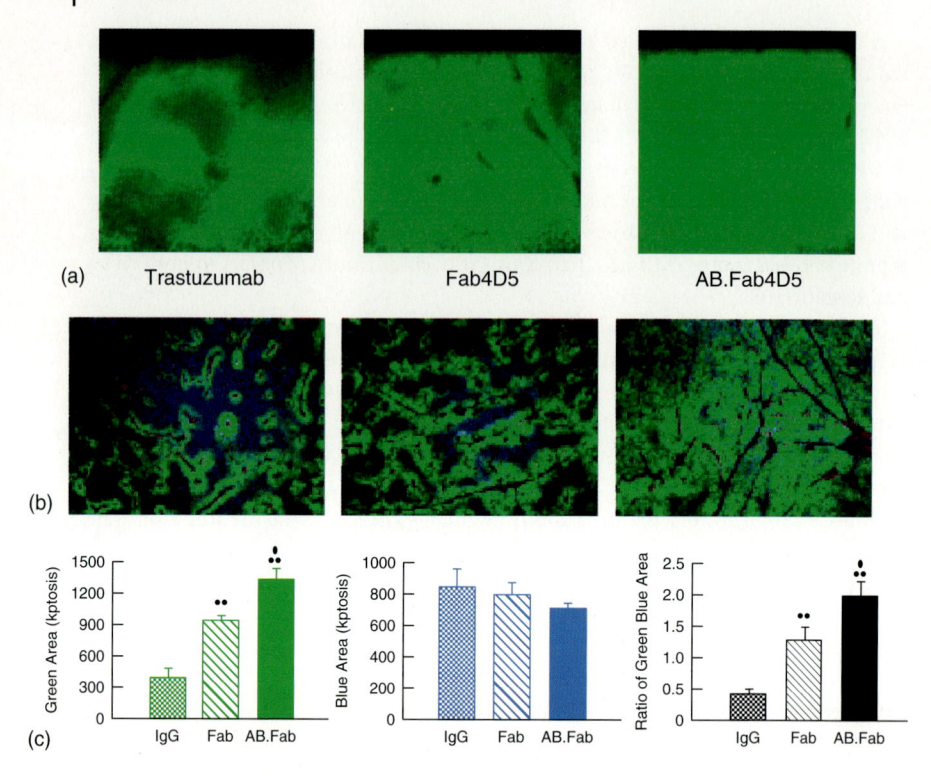

Figure 4.11 Superior tumor penetration of AB.Fab4D5. Tumor penetration was assessed at maximum tumor accumulation. Fluorescein isothiocyanate (FITC)-labeled Fab4D5 was assessed at 2 h, whereas FITC-labeled AB.Fab4D5 and trastuzumab were assessed at 24 h postinjection. (a) Representative intravital microscopy images recorded using confocal laser scanning microscopy at ×200 magnification. (b) Microscopic images of F2-1282 tumor tissue where trastuzumab, Fab4D5, or AB.Fab4D5 conjugated with FITC (green) were detected over tumor tissue and displayed a membranous staining pattern. Vasculature was visualized with an anti-mouse CD31 detected with a Cy3-conjugated secondary antibody (red). All tissues were counterstained with 4′,6-diamidino-2-phenylindole (blue) to detect nuclei. (c) Quantitative analysis using Image J software for measurement of penetrated area (green area), total area (blue area), and their ratio. $^*P < 0.05$; $^{**}P < 0.01$, compared with trastuzumab; $^{\#}P < 0.05$ compared with Fab4D5. Trastuzumab, FITC–trastuzumab ($n = 4$ mice); Fab4D5, FITC–Fab4D5 ($n = 5$ mice); AB.Fab, FITC–AB.Fab4D5 ($n = 5$ mice).

uptake in HER2-positive microxenograft mice as well as a 25-fold reduction in kidney deposition [169].

Fusion of ABD to scDbCEACD3 (59.3 kDa) retained the binding activity for all three antigens, but targeting to T-cells was to some extent reduced compared with naked scDbCEACD3 (54.5 kDa); however, the half-life of the fusion increased 5-fold in mice [167]. Interestingly, when scDbCEACD3–ABD was compared with PEGylated scDbCEACD3 they both had similar half-lives, although the ABD-fused variant showed a 2-fold favorable tumor accumulation [168].

It is of interest to address whether or not SA binds FcRn when associated with ABD. ABD shares 59% amino acid sequence similarity with a homolog from *Finegoldia magna*, which binds to a site within DII of SA as shown by X-ray crystallography [171, 172]. As the major binding site for FcRn is localized to DIII of SA, it is likely that both ABD and FcRn bind simultaneously to separate binding sites on SA. A prerequisite for FcRn-mediated recycling is that the association of ABD with SA is not disrupted by the acidic milieu within endosomes. This topic has been addressed for both scDbCEACD4–ABD and SA-binding peptides, and lowering of pH was found not to affect SA binding [162, 167]. Support for a role of FcRn in handling of ABD fusions was first obtained when a 2-fold lower half-life was measured for scDbCEACD4–ABD, while the half-life of PEGylated scDbCEACD4 was unaffected in FcRn-deficient mice [168]. The drop in half-life of the ABD fusion may be a result of a lower serum level of SA in mice lacking FcRn or lack of FcRn-mediated recycling. We recently demonstrated that ABD does not interfere with the strictly pH-dependent FcRn–SA binding kinetics, whether alone or recombinantly fused to $(Z_{HER 2:342})_2$ [173] (Figure 4.12a and b). Furthermore, FcRn binding was unaffected by the presence of IgG and the ABD fusion showed a similar biodistribution profile as rat SA in wild-type rats [173] (Figure 4.12c and d). Collectively, the studies show that ABD may be a carrier to extend the half-life of small protein drugs. In addition, ABD variants engineered to bind SA with an array of affinities open the possibility to fine-tune the pharmacokinetics of ABD-fused molecules [174].

4.8
Considering Cross-Species Binding

The first generation of monoclonal IgGs developed using hybridoma technology were all of murine origin [175, 176]. Although they showed superior activity in preclinical animal models, they failed tremendously when entering human trials as they were rapidly cleared from the circulation. At that time, this phenomenon was explained by the human anti-mouse antibody (HAMA) response. Consequently, murine sequences were genetically modified to become more human-like (humanization) as a link to reduce immunogenicity [177, 178]. Indeed, reduced HAMA effects were observed as well as increased half-life and therapeutic efficiency. However, it has now become apparent that human FcRn shows selective binding to IgG from other species; for instance, it does not bind significantly to murine IgGs – a finding that explains the disappointingly short half-life of murine IgGs in humans [179, 180]. Consistent with this is the fact that the serum level of endogenous IgG is very low in mice knocked-out for endogenous FcRn and transgenic for human FcRn [44]. On the contrary, mouse FcRn is more promiscuous and binds IgG from several species, including strong binding to human IgG at acidic pH [179]. Such differences must be considered when engineered IgGs are to be evaluated for their pharmacokinetics in mice. As extensively explored in several studies described above (Section 4.6.2), human IgG engineered to bind strongly to human FcRn

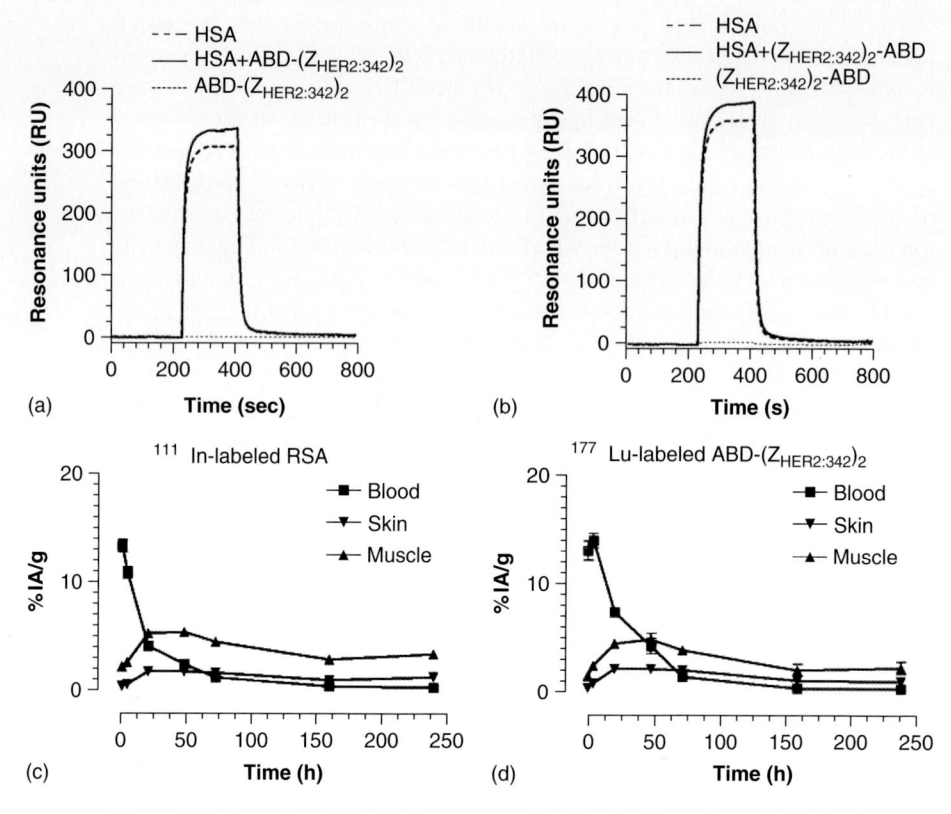

Figure 4.12 Impact on FcRn binding and *in vivo* biodistribution of ABD-fused ($Z_{HER\ 2:342}$)$_2$. Representative surface plasmon resonance showing additive binding of HSA in complex with (a) ABD–($Z_{HER\ 2:342}$)$_2$ and (b) ($Z_{HER\ 2:342}$)$_2$–ABD when injected over immobilized recombinant soluble human FcRn at pH 6.0. The blood, skin, and muscle biodistribution of (c) ^{111}In-labeled rat SA (RSA) and (d) ^{177}Lu-labeled ABD–($Z_{HER\ 2:342}$)$_2$ in a preclinical Sprague-Dawley rat model (three rats per group and time point). Organ uptake is expressed as %IA/g, and error bars indicate the standard error of the mean. (Reproduced with permission from [173].)

at pH 6.0 with retained pH dependence does not necessarily bind with the same binding kinetics to mouse FcRn [62, 118].

Preclinical evaluation to determine the pharmacokinetics of SA mutants, SA fusions, or targeting molecules are also often performed in rodents. Interestingly, human FcRn transgenic mice that lack expression of endogenous FcRn rescue MSA from degradation even in the absence of IgG binding [44]. This correlates with recent results showing that human FcRn ignores binding to mouse IgG while binding strongly to MSA [55]. Importantly, mouse FcRn binds HSA very poorly as the binding affinity for MSA is 10-fold stronger than for HSA [55]. Thus, mouse FcRn prefers to bind to MSA instead of HSA. This must necessarily affect the *in vivo* half-life of HSA-fused therapeutics in rodents as small amounts of injected fusion proteins will compete for binding to mouse FcRn in the presence of high amounts of circulating endogenous SA (40 mg/ml). This assumption is supported by the fact that HSA has a half-life of 15 h only, compared to 49 h of rat SA in rats [150]. Thus, when HSA-fused therapeutics show a moderate increase in serum half-life in rodents compared with unfused molecules, it may simply be a result of an increase in the total molecular weight of the fusion and not an effect of FcRn recycling. Thus, cross-species interactions with FcRn may have great impact on preclinical evaluations and will affect *in vivo* half-life as well as biodistribution. To fully control the impact of FcRn, one should include SA from the species used as a model, with and without fusion. It is also highly relevant that SA of small animals has a much shorter half-life than SA of larger animals (e.g., the half-life of endogenous SA in mice and rats is only about 1.5 and 2.5 days, respectively, compared to 19–21 days in humans) [1, 44, 181].

Regarding indirect targeting of FcRn via SA, cross-species SA-binding properties must be considered prior to *in vivo* evaluations. In addition, the binding properties of SA-bound complexes to FcRn must be addressed as demonstrated for the ABD-fused anti-HER2 Affibody variants. Thus, preclinical experiments performed cross-species should be carefully considered regarding FcRn binding properties.

4.9
Concluding Remarks

FcRn is a unique receptor that mediates important and versatile functions regarding handling of IgG and SA at several body sites. In addition to its key role in the transfer of maternal IgG to the fetus or neonatal, FcRn regulates the long half-life of IgG and SA via an efficient recycling pathway, in addition to being central to the clearance of the ligands in the kidneys and liver, as well as several types of immune cells. All of the functions rely on its ability to bind and transport its ligands in a strictly pH-dependent fashion within and through different cell layers of the body. Furthermore, our molecular understanding of how FcRn binds its ligands and controls their half-life has prompted engineering of IgG- and SA-based diagnostics and therapeutics to modulate their *in vivo* bioavailability. Several reports have shown that the design of such mutant IgG variants with altered FcRn binding properties holds promise in preclinical models. Modulation of the interaction with FcRn will surely generate new classes of IgG as well as SA-fused molecules with tailored pharmacokinetic properties.

Acknowledgment

J.T.A. was supported by the Norwegian Research Council (grant 179573/V40) and South-Eastern Norway Regional Health Authority (grant number 39375).

References

1. Peters, T. (1985) *Adv. Protein Chem.*, **37**, 161–245.
2. He, X.M. and Carter, D.C. (1992) *Nature*, **358**, 209–215.

3. Carter, D.C., He, X.M., Munson, S.H., Twigg, P.D., Gernert, K.M., Broom, M.B., and Miller, T.Y. (1989) *Science*, **244**, 1195–1198.
4. Curry, S., Mandelkow, H., Brick, P., and Franks, N. (1998) *Nat. Struct. Biol.*, **5**, 827–835.
5. Sugio, S., Kashima, A., Mochizuki, S., Noda, M., and Kobayashi, K. (1999) *Protein Eng.*, **12**, 439–446.
6. Deisenhofer, J. (1981) *Biochemistry*, **20**, 2361–2370.
7. Nimmerjahn, F. and Ravetch, J.V. (2008) *Nat. Rev. Immunol.*, **8**, 34–47.
8. Nimmerjahn, F. and Ravetch, J.V. (2010) *Immunol. Rev.*, **236**, 265–275.
9. Bruhns, P., Iannascoli, B., England, P., Mancardi, D.A., Fernandez, N., Jorieux, S., and Daeron, M. (2009) *Blood*, **113**, 3716–3725.
10. Nimmerjahn, F. and Ravetch, J.V. (2005) *Science*, **310**, 1510–1512.
11. Waldmann, T.A. and Strober, W. (1969) *Prog. Allergy*, **13**, 1–110.
12. Spiegelberg, H.L. and Fishkin, B.G. (1972) *Clin. Exp. Immunol.*, **10**, 599–607.
13. Simister, N.E. and Mostov, K.E. (1989) *Nature*, **337**, 184–187.
14. Martin, M.G., Wu, S.V., and Walsh, J.H. (1997) *Dig. Dis. Sci.*, **42**, 1062–1069.
15. Jakoi, E.R., Cambier, J., and Saslow, S. (1985) *J. Immunol.*, **135**, 3360–3364.
16. Brambell, F.W. (1966) *Lancet*, **2**, 1087–1093.
17. Brambell, F.W.R., Hemmings, W.A., Oakley, C.L., and Porter, R.R. (1960) *Proc. R. Soc. Lond. B*, **151**, 478–482.
18. He, W.Z., Ladinsky, M.S., Huey-Tubman, K.E., Jensen, G.J., McIntosh, J.R., and Bjorkman, P.J. (2008) *Nature*, **455**, 542–U553.
19. Hobbs, S.M., Jackson, L.E., and Peppard, J.V. (1987) *J. Biol. Chem.*, **262**, 8041–8046.
20. Fahey, J.L. and Robinson, A.G. (1963) *J. Exp. Med.*, **118**, 845–868.
21. Brambell, F.W., Hemmings, W.A., and Morris, I.G. (1964) *Nature*, **203**, 1352–1354.
22. Simister, N.E. and Rees, A.R. (1985) *Eur. J. Immunol.*, **15**, 733–738.
23. Rodewald, R. and Kraehenbuhl, J.P. (1984) *J. Cell Biol.*, **99**, 159s–164s.
24. Ghetie, V., Hubbard, J.G., Kim, J.K., Tsen, M.F., Lee, Y., and Ward, E.S. (1996) *Eur. J. Immunol.*, **26**, 690–696.
25. Borvak, J., Richardson, J., Medesan, C., Antohe, F., Radu, C., Simionescu, M., Ghetie, V., and Ward, E.S. (1998) *Int. Immunol.*, **10**, 1289–1298.
26. Junghans, R.P. and Anderson, C.L. (1996) *Proc. Natl. Acad. Sci. USA*, **93**, 5512–5516.
27. Israel, E.J., Wilsker, D.F., Hayes, K.C., Schoenfeld, D., and Simister, N.E. (1996) *Immunology*, **89**, 573–578.
28. Adamski, F.M., King, A.T., and Demmer, J. (2000) *Mol. Immunol.*, **37**, 435–444.
29. Mayer, B., Zolnai, A., Frenyo, L.V., Jancsik, V., Szentirmay, Z., Hammarstrom, L., and Kacskovics, I. (2002) *Vet. Immunol. Immunopathol.*, **87**, 327–330.
30. Kacskovics, I., Wu, Z., Simister, N.E., Frenyo, L.V., and Hammarstrom, L. (2000) *J. Immunol.*, **164**, 1889–1897.
31. Kacskovics, I., Mayer, B., Kis, Z., Frenyo, L.V., Zhao, Y., Muyldermans, S., and Hammarstrom, L. (2006) *Dev. Comp. Immunol.*, **30**, 1203–1215.
32. Sayed-Ahmed, A., Kassab, M., Abd-Elmaksoud, A., Elnasharty, M., and El-Kirdasy, A. (2010) *Acta Histochem.*, **112**, 383–391.
33. Ahouse, J.J., Hagerman, C.L., Mittal, P., Gilbert, D.J., Copeland, N.G., Jenkins, N.A., and Simister, N.E. (1993) *J. Immunol.*, **151**, 6076–6088.
34. Schlachetzki, F., Zhu, C., and Pardridge, W.M. (2002) *J. Neurochem.*, **81**, 203–206.
35. Story, C.M., Mikulska, J.E., and Simister, N.E. (1994) *J. Exp. Med.*, **180**, 2377–2381.
36. Kristoffersen, E.K. and Matre, R. (1996) *Eur. J. Immunol.*, **26**, 1668–1671.
37. Blumberg, R.S., Koss, T., Story, C.M., Barisani, D., Polischuk, J., Lipin, A., Pablo, L., Green, R., and Simister, N.E. (1995) *J. Clin. Invest.*, **95**, 2397–2402.
38. Telleman, P. and Junghans, R.P. (2000) *Immunology*, **100**, 245–251.
39. Kobayashi, K., Ogata, H., Morikawa, M., Iijima, S., Harada, N., Yoshida, T.,

Brown, W.R., Inoue, N., Hamada, Y., Ishii, H., Watanabe, M., and Hibi, T. (2002) *Gut*, **51**, 169–176.

40. Akilesh, S., Huber, T.B., Wu, H., Wang, G., Hartleben, B., Kopp, J.B., Miner, J.H., Roopenian, D.C., Unanue, E.R., and Shaw, A.S. (2008) *Proc. Natl. Acad. Sci. USA*, **105**, 967–972.
41. Sarav, M., Wang, Y., Hack, B.K., Chang, A., Jensen, M., Bao, L., and Quigg, R.J. (2009) *J. Am. Soc. Nephrol.*, **20**, 1941–1952.
42. Kim, H., Fariss, R.N., Zhang, C., Robinson, S.B., Thill, M., and Csaky, K.G. (2008) *Invest. Ophthalmol. Vis. Sci.*, **49**, 2025–2029.
43. Kim, H., Robinson, S.B., and Csaky, K.G. (2009) *Mol. Vision*, **15**, 2803–2812.
44. Chaudhury, C., Mehnaz, S., Robinson, J.M., Hayton, W.L., Pearl, D.K., Roopenian, D.C., and Anderson, C.L. (2003) *J. Exp. Med.*, **197**, 315–322.
45. Chaudhury, C., Brooks, C.L., Carter, D.C., Robinson, J.M., and Anderson, C.L. (2006) *Biochemistry*, **45**, 4983–4990.
46. Schultze, H.E. and Heremans, J.F. (1966) *Molecular Biology of Human Proteins: with Special Reference to Plasma Proteins.*, Nature and Metabolism of Extracellular Proteins, Vol. 1, Elsevier.
47. Burmeister, W.P., Huber, A.H., and Bjorkman, P.J. (1994) *Nature*, **372**, 379–383.
48. Burmeister, W.P., Gastinel, L.N., Simister, N.E., Blum, M.L., and Bjorkman, P.J. (1994) *Nature*, **372**, 336–343.
49. West, A.P. Jr. and Bjorkman, P.J. (2000) *Biochemistry*, **39**, 9698–9708.
50. Kim, J.K., Tsen, M.F., Ghetie, V., and Ward, E.S. (1994) *Eur. J. Immunol.*, **24**, 2429–2434.
51. Kim, J.K., Tsen, M.F., Ghetie, V., and Ward, E.S. (1994) *Scand. J. Immunol.*, **40**, 457–465.
52. Kim, J.K., Tsen, M.F., Ghetie, V., and Ward, E.S. (1994) *Eur. J. Immunol.*, **24**, 542–548.
53. Montoyo, H.P., Vaccaro, C., Hafner, M., Ober, R.J., Mueller, W., and Ward, E.S. (2009) *Proc. Natl. Acad. Sci. USA*, **106**, 2788–2793.
54. Andersen, J.T., Dee Qian, J., and Sandlie, I. (2006) *Eur. J. Immunol.*, **36**, 3044–3051.
55. Andersen, J.T., Daba, M.B., Berntzen, G., Michaelsen, T.E., and Sandlie, I. (2010) *J. Biol. Chem.*, **285**, 4826–4836.
56. Andersen, J.T., Daba, M.B., and Sandlie, I. (2010) *Clin. Biochem.*, **43**, 367–372.
57. Andersen, J.T. and Sandlie, I. (2007) *Clin. Chem.*, **53**, 2216.
58. Medesan, C., Radu, C., Kim, J.K., Ghetie, V., and Ward, E.S. (1996) *Eur. J. Immunol.*, **26**, 2533–2536.
59. Kim, J., Mohanty, S., Ganesan, L.P., Hua, K., Jarjoura, D., Hayton, W.L., Robinson, J.M., and Anderson, C.L. (2009) *J. Immunol.*, **182**, 2583–2589.
60. Leach, J.L., Sedmak, D.D., Osborne, J.M., Rahill, B., Lairmore, M.D., and Anderson, C.L. (1996) *J. Immunol.*, **157**, 3317–3322.
61. Firan, M., Bawdon, R., Radu, C., Ober, R.J., Eaken, D., Antohe, F., Ghetie, V., and Ward, E.S. (2001) *Int. Immunol.*, **13**, 993–1002.
62. Vaccaro, C., Bawdon, R., Wanjie, S., Ober, R.J., and Ward, E.S. (2006) *Proc. Natl. Acad. Sci. USA*, **103**, 18709–18714.
63. Grubb, J.H., Vogler, C., Tan, Y., Shah, G.N., MacRae, A.F., and Sly, W.S. (2008) *Proc. Natl. Acad. Sci. USA*, **105**, 8375–8380.
64. Chen, P., Li, C., Lang, S., Zhu, G., Reheman, A., Spring, C.M., Freedman, J., and Ni, H. (2010) *Blood*, **116**, 3660–3668.
65. Mezo, A.R., McDonnell, K.A., Hehir, C.A., Low, S.C., Palombella, V.J., Stattel, J.M., Kamphaus, G.D., Fraley, C., Zhang, Y., Dumont, J.A., and Bitonti, A.J. (2008) *Proc. Natl. Acad. Sci. USA*, **105**, 2337–2342.
66. Anderson, C.L., Chaudhury, C., Kim, J., Bronson, C.L., Wani, M.A., and Mohanty, S. (2006) *Trends Immunol.*, **27**, 343–348.
67. Gitlin, D., Kumate, J., Urrusti, J., and Morales, C. (1964) *J. Clin. Invest.*, **43**, 1938–1951.
68. Lyden, T.W., Robinson, J.M., Tridandapani, S., Teillaud, J.L., Garber, S.A., Osborne, J.M., Frey, J., Budde, P.,

and Anderson, C.L. (2001) *J. Immunol.*, **166**, 3882–3889.
69. Takizawa, T., Anderson, C.L., and Robinson, J.M. (2005) *J. Immunol.*, **175**, 2331–2339.
70. Simister, N.E. (2003) *Vaccine*, **21**, 3365–3369.
71. Mohanty, S., Kim, J., Ganesan, L.P., Phillips, G.S., Hua, K., Jarjoura, D., Hayton, W.L., Robinson, J.M., and Anderson, C.L. (2010) *J. Reprod. Immunol.*, **84**, 133–144.
72. Israel, E.J., Taylor, S., Wu, Z., Mizoguchi, E., Blumberg, R.S., Bhan, A., and Simister, N.E. (1997) *Immunology*, **92**, 69–74.
73. Dickinson, B.L., Badizadegan, K., Wu, Z., Ahouse, J.C., Zhu, X., Simister, N.E., Blumberg, R.S., and Lencer, W.I. (1999) *J. Clin. Invest.*, **104**, 903–911.
74. Spiekermann, G.M., Finn, P.W., Ward, E.S., Dumont, J., Dickinson, B.L., Blumberg, R.S., and Lencer, W.I. (2002) *J. Exp. Med.*, **196**, 303–310.
75. Yoshida, M., Claypool, S.M., Wagner, J.S., Mizoguchi, E., Mizoguchi, A., Roopenian, D.C., Lencer, W.I., and Blumberg, R.S. (2004) *Immunity*, **20**, 769–783.
76. Johansen, F.E., Pekna, M., Norderhaug, I.N., Haneberg, B., Hietala, M.A., Krajci, P., Betsholtz, C., and Brandtzaeg, P. (1999) *J. Exp. Med.*, **190**, 915–922.
77. Ghetie, V., Popov, S., Borvak, J., Radu, C., Matesoi, D., Medesan, C., Ober, R.J., and Ward, E.S. (1997) *Nat. Biotechnol.*, **15**, 637–640.
78. Roopenian, D.C., Christianson, G.J., Sproule, T.J., Brown, A.C., Akilesh, S., Jung, N., Petkova, S., Avanessian, L., Choi, E.Y., Shaffer, D.J., Eden, P.A., and Anderson, C.L. (2003) *J. Immunol.*, **170**, 3528–3533.
79. Qiao, S.W., Kobayashi, K., Johansen, F.E., Sollid, L.M., Andersen, J.T., Milford, E., Roopenian, D.C., Lencer, W.I., and Blumberg, R.S. (2008) *Proc. Natl. Acad. Sci. USA*, **105**, 9337–9342.
80. Akilesh, S., Christianson, G.J., Roopenian, D.C., and Shaw, A.S. (2007) *J. Immunol.*, **179**, 4580–4588.
81. Wani, M.A., Haynes, L.D., Kim, J., Bronson, C.L., Chaudhury, C., Mohanty, S., Waldmann, T.A., Robinson, J.M., and Anderson, C.L. (2006) *Proc. Natl. Acad. Sci. USA*, **103**, 5084–5089.
82. Ward, E.S. and Ober, R.J. (2009) *Adv. Immunol.*, **103**, 77–115.
83. Zhu, X., Meng, G., Dickinson, B.L., Li, X., Mizoguchi, E., Miao, L., Wang, Y., Robert, C., Wu, B., Smith, P.D., Lencer, W.I., and Blumberg, R.S. (2001) *J. Immunol.*, **166**, 3266–3276.
84. Kobayashi, K., Qiao, S.W., Yoshida, M., Baker, K., Lencer, W.I., and Blumberg, R.S. (2009) *Gastroenterology*, **137**, 1746–1756, e1741.
85. Vidarsson, G., Stemerding, A.M., Stapleton, N.M., Spliethoff, S.E., Janssen, H., Rebers, F.E., de Haas, M., and van de Winkel, J.G. (2006) *Blood*, **108**, 3573–3579.
86. Mi, W., Wanjie, S., Lo, S.T., Gan, Z., Pickl-Herk, B., Ober, R.J., and Ward, E.S. (2008) *J. Immunol.*, **181**, 7550–7561.
87. Deane, R., Sagare, A., Hamm, K., Parisi, M., LaRue, B., Guo, H., Wu, Z., Holtzman, D.M., and Zlokovic, B.V. (2005) *J. Neurosci.*, **25**, 11495–11503.
88. Garg, A. and Balthasar, J.P. (2009) *AAPS J.*, **11**, 553–557.
89. Zhang, Y. and Pardridge, W.M. (2001) *J. Neuroimmunol.*, **114**, 168–172.
90. Wang, W., Wang, E.Q., and Balthasar, J.P. (2008) *Clin. Pharmacol. Ther.*, **84**, 548–558.
91. Kim, J., Bronson, C.L., Hayton, W.L., Radmacher, M.D., Roopenian, D.C., Robinson, J.M., and Anderson, C.L. (2006) *Am. J. Physiol.*, **290**, G352–G360.
92. Kenanova, V., Olafsen, T., Williams, L.E., Ruel, N.H., Longmate, J., Yazaki, P.J., Shively, J.E., Colcher, D., Raubitschek, A.A., and Wu, A.M. (2007) *Cancer Res.*, **67**, 718–726.
93. Olafsen, T., Kenanova, V.E., Sundaresan, G., Anderson, A.L., Crow, D., Yazaki, P.J., Li, L., Press, M.F., Gambhir, S.S., Williams, L.E., Wong, J.Y., Raubitschek, A.A., Shively, J.E., and Wu, A.M. (2005) *Cancer Res.*, **65**, 5907–5916.
94. Weiner, L.M. and Carter, P. (2005) *Nat. Biotechnol.*, **23**, 556–557.

95. Wark, K.L. and Hudson, P.J. (2006) *Adv. Drug. Deliv. Rev.*, **58**, 657–670.
96. Beck, A., Wurch, T., Bailly, C., and Corvaia, N. (2010) *Nat. Rev. Immunol.*, **10**, 345–352.
97. Weiner, L.M., Surana, R., and Wang, S. (2010) *Nat. Rev. Immunol.*, **10**, 317–327.
98. Huang, C. (2009) *Curr. Opin. Biotechnol.*, **20**, 692–699.
99. Jazayeri, J.A. and Carroll, G.J. (2008) *BioDrugs*, **22**, 11–26.
100. Binz, H.K., Amstutz, P., and Pluckthun, A. (2005) *Nat. Biotechnol.*, **23**, 1257–1268.
101. McGregor, D.P. (2008) *Curr. Opin. Pharmacol.*, **8**, 616–619.
102. Nelson, A.L. and Reichert, J.M. (2009) *Nat. Biotechnol.*, **27**, 331–337.
103. Ducharme, E. and Weinberg, J.M. (2008) *Expert Opin. Biol. Ther.*, **8**, 491–502.
104. Frampton, J.E. and Lyseng-Williamson, K.A. (2009) *Drugs*, **69**, 307–317.
105. Strober, B.E. and Menon, K. (2007) *Dermatol. Ther.*, **20**, 270–276.
106. Korhonen, R. and Moilanen, E. (2009) *Basic Clin. Pharmacol. Toxicol.*, **104**, 276–284.
107. Kim, J.K., Firan, M., Radu, C.G., Kim, C.H., Ghetie, V., and Ward, E.S. (1999) *Eur. J. Immunol.*, **29**, 2819–2825.
108. Suzuki, T., Ishii-Watabe, A., Tada, M., Kobayashi, T., Kanayasu-Toyoda, T., Kawanishi, T., and Yamaguchi, T. (2010) *J. Immunol.*, **184**, 1968–1976.
109. Dumont, J.A., Low, S.C., Peters, R.T., and Bitonti, A.J. (2006) *BioDrugs*, **20**, 151–160.
110. Bitonti, A.J., Dumont, J.A., Low, S.C., Peters, R.T., Kropp, K.E., Palombella, V.J., Stattel, J.M., Lu, Y., Tan, C.A., Song, J.J., Garcia, A.M., Simister, N.E., Spiekermann, G.M., Lencer, W.I., and Blumberg, R.S. (2004) *Proc. Natl. Acad. Sci. USA*, **101**, 9763–9768.
111. Peters, R.T., Low, S.C., Kamphaus, G.D., Dumont, J.A., Amari, J.V., Lu, Q., Zarbis-Papastoitsis, G., Reidy, T.J., Merricks, E.P., Nichols, T.C., and Bitonti, A.J. (2010) *Blood*, **115**, 2057–2064.
112. Kenanova, V., Olafsen, T., Crow, D.M., Sundaresan, G., Subbarayan, M., Carter, N.H., Ikle, D.N., Yazaki, P.J., Chatziioannou, A.F., Gambhir, S.S., Williams, L.E., Shively, J.E., Colcher, D., Raubitschek, A.A., and Wu, A.M. (2005) *Cancer Res.*, **65**, 622–631.
113. Dall'Acqua, W.F., Kiener, P.A., and Wu, H. (2006) *J. Biol. Chem.*, **281**, 23514–23524.
114. Hinton, P.R., Johlfs, M.G., Xiong, J.M., Hanestad, K., Ong, K.C., Bullock, C., Keller, S., Tang, M.T., Tso, J.Y., Vasquez, M., and Tsurushita, N. (2004) *J. Biol. Chem.*, **279**, 6213–6216.
115. Hinton, P.R., Xiong, J.M., Johlfs, M.G., Tang, M.T., Keller, S., and Tsurushita, N. (2006) *J. Immunol.*, **176**, 346–356.
116. Datta-Mannan, A., Witcher, D.R., Tang, Y., Watkins, J., and Wroblewski, V.J. (2007) *J. Biol. Chem.*, **282**, 1709–1717.
117. Datta-Mannan, A., Witcher, D.R., Tang, Y., Watkins, J., Jiang, W., and Wroblewski, V.J. (2007) *Drug Metab. Dispos.*, **35**, 86–94.
118. Petkova, S.B., Akilesh, S., Sproule, T.J., Christianson, G.J., Al Khabbaz, H., Brown, A.C., Presta, L.G., Meng, Y.G., and Roopenian, D.C. (2006) *Int. Immunol.*, **18**, 1759–1769.
119. Zalevsky, J., Chamberlain, A.K., Horton, H.M., Karki, S., Leung, I.W., Sproule, T.J., Lazar, G.A., Roopenian, D.C., and Desjarlais, J.R. (2010) *Nat. Biotechnol.*, **28**, 157–159.
120. Sesarman, A., Vidarsson, G., and Sitaru, C. (2010) *Cell Mol. Life Sci.*, **67**, 2533–2550.
121. Akilesh, S., Petkova, S., Sproule, T.J., Shaffer, D.J., Christianson, G.J., and Roopenian, D. (2004) *J. Clin. Invest.*, **113**, 1328–1333.
122. Li, N., Zhao, M., Hilario-Vargas, J., Prisayanh, P., Warren, S., Diaz, L.A., Roopenian, D.C., and Liu, Z. (2005) *J. Clin. Invest.*, **115**, 3440–3450.
123. Hansen, R.J. and Balthasar, J.P. (2002) *Thromb. Haemost.*, **88**, 898–899.
124. Jaggi, J.S., Carrasquillo, J.A., Seshan, S.V., Zanzonico, P., Henke, E., Nagel, A., Schwartz, J., Beattie, B., Kappel, B.J., Chattopadhyay, D., Xiao, J., Sgouros, G., Larson, S.M., and Scheinberg, D.A. (2007) *J. Clin. Invest.*, **117**, 2422–2430.

125. Vaccaro, C., Zhou, J., Ober, R.J., and Ward, E.S. (2005) *Nat. Biotechnol.*, **23**, 1283–1288.
126. Peters, T. Jr. (1985) *Adv. Protein Chem.*, **37**, 161–245.
127. Stehle, G., Sinn, H., Wunder, A., Schrenk, H.H., Stewart, J.C., Hartung, G., Maier-Borst, W., and Heene, D.L. (1997) *Crit. Rev. Oncol. Hematol.*, **26**, 77–100.
128. Bolling, C., Graefe, T., Lubbing, C., Jankevicius, F., Uktveris, S., Cesas, A., Meyer-Moldenhauer, W.H., Starkmann, H., Weigel, M., Burk, K., and Hanauske, A.R. (2006) *Invest. New Drugs*, **24**, 521–527.
129. Kratz, F., Abu Ajaj, K., and Warnecke, A. (2007) *Expert Opin. Invest. Drugs*, **16**, 1037–1058.
130. Wunder, A., Muller-Ladner, U., Stelzer, E.H., Funk, J., Neumann, E., Stehle, G., Pap, T., Sinn, H., Gay, S., and Fiehn, C. (2003) *J. Immunol.*, **170**, 4793–4801.
131. Miele, E., Spinelli, G.P., Tomao, F., and Tomao, S. (2009) *Int. J. Nanomed.*, **4**, 99–105.
132. Petrelli, F., Borgonovo, K., and Barni, S. (2010) *Expert Opin. Pharmacother.*, **11**, 1413–1432.
133. Giannoukakis, N. (2003) *Curr. Opin. Invest. Drugs*, **4**, 1245–1249.
134. Xie, D., Yao, C., Wang, L., Min, W., Xu, J., Xiao, J., Huang, M., Chen, B., Liu, B., Li, X., and Jiang, H. (2010) *Antimicrob. Agents Chemother.*, **54**, 191–196.
135. Schulte, S. (2009) *Thromb. Res.*, **124** (Suppl. 2), S6–S8.
136. Schulte, S. (2008) *Thromb. Res.*, **122** (Suppl. 4), S14–S19.
137. Weimer, T., Wormsbacher, W., Kronthaler, U., Lang, W., Liebing, U., and Schulte, S. (2008) *Thromb. Haemost.*, **99**, 659–667.
138. Chen, J.H., Zhang, X.G., Jiang, Y.T., Yan, L.Y., Tang, L., Yin, Y.W., Cheng, D.S., Chen, J., and Wang, M. (2010) *Cancer Immunol. Immunother.*, **59**, 1335–1345.
139. Yeh, C., Altaf, S.A., and Hoag, S.W. (1997) *Pharm. Res.*, **14**, 1161–1170.
140. Syed, S., Schuyler, P.D., Kulczycky, M., and Sheffield, W.P. (1997) *Blood*, **89**, 3243–3252.
141. Halpern, W., Riccobene, T.A., Agostini, H., Baker, K., Stolow, D., Gu, M.L., Hirsch, J., Mahoney, A., Carrell, J., Boyd, E., and Grzegorzewski, K.J. (2002) *Pharm. Res.*, **19**, 1720–1729.
142. Osborn, B.L., Sekut, L., Corcoran, M., Poortman, C., Sturm, B., Chen, G., Mather, D., Lin, H.L., and Parry, T.J. (2002) *Eur. J. Pharmacol.*, **456**, 149–158.
143. Duttaroy, A., Kanakaraj, P., Osborn, B.L., Schneider, H., Pickeral, O.K., Chen, C., Zhang, G., Kaithamana, S., Singh, M., Schulingkamp, R., Crossan, D., Bock, J., Kaufman, T.E., Reavey, P., Carey-Barber, M., Krishnan, S.R., Garcia, A., Murphy, K., Siskind, J.K., McLean, M.A., Cheng, S., Ruben, S., Birse, C.E., and Blondel, O. (2005) *Diabetes*, **54**, 251–258.
144. Bain, V.G., Kaita, K.D., Yoshida, E.M., Swain, M.G., Heathcote, E.J., Neumann, A.U., Fiscella, M., Yu, R., Osborn, B.L., Cronin, P.W., Freimuth, W.W., McHutchison, J.G., and Subramanian, G.M. (2006) *J. Hepatol.*, **44**, 671–678.
145. Subramanian, G.M., Fiscella, M., Lamouse-Smith, A., Zeuzem, S., and McHutchison, J.G. (2007) *Nat. Biotechnol.*, **25**, 1411–1419.
146. Sung, C., Nardelli, B., LaFleur, D.W., Blatter, E., Corcoran, M., Olsen, H.S., Birse, C.E., Pickeral, O.K., Zhang, J., Shah, D., Moody, G., Gentz, S., Beebe, L., and Moore, P.A. (2003) *J. Interferon Cytokine Res.*, **23**, 25–36.
147. Glue, P., Fang, J.W., Rouzier-Panis, R., Raffanel, C., Sabo, R., Gupta, S.K., Salfi, M., and Jacobs, S. (2000) *Clin. Pharmacol. Ther.*, **68**, 556–567.
148. Schrama, D., Reisfeld, R.A., and Becker, J.C. (2006) *Nat. Rev. Drug Discov.*, **5**, 147–159.
149. Chapman, A.P., Antoniw, P., Spitali, M., West, S., Stephens, S., and King, D.J. (1999) *Nat. Biotechnol.*, **17**, 780–783.
150. Smith, B.J., Popplewell, A., Athwal, D., Chapman, A.P., Heywood, S., West, S.M., Carrington, B., Nesbitt, A.,

Lawson, A.D., Antoniw, P., Eddelston, A., and Suitters, A. (2001) *Bioconjug. Chem.*, **12**, 750–756.

151. Muller, D. and Kontermann, R.E. (2007) *Curr. Opin. Mol. Ther.*, **9**, 319–326.

152. Muller, D., Karle, A., Meissburger, B., Hofig, I., Stork, R., and Kontermann, R.E. (2007) *J. Biol. Chem.*, **282**, 12650–12660.

153. Yazaki, P.J., Kassa, T., Cheung, C.W., Crow, D.M., Sherman, M.A., Bading, J.R., Anderson, A.L., Colcher, D., and Raubitschek, A. (2008) *Nucl. Med. Biol.*, **35**, 151–158.

154. Klein, O., Lynge, J., Endahl, L., Damholt, B., Nosek, L., and Heise, T. (2007) *Diabetes Obes. Metab.*, **9**, 290–299.

155. Koehler, M.F., Zobel, K., Beresini, M.H., Caris, L.D., Combs, D., Paasch, B.D., and Lazarus, R.A. (2002) *Bioorg. Med. Chem. Lett.*, **12**, 2883–2886.

156. Zobel, K., Koehler, M.F., Beresini, M.H., Caris, L.D., and Combs, D. (2003) *Bioorg. Med. Chem. Lett.*, **13**, 1513–1515.

157. Hermansen, K., Davies, M., Derezinski, T., Martinez Ravn, G., Clauson, P., and Home, P. (2006) *Diabetes Care*, **29**, 1269–1274.

158. Home, P. and Kurtzhals, P. (2006) *Expert Opin. Pharmacother.*, **7**, 325–343.

159. Trussel, S., Dumelin, C., Frey, K., Villa, A., Buller, F., and Neri, D. (2009) *Bioconjug. Chem.*, **20**, 2286–2292.

160. Holt, L.J., Basran, A., Jones, K., Chorlton, J., Jespers, L.S., Brewis, N.D., and Tomlinson, I.M. (2008) *Protein Eng. Des. Sel.*, **21**, 283–288.

161. Walker, A., Dunlevy, G., Rycroft, D., Topley, P., Holt, L.J., Herbert, T., Davies, M., Cook, F., Holmes, S., Jespers, L., and Herring, C. (2010) *Protein Eng. Des. Sel.*, **23**, 271–278.

162. Dennis, M.S., Zhang, M., Meng, Y.G., Kadkhodayan, M., Kirchhofer, D., Combs, D., and Damico, L.A. (2002) *J. Biol. Chem.*, **277**, 35035–35043.

163. Nguyen, A., Reyes, A.E. II, Zhang, M., McDonald, P., Wong, W.L., Damico, L.A., and Dennis, M.S. (2006) *Protein Eng. Des. Sel.*, **19**, 291–297.

164. Dennis, M.S., Jin, H., Dugger, D., Yang, R., McFarland, L., Ogasawara, A., Williams, S., Cole, M.J., Ross, S., and Schwall, R. (2007) *Cancer Res.*, **67**, 254–261.

165. Wu, A.M. and Senter, P.D. (2005) *Nat. Biotechnol.*, **23**, 1137–1146.

166. Schlapschy, M., Theobald, I., Mack, H., Schottelius, M., Wester, H.J., and Skerra, A. (2007) *Protein Eng. Des. Sel.*, **20**, 273–284.

167. Stork, R., Muller, D., and Kontermann, R.E. (2007) *Protein Eng. Des. Sel.*, **20**, 569–576.

168. Stork, R., Campigna, E., Robert, B., Muller, D., and Kontermann, R.E. (2009) *J. Biol. Chem.*, **284**, 25612–25619.

169. Tolmachev, V., Orlova, A., Pehrson, R., Galli, J., Baastrup, B., Andersson, K., Sandstrom, M., Rosik, D., Carlsson, J., Lundqvist, H., Wennborg, A., and Nilsson, F.Y. (2007) *Cancer Res.*, **67**, 2773–2782.

170. Nord, K., Gunneriusson, E., Ringdahl, J., Stahl, S., Uhlen, M., and Nygren, P.A. (1997) *Nat. Biotechnol.*, **15**, 772–777.

171. Johansson, M.U., Frick, I.M., Nilsson, H., Kraulis, P.J., Hober, S., Jonasson, P., Linhult, M., Nygren, P.A., Uhlen, M., Bjorck, L., Drakenberg, T., Forsen, S., and Wikstrom, M. (2002) *J. Biol. Chem.*, **277**, 8114–8120.

172. Lejon, S., Frick, I.M., Bjorck, L., Wikstrom, M., and Svensson, S. (2004) *J. Biol. Chem.*, **279**, 42924–42928.

173. Andersen, J.T., Pehrson, R., Tolmachev, V., Bekele, M.D., Abrahmsen, L., and Ekblad, C. (2011) *J. Biol. Chem.*, **286**, 5234–5241.

174. Linhult, M., Binz, H.K., Uhlen, M., and Hober, S. (2002) *Protein Sci.*, **11**, 206–213.

175. Kohler, G. and Milstein, C. (1975) *Nature*, **256**, 495–497.

176. Reichert, J.M. (2001) *Nat. Biotechnol.*, **19**, 819–822.

177. Boulianne, G.L., Hozumi, N., and Shulman, M.J. (1984) *Nature*, **312**, 643–646.

178. Jones, P.T., Dear, P.H., Foote, J., Neuberger, M.S., and Winter, G. (1986) *Nature*, **321**, 522–525.
179. Ober, R.J., Radu, C.G., Ghetie, V., and Ward, E.S. (2001) *Int. Immunol.*, **13**, 1551–1559.
180. Zhou, J., Mateos, F., Ober, R.J., and Ward, E.S. (2005) *J. Mol. Biol.*, **345**, 1071–1081.
181. Zhou, J., Pop, L.M., and Ghetie, V. (2005) *Lupus*, **14**, 458–466.

5
Development of Cancer-Targeting Ligands and Ligand–Drug Conjugates
Ruiwu Liu, Kai Xiao, Juntao Luo, and Kit S. Lam

5.1
Introduction

Cytotoxic chemotherapy is effective against some cancers, but is very toxic and cancer patients receiving such drugs often experience significant side-effects, such as neutropenia, thrombocytopenia, anemia, nausea, and vomiting. Some chemotherapeutic drugs can also elicit additional organ-specific major side-effects. For example, cardiomyopathy can result from doxorubicin (DOX), pulmonary fibrosis from bleomycin, renal failure from cisplatin, and peripheral neuropathy from vincristine or paclitaxel. In the last decade, many new drugs have been approved by the US Food and Drug Administration (FDA) for cancer treatment. Some of these drugs are small molecules that aim at specific molecular targets such as imatinib against Bcr–Abl tyrosine kinase in chronic myelogenic leukemia, erlotinib against epidermal growth factor receptor (EGFR) tyrosine kinase, sorafenib against RAF kinase and the vascular endothelial growth factor receptor (VEGFR) 2/platelet-derived growth factor receptor-β signaling cascade, and bortezomib against proteasome and the NF-κB pathway. While clinically useful, the duration of clinical response for many of these drugs is rather short lasting and resistant tumor cells often emerge. Some other newer drugs are monoclonal antibodies (mAbs) that target cancer cell surface receptors. The antitumor effects of some of these antibodies (e.g., anti-EGFR or anti-HER2/*neu*) are probably due to the blockage of the promitogenic function of circulating growth factors. Some of these antibodies (e.g., anti-CD20) inhibit tumor growth through antibody-dependent cellular cytotoxicity effects. Others use cell surface targeting antibody as a vehicle to deliver radionuclides (e.g., Zevalin® or Bexxar®, anti-CD20 antibody loaded with ^{90}Y or ^{131}I, respectively), toxin (e.g., Mylotarg®, anti-CD33 antibody conjugated to calicheamicin), or cytotoxic chemotherapeutic agents to the cancer cells. Cancer-targeting antibodies utilizing this latter mechanism are problematic because (i) antibodies to the cancer cells have difficulty infiltrating the entire tumor mass due their large size (MW $\sim$ 160 000) and (ii) the Fc region of the antibody binds to the reticuloendothelial system, resulting in high uptake of radionuclides, cytotoxic drugs, or toxins into bone marrow, liver, and spleen, leading to severe toxicities. To overcome these problems,

Drug Delivery in Oncology: From Basic Research to Cancer Therapy, First Edition.
Edited by Felix Kratz, Peter Senter, and Henning Steinhagen.
© 2012 Wiley-VCH Verlag GmbH & Co. KGaA. Published 2012 by Wiley-VCH Verlag GmbH & Co. KGaA.

many investigators are exploring the use of antibody fragments or smaller antibody constructs such as the minibody and diabody [1, 2].

Peptides, peptidomimetics, or small molecules are alternative and possibly more effective targeting agents against cancer. These molecules are smaller (MW < 1500), chemically stable, easy to synthesize in large scale, and can be readily conjugated to radionuclides, cytotoxic drugs, or toxins. Peptides that are N- and C-terminally blocked, cyclized, and/or contain D-amino acid and unnatural amino acids are generally very stable to proteolysis. They could serve as efficient vehicles to deliver high-dose toxic therapeutic payloads to the tumor site while sparing normal tissues. Therapeutic indices of these targeting drug conjugates are expected to be significantly higher than those of corresponding free-circulating drugs. In this chapter, we shall discuss the development of such cancer cell surface-targeting ligand–drug conjugates for cancer therapy.

5.2
Overview of Cancer-Targeting Ligand–Drug Conjugates

Cytotoxic chemotherapeutic agents, despite their toxic side-effects, have been useful for the treatment of many cancers. Cancer recurrence after such treatments is due to the emergence of drug-resistant cells or the presence of drug-resistant cancer stem cells. In refractory leukemia and lymphoma, the only curative option for most patients is hematopoietic stem cell transplantation in which the patient will receive a very high dose of chemotherapy (melphalan, cytoxan, or thiotepa) with or without radiation, followed by hematopoietic stem cell infusion 24–72 h later. A fraction of these patients do enjoy long-term survival of their diseases. However, this treatment is extremely toxic and some patients can die from the treatment. In principle, if the highly toxic chemotherapeutic drugs can be delivered systematically at high level to all tumor sites while sparing normal tissues, particularly the bone marrow, more patients will be cured. Such differential delivery of cancer drugs to the tumor sites can potentially be achieved with cancer-targeting ligand–drug conjugates. Figure 5.1 summarizes the design of many of such conjugates, which comprise of the tumor-targeting ligand covalently attached to the therapeutic payload via a linker. These targeting ligand–drug conjugates can be considered as a unique class of prodrug that can be delivered to and activated at the tumor site or inside the tumor cells where the active anticancer drugs are released to exert their antitumor effects.

The tumor-targeting ligands generally target one of the following three sites: (i) cancer cell surface receptors, (ii) tumor endothelial cell surface receptors, and (iii) the tumor's extracellular matrix. These ligands can be proteins, peptides, glycopeptides, peptidomimetics, small molecules, or nucleic acid aptamers. The most common protein targeting ligands are mAbs, which target specific tumor-associated proteins on the tumor cell surface. Cytokines (e.g., interleukin (IL)-2) and growth factors are examples of other protein-targeting ligands. Peptides are attractive alternative cancer-targeting ligands. There are numerous known

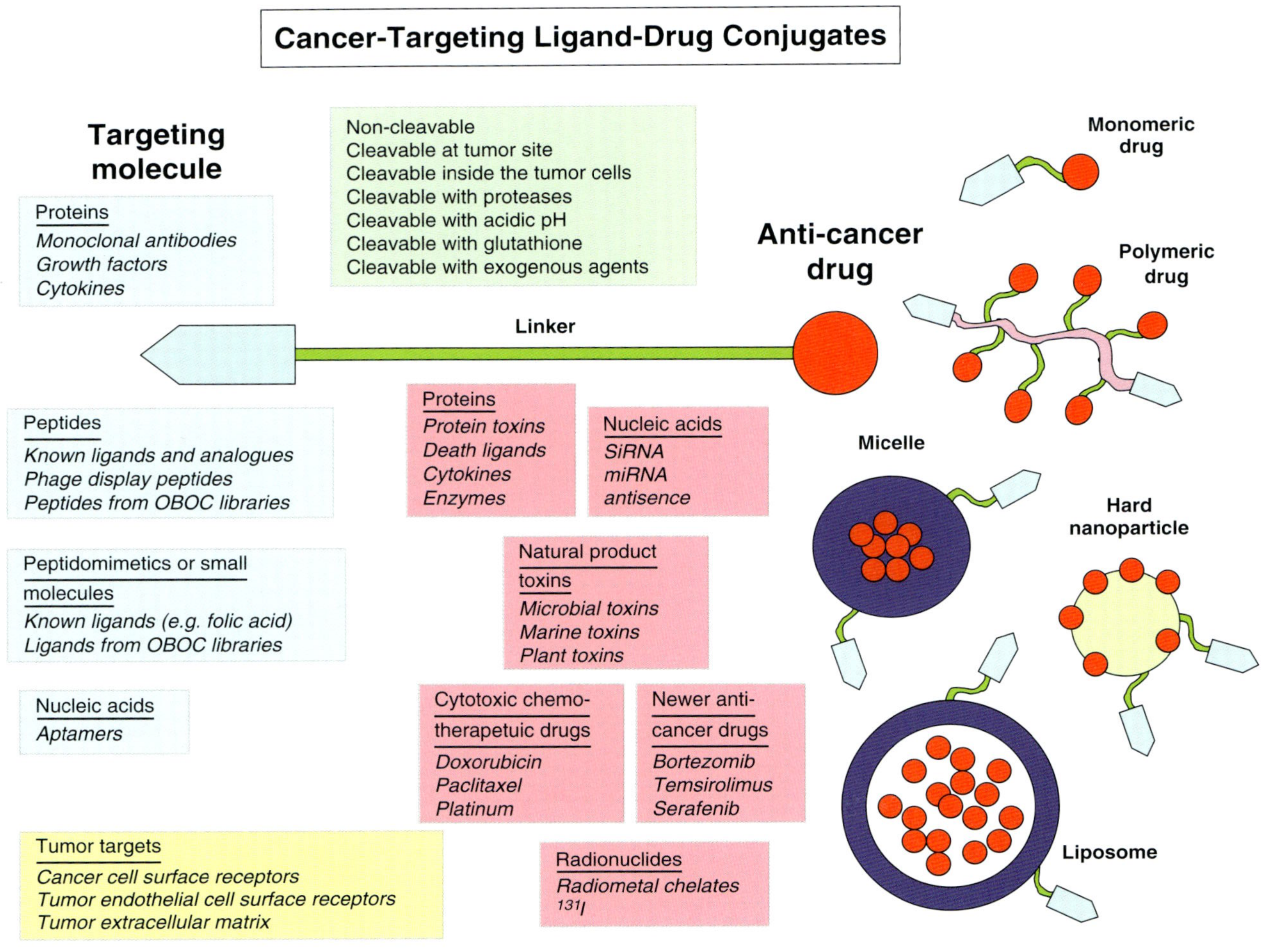

5.2 Overview of Cancer-Targeting Ligand–Drug Conjugates

Cancer-Targeting Ligand-Drug Conjugates

Targeting molecule

Proteins
Monoclonal antibodies
Growth factors
Cytokines

Peptides
Known ligands and analogues
Phage display peptides
Peptides from OBOC libraries

Peptidomimetics or small molecules
Known ligands (e.g. folic acid)
Ligands from OBOC libraries

Nucleic acids
Aptamers

Linker

Non-cleavable
Cleavable at tumor site
Cleavable inside the tumor cells
Cleavable with proteases
Cleavable with acidic pH
Cleavable with glutathione
Cleavable with exogenous agents

Anti-cancer drug

Proteins
Protein toxins
Death ligands
Cytokines
Enzymes

Nucleic acids
SiRNA
miRNA
antisense

Natural product toxins
Microbial toxins
Marine toxins
Plant toxins

Cytotoxic chemo-therapeutic drugs
Doxorubicin
Paclitaxel
Platinum

Newer anti-cancer drugs
Bortezomib
Temsirolimus
Serafenib

Radionuclides
Radiometal chelates
131I

Tumor targets
Cancer cell surface receptors
Tumor endothelial cell surface receptors
Tumor extracellular matrix

Monomeric drug
Polymeric drug
Hard nanoparticle
Micelle
Liposome

Figure 5.1 Summary of various cancer-targeting ligand–drug conjugates.

peptide hormones, some of which have already been used for cancer targeting. For example, octreotide, a cyclic octapeptide analog of somatostatin (SST), has been used for radiotargeting of neuroendocrine tumor [3]. More recently, AN-152, a linear peptide analog of luteinizing hormone-releasing hormone (LHRH; also known as gonadotropin-releasing hormone), has been used to target ovarian cancer, breast cancer, and prostate cancer [4]. Cancer-targeting peptides can also be discovered by using live cancer cells as probes to screen phage-display or one-bead/one-compound (OBOC) combinatorial peptide libraries. These methods will be detailed in Section 5.3. Naturally occurring small molecules such as folic acid have also been used as delivery vehicles for many cancer types. Since the OBOC method is synthetic-based, it can also be used to discover small molecules, peptidomimetics, and macrocyclic molecules for cancer targeting. Another class of targeting molecule is the nucleic acid aptamers developed through systematic evolution of ligands by exponential enrichment (SELEX) [5].

The linker that covalently joins the targeting molecule and the therapeutic payload together can be either cleavable or noncleavable. Many linkers cleavable under various conditions have been developed. Some take advantage of the reductive and acidic condition at the tumor site or inside the tumor cells. Some are labile to enzymes such as esterases and specific proteases at the tumor site or inside the tumor cells. Some are susceptible to cleavage by exogenous chemicals or enzymes given intravenously on-demand at the desired time.

Regarding therapeutic payload, many different drugs are possible. These include protein drugs such as *Pseudomonas* toxin, Fas ligand, cytokines, and enzymes. Others are highly potent small-molecule or natural product toxins such as duocarmycin A and calicheamicin. Standard chemotherapeutic drugs have also been used; however, because of their modest potency, often more than one drug molecule is needed per drug conjugate, as the polymeric drug conjugates illustrate. To further increase the quantity of therapeutic payload per drug conjugate, drugs can be loaded into nanoparticles such as liposomes, micelles, and dendrimers. In addition to the standard cytotoxic chemotherapeutic agents, newer and more target-specific cancer drugs such as bortezomib (a proteasome inhibitor), temsirolimus (a mammalian target of rapamycin (mTOR) inhibitor), and sorafenib (a protein kinase inhibitor) can also be readily packaged into micelles for cancer therapy. One unique therapeutic payload involves the antibody-directed enzyme prodrug therapy (ADEPT) in which the antibody delivers an exogenous enzyme to the tumor site after which a small-molecule prodrug is administered systemically. The small-molecule prodrug will then be activated at the tumor site by the targeted enzyme for its anticancer effects. Radionuclides such as ^{131}I and ^{90}Y have been used as therapeutic payloads in radioimmunotherapy [6] or in peptide-mediated radiotherapy [7]. In recent years, short nucleic acid molecules such as small interfering RNA and microRNA have been recognized as potential highly specific therapeutics for cancer. The major hurdle, however, is to be able to deliver these RNA molecules into the target cells efficiently.

5.3
Cancer-Targeting Ligands

5.3.1
Introduction

As already mentioned, cancer-targeting ligands can be peptides, glycopeptides, peptidomimetics, small molecules, proteins, nucleic acid aptamers, and antibodies. Many of these targeting molecules can be developed through (i) the use of native ligands or their analogs such as octreotide against SST receptor, bradykinin analogs against bradykinin receptor, AN-152 against LHRH receptor, and folic acid against the folate receptor, (ii) molecular modeling if the X-ray structure of the cancer-associated receptor or related receptor is known, and/or (iii) screening combinatorial libraries.

The combinatorial library method is an enabling tool that allows efficient identification of targeting ligands against known or unknown cancer-associated receptors. Of the six combinatorial methods reported so far [8], the biological library method (e.g., phage-display library) and the OBOC library method are the two most popular approaches that have been successfully applied to the discovery of cancer-targeting ligands. Both of these methods use cancer-related proteins or live cancer cells as the screening probes. Library screening with living cells has several advantages: (i) the cell surface receptors are presented in their native conformation; (ii) cloning, expression, and purification of membrane-bound targets are not needed; (iii) ligands for binding and/or internalization into the cells can be identified, selection of a cell surface binding phage as opposed to an internalized phage can be accomplished by modifying the washing techniques, and endocytic ligands can be identified from an OBOC library with a cleavable linker; (iv) the cell surface target can be an unknown receptor; and (v) functional ligands that elicit downstream signaling can be readily identified, particularly with the OBOC method.

5.3.2
Phage-Display Library Approach

Bacteriophages (phages) are single-stranded DNA viruses that infect bacteria. In 1985, Smith first developed the "fusion phage" by inserting foreign DNA fragments into the encoding gene of the pIII protein [9]. About five copies of the pIII protein are displayed on the infectious end of the virus. This technology enables the expression of protein or L-amino acid-containing peptide on the virion surface without affecting the viral infectivity. A phage-display library is comprised of a heterogeneous mixture of phage clones, each carrying a different foreign DNA insert and therefore displaying a different peptide or protein on its surface. The M13 phage is the most widely used phage-display system because it has a high capacity for replication and is able to receive large DNA inserts into its genome. Phage-display technology is a very efficient approach to generate large numbers of diverse peptides and proteins, presented as fusion proteins on the viral capsid. The use of phage-displayed peptide libraries to develop tumor-targeting ligands has been extensively reviewed [8, 10, 11].

The phage-display library method has several advantages: (i) it can display combinatorial protein (e.g., antibody, protein domain) or peptide libraries; (ii) the size of the grafted peptide or protein is not limited by the constraints of synthetic chemistry, as in the case of the synthetic peptide library; (iii) it can take advantage of known protein folds (e.g., zinc-finger fold, immunoglobulin fold, or conotoxin fold) by grafting random oligopeptides on such tertiary folds; (iv) the method is highly efficient, inexpensive, amenable to both short and long peptides, linear and simple cyclic peptides (disulfide formation with two L-cysteines), and can be carried out in most molecular biology laboratories; (v) phage-display peptide libraries are commercially available; and (vi) phage-displayed libraries can be screened with *in vivo* selection techniques in xenograft models or in human cancer patients. However, despite of the many advantages, this biologic library approach suffers some important limitations: (i) only the natural L-amino acid peptide libraries (comprised of 20 eukaryotic amino acids) can be incorporated into the phages (such peptides are generally susceptible to proteolysis particularly if the N- and C-termini are not blocked); (ii) screening assays of the phage-display libraries are generally limited to the binding assays (e.g., biopanning) and some functional assays such as protease substrate determination; (iii) complicated bicyclic, compact scaffolding, branched structures, or molecules with special cyclization chemistry are impossible with this method; and (iv) optimizing a phage-display peptide into a proteolytic stable molecule while still retaining a high binding activity and specificity to the cell surface receptor is not trivial.

Phage-display libraries are commercially available, such as Ph.D.-7, Ph.D.-12, and Ph.D.-C7C (cyclic with a disulfide bond) libraries that can be purchased from New England Biolabs (Ipswich, MA). The Ph.D.-12 library is based on a combinatorial library of random dodecapeptides fused to a minor coat protein (pIII) of M13 phage. The displayed peptide (12mer) is expressed at the N-terminus of pIII (i.e., the first residue of the mature protein is the first randomized position). The peptide is followed by a short spacer (-GGGS-) and then the wild-type pIII sequence. The library consists of approximately 2.7×10^9 unique phages. Phage-display libraries can also be constructed according to different needs. Shukla and Krag recently reported a new kind of phage-display library in which the linear or cysteine-constrained random peptides were fused, at their N-termini, to a catalytically active P99 β-lactamase (β-lactam hydrolase, EC 3.5.2.6) [12]. Using this system, several cancer cell-specific binding and internalizing β-lactamase–peptide fusion ligands were isolated by screening these libraries against live BT-474 human breast cancer cells. β-Lactamase is an excellent reporter that helps the tracking of fusion peptide ligands in their cell binding and internalizing screenings. The β-lactamase fusion made the whole process of clone screening simple yet efficient. The β-lactamase–peptide ligands selected from such libraries do not require peptide synthesis and modifications. Such ligands have a potential for their direct use in targeted enzyme prodrug therapy as well as targeted delivery of chemotherapeutic agents. This is the first report on the selection of cell-internalized enzyme conjugates using phage-display technology.

5.3.2.1 Phage-Display Library Screening and Decoding

The process of selecting phage clones that bind a specific target is called "biopanning." A step-by-step screening protocol can be found in an article written by Kay et al. [13]. There are several factors that need to be taken into account when screening phage-display libraries: the number of phages used, stringency of selection process, competitive selection, and subtractive panning. The four general methods for targeting ligand discovery via screening phage-display libraries are [14]:

In vitro selection: a phage-displayed peptide or antibody library is incubated with purified protein of interest or live cancer cell lines.

In vivo selection in mouse: phages are injected to xenograft mouse models, transgenic or other clinically relevant models.

In vivo selection from cancer patients: in this case, patients with late stage cancers are infused with random phage-display peptide or antibody library in either a single or multiple panning experiments.

Ex vivo selection: dissociated cells obtained from biopsy lesions are used for *ex vivo* panning.

In principle, phage-display libraries can also be screened by perfusing isolated organs or tumors through the big vessels in a much more controlled fashion, such as adding high concentration of blocking agents against certain receptors, and in the absence of blood cells or plasma. Among these methods, *in vitro* screening of phage-displayed libraries with live cancer cells is the most popular approach to identify cancer-targeting peptides or antibodies. In order to achieve high binding specificity, several rounds of selection are needed. After several round of biopanning, captured phages are cloned so that the displayed peptides responsible for binding can be studied individually. The amino acid sequence of the peptide can be easily obtained (via the genetic code) by sequencing of the viral DNA.

5.3.2.2 Examples

Phage-display antibody and peptide libraries have been widely used in targeting ligand selection for a variety of tumor types: breast, lung, osteosarcomas, pancreatic ductal adenocarcinomas, thyroid, head and neck, squamous cell carcinomas (SCCs), liver, prostate, bladder, colon, and gastric cancers. Here, we will focus on peptide ligands identified using the phage-display library approach. Unbiased biopanning of phage-displayed peptide libraries has yielded a myriad of peptides that bind cancer cells and cancer-associated antigens. Examples of some of these peptide ligands are shown in Table 5.1.

5.3.2.2.1 *In Vitro* **Selection of Tumor Cell-Targeting Phages (Ligands)** Phage-display technology has been widely used for *in vitro* selection of cancer-targeting ligands via screening phage-display peptide libraries against cancer cells (Table 5.1). For

Table 5.1 Examples of cancer-targeting peptides identified by the phage-display library method [8].

	Ligand sequence	Phage selection[a]
Ligands to specific tumor cells		
Melanoma patient [15]	MRIRCAAAWRATGTHCSLRA	c
Breast cancer patient [15]	GSPQCPGGFNCPRCDCGAGY	c
Breast cancer	ASANPFPTKALL [16]	b
	CASPSGALRSC (internalized) [17]	
Squamous cell carcinoma	CDTRL, CGKRK	d → b
Lung cancer	EHMALTYPFRPP (ZS-1) [18]	a
	TDSILRSYDWTY (SP5-2) [19]	
Bladder cancer	CXNXDXR(X)/(R)C, CSNRDARRC	a
Neuroblastoma [20]	HLQIQPWYPQIS, VPWMEPAYQRFL	a
Medullary thyroid cancer	SRESPHP	b
Pancreatic islet cell carcinoma [21]	CRSRKG, CKAAKNK, CRGRRST	d → b
Colon carcinoma	VHLGYAT	a
Invasive colon cancer	CPIEDRPMC	a
Hepatocellular carcinoma [22]	FLLEPHLMDTSM, FQHPSFI	a
LNCaP prostate cancer	DPRATPGS	a
CEN-1 human nasopharyngeal carcinoma [23]	EDIKPKTSLAFR	b
Head and neck carcinoma	SPRGDLAVLGHKY (HBP1) [24]	a
	CRGDLASLC (Peptide-29) [25]	
Ligands to specific proteins		
B-cell-associated immunoglobulin [26]	AIMASGQWL, QILASGRWL, LVRSTGQFV, LVSPSGSWT, ALRPSGEWL, RRPSHAMAR	a
$\alpha_5\beta_1$	GACRGDCLGA	a
$\alpha_6\beta_1$	FGRIPSPLAYTYSFR, HRWMPHVFAVRQGAS, VSWFSRHRYSPFAVS	a
$\alpha_v\beta_6$ [25]	CRGDLASLC (peptide-29)	a
$\alpha_v\beta_3$ [27]	CDCRGDCFC (RGD-4C)	b
CD-21	GRVPSMFGGHFFFSR, RMWPSSTVNLSAGRR, PNLDFSPTCSFRFGC	a
VEGFR1	ASSSYPLIHWRPWAR, ATWLPPR	a
IgM λ receptor of the human Burkitt lymphoma cell line SUP-B8 [28]	KNGPWYAYTGRO, NWAVWXKR, YXXEDLRRR, XXPVDHGL	a
Fibroblast growth factor receptor	AESGDDYCVLVFTDSAWTKICDWSHFRN	a
Aminopeptidase P	CPGPEGAGC	b
hVEGFR3 [29]	CSDSWHYWC (P1)	a
Galectin-3 [30]	ANTPCGPYTHDCPVKR (G3-C12)	b
E-selectin [31]	IELLQAR	a

Table 5.1 (continued).

	Ligand sequence	Phage selection[a]
Ligands to vasculature		
Angiogenic vessel-homing peptide (B16BL6 melanoma, Meth A sarcoma) [32]	APRPG, PRPGAPLAGSWPGTS, DRWRPALPVVLFPLH, ASSSYPLIHWRPWAR	b
Vasculature of various tumors (carcinoma, sarcoma, and melanoma) [27]	CDCRGDCFC (RGD-4C), CNGRCVSGCAGRC	b
Vasculature of human colon cancer [33]	CPHSKPCLC	b
Vasculature of human gastric cancer [34]	CGNNSNPKSC (GX1)	b
Vasculature in the angiogenic stages of pancreatic islet carcinogenesis [21]	CRSRKG, CKAAKNK, CRGRRST	d → b

[a] a, *in vitro* selection; b, *in vivo* selection from xenograft model; c, *in vivo* selection from cancer patients; d, *ex vivo* selection.

example, Tu *et al.* recently reported the discovery of a peptide, ZT-1 (sequence QQMHLMSYAPGP), that specifically targeted NCI-H1299 cells (non-small-cell lung cancer (NSCLC) cell line) using phage-display technology [35]. In their study, the NCI-H1299 and the normal lung small airway epithelial cell lines were used for subtractive screening *in vitro* with a phage-display 12mer peptide library. After three rounds of panning, a group of peptides capable of binding specifically to NCI-H1299 cells was obtained, and the affinity of these peptides bind to the targeted cells and tissues was studied. Through cell-based enzyme-linked immunosorbent assay (ELISA), immunocytochemical staining, immunohistochemical staining, and immunofluorescence, an M13 phage displaying ZT-1 peptide was isolated. ZT-1 was found to bind to NCI-H1299 and A549 lung cancer cells and biopsy specimens, but not to normal lung tissue samples, other cancer cells, or nontumor adjacent lung tissues. In another study, Lee *et al.* screened a Ph.D.-C7C (cyclic with a disulfide bond) with cells isolated from a human bladder cancer (HT-1376) xenograft [36]. The selected peptide "CSNRDARRC" was able to bind to bladder cancer cells isolated from a xenograft tumor and carcinogen-induced bladder tumors, but not to normal mouse bladder cells, human umbilical vein endothelial cells, or normal rat kidney cells. Selectivity of this peptide for tumor cells was also validated by testing primary tissue samples from patients with urothelial tumors. This peptide was also found to bind to exfoliated cells isolated from the urine of bladder cancer patient.

In vitro screening of phage-displayed peptide libraries has also been used to identify ligands that bind cancer-associated proteins (Table 5.1). For example,

Qin et al. reported the identification of a novel peptide ligand P1 (CSDSWHYWC) of hVEGFR3 via *in vitro* selection [29]. VEGFR3 is upregulated in a variety of human cancers and is a potentially rational target for drug delivery. A total of three successive rounds of panning with hVEGFR3 ectodomain Fc fusion protein were performed with a random Ph.D.-C7C library. The phage-display peptide P1 exhibited the highest affinity to VEGFR3 in phage ELISA. Peptide P1 could bind to VEGFR3 and to VEGFR3-positive carcinoma cells with high specificity.

5.3.2.2.2 *In Vivo* Selection of Tumor-Targeting Phages (Ligands) Using Xenograft Models *In vitro* screening of phage-display libraries has yielded numerous binding peptides against many different cell lines, but few of them have been demonstrated to have good *in vivo* targeting efficacy. Some investigators believe that *in vivo* panning of phage-display libraries in tumor-bearing animals may lead to peptides with optimal stability and targeting properties *in vivo*. A notable success of this approach is the identification of vascular-targeting peptides (see Table 5.1), such as those with an RGD motif that bind $\alpha_v\beta_3$ integrin, via *in vivo* selections. The success may be due to the abundance and expression patterns of integrins in tumors and supporting vasculature. In a recent *in vivo* selection study, Du et al. identified a hepatocarcinoma-specific binding peptide from a hepatocellular carcinoma BEL-7402 xenograft [37]. After three rounds of biopanning, a dipeptide motif of Pro–Ser was found. Of all the 130 clones tested, phage A54 (sequence AGKGTPSLETTP) was found to have the highest binding affinity and specificity against liver cancer cells. *In vivo* biodistribution studies of A54 in xenograft-bearing mice demonstrated phage enrichment in tumor tissues and normal liver. In *in vivo* therapeutic studies, mice treated with A54 peptide–DOX resulted in tumor reduction and prolonged survival, when compared to mice treated with free DOX.

Recently, Ruoshlahti et al. reported *in vivo* screening of cyclic peptide phage-display libraries with a transgenic mouse model of SCC [14]. Unlike a xenograft model in which the tumor is comprised of human tumor cells and host blood vessels and extracellular matrix, the transgenic model is spontaneous and the entire tumor, including tumor blood vessels, is of murine origin. One peptide, CSRPRRSEC, was found to bind specifically to dysplastic/premalignant skin lesions. Two other peptides, CGKRK and CDTRL, were found to bind to malignant SCC tumors. In order to optimize clinical phage screening techniques, Kolonin et al. developed a new *in vivo* phage screening technique named "synchronous selection" [38]. In this method, biopanning for multiple organs was done simultaneously and the data subjected to complex statistical analysis to identify tripeptide motifs that bind selectively to each organ. Newton et al. described a different *in vivo* selection approach termed the "micropanning assay" to select for phages that extravasate and bind human PC3 prostate carcinoma xenografts in SCID mice [39]. This assay is able to distinguish phage with high affinity for prostate tumor tissues/heterotransplanted cell lines relative to normal host tissues. The isolated phage clone (G-1) with the sequence "IAGLATPGWSHWLAL" was fluorescently labeled with near-IR fluorescent dye AlexaFluor® 680, and was demonstrated to be able to bind to PC3 cells *in vitro* and to target PC3 xenograft *in vivo*.

5.3.2.2.3 *In Vivo* **Selection of Phages (Ligands) in Patients with Cancers** Direct screening of phage-displayed peptide libraries in patients may allow the identification of ligands that target biochemical differences in the endothelium of blood vessels. In 2006, Krag *et al.* published a phase I clinical report of bacteriophage library infusions in human cancer patients [15]. Eight patients with late-stage breast, melanoma, and pancreatic cancer were infused with random phage-display peptide libraries or phage-display short-chain Fv antibodies in either a single or multiple *in vivo* panning experiments. No serious side-effects, including allergic reactions, were observed with up to three infusions. In one of the breast cancer patients, one of the peptides identified, GSPQCPGGFNCPRCDCGAGY, occurred with very high frequency. One peptide clone with the sequence MRIRCAAAWRATGTHCSLRA identified from a melanoma patient appeared to be specific to that individual patient's tumor, but did not bind human melanocytes and other melanoma cell lines except for weak binding to SK-MEL-5 melanoma cell line. This peptide shares a significant motif with human multiple EGF-like domain protein 7. This *in vivo* human experiment has demonstrated the feasibility of phage panning in cancer patients for the identification of customized patient tumor-binding ligands, leading to "personalized" therapeutics. However, performing pharmacology–toxicology studies on each peptide isolated for each patient will pose tremendous cost as well as logistic and regulatory problems.

In another phage-display peptide library panning experiment performed in a patient, Zurita *et al.* identified a mimic motif of IL-11 from prostate biopsies [40]. The IL-11 peptide mimic (cyclic nonapeptide CGRRAGGSC) bound specifically to a corresponding IL-11 receptor (IL $-$ 11Rα) which is a potential therapeutic target for human prostate cancer. When linked to a proapoptotic peptide, CGRRAGGSC, the peptide was able to induce dose-dependent apoptosis in an IL-11Rα-positive cell line. Their results illustrate the ability of direct combinatorial screening systems in cancer patients for identification of relevant targets in the context of human diseases.

5.3.2.2.4 *Ex Vivo* **Selection of Tumor-Binding Phages (Ligands)** Screening of phage-displayed libraries with dissociated cells obtained from biopsy lesions has been referred as *ex vivo* biopanning [14]. Phage-display peptide libraries have been used for *ex vivo* selection of tumor-binding ligands. Maruta *et al.* reported an *ex vivo*, intra-arterial method for biopanning in freshly resected human tumors, enabling reiterative selection of oligopeptide sequences capable of intravascular targeting to human colorectal tumors [41]. Significant consensus was observed after two rounds of panning in tumors from different patients and lead sequences demonstrated tumor targeting in samples from unrelated patients.

5.3.3
OBOC Combinatorial Library Approach

An OBOC library is comprised of a large number of compound-beads that can be generated concurrently by a "split-mix" synthesis method [42]. Each 80- to

100-μm bead displays only one chemical entity, but contains approximately 100 pmol of the same compound. The length of the amino acid chain in the peptide library and the number of amino acids used in each coupling cycle determine the permutation or diversity that can exist within the library. For example, a hexamer peptide library synthesized with 30 possible amino acids in each position has 30^5 or 2.43×10^7 permutations. Lam et al. first reported the OBOC technology in 1991 that involved short linear peptide libraries [42]; since then, the technology has been expanded to cyclic and branched peptides, glycopeptides, peptidomimetics, and small molecules. The main advantages of the OBOC method are: (i) a large number (10^6–10^8) of compounds can be synthesized and screened within a short period of time (e.g., 1–2 weeks); (ii) unlike phage-display peptide libraries, unnatural amino acids, or building blocks such as monosaccharides, nucleotides, lipids, or even small organic moieties, can be easily incorporated into the OBOC libraries; (iii) complicate bicyclic, compact scaffolding, branched structures, or molecules with special cyclization chemistry are feasible with OBOC method; and (iv) ligands identified from the OBOC method have a built-in poly(ethylene glycol) (PEG) handle to link the cancer-targeting ligand to the therapeutic payload, which has proven to be extremely beneficial for the development of targeting drug conjugates [43].

5.3.3.1 OBOC Library Design

An OBOC library can be liberally designed according to different applications: general use versus specific project, hits identification versus optimization, on-bead screening versus releasable assay, as well as preferred types of library, and so on. Different synthetic approaches will be needed accordingly. In order to maximize the chance of identifying good hits as well as obtain structure–activity relationship (SAR) information during the initial screening, we have started to use many diverse building blocks (hydrophobic/hydrophilic, polar/nonpolar, positive/negative charge, and L-/D-amino acids) to make OBOC peptide libraries. Table 5.2 shows a list of L/D and natural/unnatural amino acids selected for an OBOC peptide library, which can be decoded with either microsequencing (by different retention times in sequencing high-performance liquid chromatography) or mass spectrometry (MS) (by different MW) (see below). For small molecules or peptidomimetic compounds, we generally incorporate three-point diversities into a fixed chemical scaffold, which can be premade or formed as the building blocks are being incorporated.

The surface of a living cell is generally negatively charged due to the sialic acids and phosphorylic moiety of the phospholipids. In order to avoid nonspecific anionic–cationic interactions between the cells and the peptide present on the bead surface, we often purposely lower the relative amount of basic amino acids (lysine and arginine) in our library construction. However, we generally do not eliminate these basic residues totally because a basic residue may be required for binding. This is certainly true for the RGD motif for $\alpha_v\beta_3$ integrin. Upon further optimization of lead compounds with focused OBOC libraries, we will add unnatural amino acids and/or organic moieties to the libraries, which often leads to the development of ligands with higher affinity and specificity as well as proteolytic stability. The

Table 5.2 Thirty amino acids for both sequencing and MS decoding OBOC peptide libraries.

No.	Amino acid	Accurate MW	No.	Amino acid	Accurate MW
1	G	75.03	16	H	155.07
2	A	89.05	17	Chg	157.11
3	Acpc	101.05	18	Aad	161.07
4	Dpr	104.06	19	f	165.08
5	S	105.04	20	D-3-Pal	166.07
6	P	115.06	21	Thi	171.04
7	v	117.08	22	R	174.11
8	t	119.06	23	Aic	177.08
9	I	131.09	24	Phe(4-Me)	179.09
10	N	132.05	25	Y	181.07
11	D	133.04	26	HCit	189.11
12	Ach	143.09	27	D-Tyr(Me)	195.09
13	q	146.07	28	W	204.09
14	e	147.05	29	Nal-1	215.09
15	Phg	151.06	30	Bpa	269.11

Standard single-letter codes are used for natural amino acids and small letters represent their D-isomers. Codes for unnatural amino acids: Acpc, 1-aminocyclopropane-1-carboxylic acid; Dpr, L-2,3-diaminopropionic acid; Ach, 1-amino-1-cyclohexane carboxylic acid; Phg, L-Phenylglycine; Chg, L-2-cyclohexylglycine; Aad, L-2-aminohexanedioic acid; D-3-Pal, D-3-(3-pyridyl)alanine; Thi, L-3-(2-thienyl)alanine; Aic, 2-aminoindane-2-carboxylic acid; Phe(4-Me), L-4-methylphenylalanine; HCit, L-homocitrulline; D-Tyr(Me), D-O-methyltyrosine; Nal-1, L-3-(1-naphthyl)alanine; Bpa, L-4-benzoylphenylalanine.

OBOC approach can also be used to optimize peptide ligands identified from phage-display peptide libraries. For example, based on alanine-walk studies (i.e., replacing each amino acid of the parent peptide with one alanine at a time), the critical contact residues of the phage-display ligand can be determined, and focused OBOC libraries with fixed contact residues and randomized natural and unnatural building blocks can be designed for further optimization of the phage-display leads. The resulting ligands comprised of both natural and unnatural amino acids will likely to be more stable to proteolysis.

The OBOC method is highly versatile and allows one to design peptide libraries with cyclic, bicyclic, or branch structures (Table 5.3). Simple cyclization can be achieved with (i) a disulfide bond between two flanking cysteines, (ii) lactam bond formation between the N-terminus and the side-chain of Asp or Glu, (iii) cycloaddition ("click" chemistry) between the alkyne side-chain of propargylglycine and azide group added to the N-terminus, or (iv) olefin metathesis cyclization using the ruthenium-catalyzed ring-closing metathesis reaction of Grubbs. An allyl group can be introduced in the peptide using commercial available allylglycine. For bicyclic peptides such as one with a conotoxin motif, a linear peptide with a GCXXXXXEXXXXC-bead library can be constructed using two orthogonal cyclization strategies: lactam and disulfide bond formation. Branched peptides can be

Table 5.3 Examples of OBOC peptide libraries.

Linear	Cyclic	Bicyclic	Branch

Linear	Cyclic	Bicyclic	Branch
xxxxxx—○	GPxxxxG—○ cyclized, with xxxxx coding tag	GCxxxxxExxxxC—○ (S–S bridge), xxxxxxxxxC coding tag	$X_6X_5X_4$ branch; $X_6X_5X_4KX_3X_2X_1$; $X_6X_5X_4X_3X_2X_1$ coding tag
xUXxxUx—○	xxxxxxxE cyclic with xxxxxxx coding tag	cXUxxUc—○ (S–S)	$X_9X_8X_7$ branch; $X_6X_5X_4FX_3X_2X_1$; $X_9X_8X_7X_6X_5X_4X_3X_2X_1$ coding tag
xxxXxxx—○	xxxxxxxPra (triazole cyclic) with xxxxxxx coding tag		
XXXBXX XXXX$_B$XX—○ Coding tag			

X, natural amino acids except cysteine; x, 19 D-isomers; U, sequenceable unnatural α-amino acids; B, unsequenceable building blocks that are coded with sequenceable amino acid X_B; Pra, propargylglycine.

easily made using lysine, ornithine, or nitrophenylalanine as the branch point. The latter requires reduction of the NO_2 group to primary amine prior to construction of the branch.

5.3.3.2 OBOC Library Construction

There are many different types of resin beads on the market. For the construction of OBOC libraries used for on-bead binding assays (e.g., whole-cell binding as described below), we select TentaGel™ resin (Rapp Polymere, Tübingen, Germany) as the solid support because it is uniform in size, nonsticky, and suitable in a wide range of organic solvents and water. For construction of the OBOC libraries to identify protease substrates, highly porous resins such as PEG acrylamide (PEGA) beads (Calbiochem-Novabiochem, San Diego, CA) were used because these allowed the enzyme to gain access to the bead interior. In those libraries, a fluorescent (donor) molecule (e.g., 2-aminobenzoic acid) is attached to the C-terminal through a lysine side-chain. The last amino acid in this library should be a quencher (acceptor), such as 3-nitrotyrosine. We and others have successfully identified protease substrates that can be used as cleavage linkers for ligand–drug conjugates [44, 45].

For the OBOC peptide libraries that are comprised of sequenceable α-amino acids (including 20 eukaryotic amino acids, many unnatural amino acids, and amino acid derivatives), the construction can be easily achieved through the "split-mix" synthesis strategy and standard solid-phase peptide synthesis method employing Fmoc chemistry. In brief, beads are split into separate reaction vessels and each portion of beads receives only one amino acid. After the amino acid coupling reaction is done, the beads are combined and mixed, Fmoc-deprotected, then split again for a second coupling cycle. This process is continued until the last cycle of coupling is done. To synthesize "nonsequenceable" peptides (e.g., with nonsequenceable building blocks, without a free N-terminus, or branched peptides), peptidomimetic, and small-molecule OBOC libraries, chemical encoding (to record the synthesis history) is needed because the structure of compound on a single beads cannot be directly determined with conventional spectrometry methods. We have successfully developed several encoding methods employing topologically segregated bilayer beads [46–48]. In our encoding systems, the library compounds display on the outer layer of the bead and the coding tags reside in the bead interior. Such bead configuration minimizes interference of the coding tags with the screening probe. After screening, the coding tag(s) on positive beads can then be decoded by either Edman microsequencing or MS (see Section 5.3.3.4).

The synthetic and encoding approach of a peptide-encoded glycopeptide library is shown in Scheme 5.1 as an example. In this tripeptide-based glycopeptide library, bilayer beads are formed during the synthesis, which allows the glycopeptides (library molecules) to be generated on the outer layer only. The sugar building blocks, which are coded with sequenceable amino acids, are linked to the peptide via click chemistry. The coding tag is a tetrapeptide that resides in the bead interior and can be readily decoded with microsequencing.

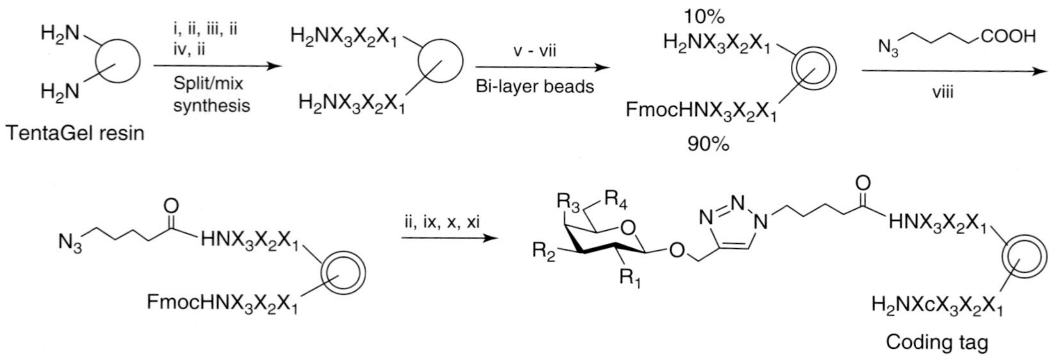

Scheme 5.1 Synthesis of an encoded OBOC glycopeptide library. X_1, X_2, X_3 and X_C stand for sequenceable amino acids. X_C codes for different sugars. Reagents and conditions: (i) split beads, then Fmoc-X_1, HOBt, DIC; (ii) combine beads, then 20% Piperidine/DMF; (iii) spilt beads, then Fmoc-X_2, HOBt, DIC; (iv) split beads, then Fmoc-X_3, HOBt, DIC (v) prepare bilayer beads: swell beads in water, 24 h, then AllocOSu (0.1 eq. to bead loading), DIEA, DCM/diethyl ether (55/45, v/v), 30 min; (vi) Fmoc-OSu (3 eq.), DIEA, DMF, 30 min; (vii) Pd(PPh$_3$)$_4$, PhSiH$_3$, DCM, 30 min; (viii) N$_3$(CH$_2$)$_4$COOH, HOBt, DIC; (ix) Split beads, then Boc-X_C, HOBt, DIC; (x) Click reaction, sugar-alkyn, CuI, DIEA, DMF; (xi) Combine beads, then TFA:phenol:thioanisole:water:triisopropylsilane (82.5:5:5:2.5, v/v). HOBt = N-hydroxybenzotriazole, DIC = N,N′-diisopropylcarbodiimide, DIEA = N,N-diisopropylethylamine, AllocOSu = allyloxycarbonyl-N-hydroxysuccinimide, DCM = dichloromethane, FmocOSu = 9-fluorenylmethyloxycarbonyl-N-hydroxysuccinimide, DMF = N,N-dimethylformamide, TFA = trifluoroacetic acid.

5.3.3.3 OBOC Library Screening

Whole-cell on-bead binding screening of OBOC libraries is widely used to identify cancer-targeting ligands against cell surface receptors. In this assay, living cells are incubated with an OBOC library of beads for a period of time (15 min to 24 h). Beads covered with a monolayer of cancer cells are considered as positive beads (hits) (Figure 5.2). Such beads can be identified and picked up manually under a microscope with a micropipette. In order to identify targeting ligands that specifically bind to cancer cells but not normal cells, we have developed two "subtraction screening" methods. In the first method, we first screen the OBOC library with cancer cells, isolate the beads coated with cancer cells, and strip the cells off the beads with 6 M guanidine chloride aqueous solution followed by thorough washing with water and medium. The recycled beads are then tested for binding with normal cells. Those beads that bind to only cancer cells but not normal cell types are considered "true positive" of interest. The second method is called the "dual-color screening method," which involves tagging the cancer cells with a fluorochrome (e.g., calcein AM) and mixing them with unlabeled normal cells. The cell mixtures are coincubated with library beads. Those beads that only bind to the fluorescent cells are considered "true-positive" beads. In addition to screening for cell binding ligands, one may also screen OBOC libraries for both cell attachment and cell function. We have screened for peptides that induce specific cell function such as apoptosis or cell signaling. For the discovery of proapoptotic peptides, we may add caspase-3 fluorescent substrate to the bead library to identify beads coated with cells that are undergoing apoptosis. For cell signaling, we may use a Green Fluorescent Protein (GFP)-transfected cell line in which GFP will be expressed upon activation of a specific cell signaling pathway or use an on-bead immunohistochemical method to stain a specific phosphorylation site of a cell signaling protein.

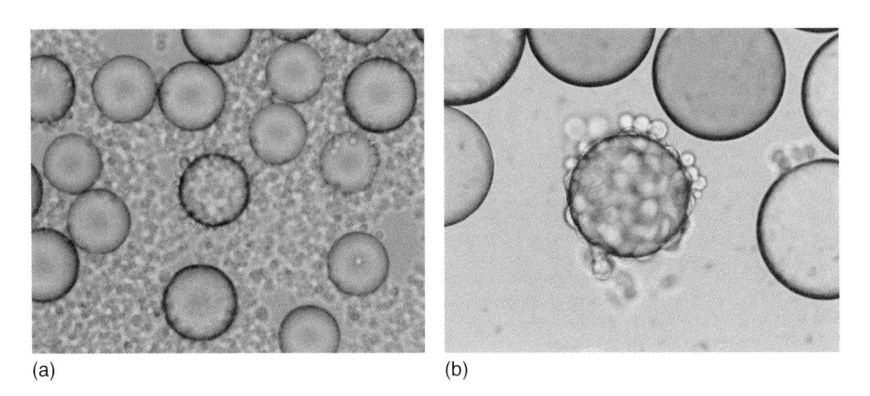

Figure 5.2 Photomicrographs of positive beads ("hit") identified from screening random OBOC combinatorial peptide libraries. (a) A positive bead in the middle of the field. (b) Many of the cells on the positive bead flatten out after incubation.

OBOC on-bead cell binding can be applied to both suspension and adherent cell cultures. Trypsin is often used to strip the adherent cells off the culture flask. However, it is important to minimize the exposure time of the cells to the enzyme to avoid damaging some cell surface receptors that are required for ligand binding. The OBOC library approach can also be applied to fresh cancer cells isolated from patient blood, biopsy specimens, pleural fluid, or ascite fluid.

5.3.3.4 OBOC Library Decoding

The two general and reliable decoding methods for OBOC libraries are microsequencing (using Edman chemistry) and MS. An automatic protein sequencer is routinely used in our laboratory to determine the amino acid sequence of OBOC peptide libraries that are comprised of α-amino acids or their derivatives (with a predetermined sequencing profile) and peptoids (N-substituted oligoglycine). We have reported an improved microsequencing method that can sequence both natural amino acids and many α-unnatural amino acids as well as α-amino acid derivatives (generated from side-chain derivatization) [49]. Microsequencing can also be applied to peptide-encoded nonsequenceable peptide OBOC libraries, peptidomimetic libraries, and small-molecule OBOC libraries [46]. The advantage of microsequencing decoding is that no cleavage and retrieval of coding tags is needed, and it usually gives more unambiguous results especially for difficult-to-make molecules because it gives only one residue (one major peak) at a sequencing cycle (all peaks including impurity peaks coexist as in MS decoding). However, microsequencing is expensive and time-consuming, especially when unnatural amino acids or amino acid derivatives are involved because an external standard has to be developed. In addition, microsequencing may not be as readily available for many laboratories as MS is. To date, there are five MS decoding methods for OBOC libraries reported in the literature [8, 50]. The "ladder sequencing" method is restricted to libraries with sequenceable peptides or peptoids. The "ladder synthesis" method reported originally presents peptide ladders on the bead surface, which could interfere with biological screening. In order to overcome this shortcoming, we have since reported an improved ladder synthesis approach that applies both the ladder synthesis and bilayer bead concepts to encode OBOC nonsequenceable peptide and peptidomimetic libraries. An additional advantage is that only a single building block is used for coupling during each coupling step, therefore eliminating the problems caused by the differential coupling rates of two different building blocks (as in "ladder synthesis"). Using the bilayer bead approach, Pei's group reported another MS decoding method called "partial Edman degradation". In this method, Edman degradation chemistry was used to form a ladder of truncated peptide-coding tags from the N-terminus. For a more detailed comparison of the above-mentioned four methods, please refer to our review [8]. Recently Amadei et al. reported "on-target sequence deconvolution" using matrix-assisted laser desorption/ionization time-of-flight/time-of-flight (MALDI-TOF/TOF) instrumentation [50]. In this method, short peptides (MW < 2000 Da), covalently attached to TentaGel beads through a photolabile linker, were placed onto the MALDI target, apportioned with suitable matrix (2,5-dihydroxybenzoic acid), and then excited with a laser (Nd:YAG, 355 nm). This induced easy and highly reproducible photochemical cleavage, desorption (MS mode), and fragmentation (MS/MS mode). Peptide fragments were identified with a mass accuracy of 0.1 Da of the expected values. This technique significantly accelerates the sequence detection of positive peptide hits obtained from random combinatorial libraries when screening against biological targets. Please note, extra attention is needed to avoid light exposure during peptide library construction.

It is important to realize that the physical partition method for making bilayer beads can be applied at any step during library construction, thus allowing us to construct a linear coding peptide tag to encode complex bicyclic or branch structures (see Table 5.3). This coding tag can be readily decoded with one of the several methods mentioned above.

5.3.3.5 Ligand Optimization

The OBOC library approach is not only an efficient way of hit identification, but also a powerful tool for hit optimization. Initial ligands identified through screening diverse OBOC libraries often do not exhibit the desired binding affinity and specificity. To optimize such ligand hits, we often need to synthesize and screen OBOC focused libraries. In order to determine the critical residues or secondary structures that are required for binding, simple SAR studies on hits will be performed, which include "alanine walk," "deletion studies" (i.e., truncate the peptide from the N-terminus or from the C-terminus, one amino acid at a time), and "enantiomer replacement" (i.e., each amino acid is replaced with its enantiomer one at a time). Based on the motif and SAR information, one can design OBOC focused libraries in which critical building blocks found in lead compounds at specific positions will be used to couple a larger portion of the resin beads at that cycle, or if equal portions of beads were used for each amino acid, more analogs of that specific amino acid will be used for library construction. As a result, the library will be biased toward analogs related to the lead compounds. Another type of focused library is to fix the active motif and extend the C- and/or N-terminus of the peptide with a sequence of random residues, which will enable probes for additional contact residues adjacent to the initial ligand binding site. One can also probe additional binding sites by generating a branch of random sequence at the middle of the peptide using the ε-amino group of L- or D-lysine as the branching residue. Many of these methods have already been successfully applied to the optimization of our lymphoma, breast cancer, glioblastoma, and ovarian cancer-targeting ligands.

Screening of focused library is usually performed under high stringency conditions because many of the beads are expected to bind to the target (live cells or purified proteins). In order to identify highly potent ligands, we often lower the concentration of cell numbers or target protein (probe), add soluble competing ligands in the screening buffer [51], or shorten the incubation (binding) time. An alternative is to construct the bead libraries using down-substituted beads so that a lower concentration of library compound is displayed on the bead surface [52]. In these beads, only the outer layer (library compounds) is down-substituted; the inner core of the bead (coding tag) remains 100% substituted to ensure enough material for decoding. These strategies can be employed either alone or in combination.

5.3.3.6 Examples

Using whole-cell bead-binding assays to screen OBOC libraries, many potent and specific cell surface ligands have been successfully identified against a number of different cancer cell lines, including both adherent and nonadherent cells. A variety of OBOC libraries have been used for screening, including peptide (containing all L- or D-amino acids, mixed L/D-amino acids, mixed natural/unnatural amino acids), glycopeptide, peptidomimetic, and small-molecule libraries. The cancer-targeting ligands discovered by the OBOC approach are summarized in Table 5.4. Some of them have interesting biological properties other than just cell binding.

We reported the use of the OBOC library approach to identify a high-affinity peptidomimetic ligand LLP2A (IC_{50} = 2pM) that targets activated $\alpha_4\beta_1$ of T- and B-lymphoma xenografts with high sensitivity and specificity [51]. We first screened an initial library with huge permutations (5.4×10^{10}) to narrow down preferred building blocks in each position, then designed and screened a highly focused peptidomimetic library (1560 permutations) under high stringency conditions. LLP2A is 1000-fold more potent than the initial leads. Using similar methods, we have developed two D-amino acid containing cyclic octapeptide ligands, LXY1 [53] and OAO2 [54], against $\alpha_3\beta_1$ integrin of glioblastoma and ovarian cancer, respectively. LXY1, when conjugated to Cy5.5 or AlexaFluor680 near-IR fluorescent dye, was able to image α_3 integrin-expressed U-87 MG glioblastoma xenograft in nude mice [53]. OAO2, when conjugated with 1,4,7,10-tetraazacyclododecane-1,4,7,10-tetraacetic acid (DOTA) and radiolabeled with ^{64}Cu, demonstrated good tumor targeting in ES-2 ovarian cancer xenografts in nude mice using microPET imaging [8]. We have recently reported the use of the OBOC peptide library method in combination with whole-cell binding assays to identify a novel and potent cyclic RGD peptide LXW7, cGRGDdvc (cyclized with a disulfide bond), with a build-in handle (PEG linker) at the C-terminus [43]. LXW7 has been demonstrated to possess high binding affinity and specificity against $\alpha_v\beta_3$ integrin *in vitro*. Furthermore, *in vivo* and *ex vivo* imaging experiments have indicated that the LXW7–biotin/streptavidin–Cy5.5 complex was able to target U-87 MG glioblastoma and A375M melanoma xenografts with high efficiency, but uptake of this complex into the liver was lower than the well-known RGD "head-to-tail" cyclic pentapeptide ligands reported in the literature [55]. The chemical structures of LLP2A, OA02, LXY1, and LXW7 are shown in Figure 5.3.

Johansson *et al.* recently reported the screening of a 65536-member OBOC combinatorial library of glycopeptide dendrimers for binding of Jurkat cells [56]. A lead compound, dendrimer J1 (β-Gal-GRHA)$_2$Dpr-TRHDCNH$_2$ (β-Gal = β-galactosyl-thiopropionic acid) was identified and conjugated to colchicines as a targeted therapeutic agent. The colchicine–J1 conjugate (through a cysteine-thioether) was found to be cytotoxic with a LD$_{50}$ of 1.5 µM.

Aggarwal *et al.* constructed a random OBOC library of 12-amino-acid dimeric peptides on PEGA beads (named as a one-bead/one-dimer library) [57]. This library

Table 5.4 Cancer-targeting ligands identified by the OBOC combinatorial library method [8].

Ligands to specific tumor cells	Cell surface receptors	Ligand sequence
Jurkat and Molt-4 T-cell lymphoma, Raji B-cell lymphoma [51]	activated $\alpha_4\beta_1$ integrin	Sm-K38-Aad-Ach (LLP2A) (Figure 5.3)
Jurkat T-cell lymphoma [56]	NA	(β-Gal-GRHA)2Dpr-TRHDC (J1)
Raji B-cell lymphoma	$\alpha_4\beta_1$ integrin	sppLDIn, eapLDId, fypLDFf, FSIpLDI, QSYpLDF cLDYWDc, cWDLDHHc
SKOV-3 ovarian adenocarcinoma	$\alpha_4\beta_1$ integrin	cDEL-Nle-Ewc, c-Nle-d-Nle-PhgDc, cLDI-Chg-Hyp-Yc, c-Nle-d-Chg-NDFc
Jurkat T-cell lymphoma	$\alpha_4\beta_1$ integrin	xLDFpXXX, xxxxp-Nle-DIxxxx, XXXpLDI/F/V, cLDIXXc, cXLDI/V/Fc, cXXLDIc, cWDXXXc
ES-2 ovarian adenocarcinoma	$\alpha_4\beta_1$ integrin	vqgp-Nle-DIafvl, wdinp-Nle-DIgsfn, vgnvp-Nle-DIgqea, yminp-Nle-DIdnhh, wsrip-Nle-Diqeps, c-Nle-DVDEc, c-Nle-d-Chg-YMc, cSD-Nle-d-Chg-c, c-Nle-DWEEc
Bronchioloalveolar H1650 carcinoma	$\alpha_4\beta_1$ integrin	cX-Nle-DXXXXc, c-Nle-DXXXXc
U-87 MG glioblastoma [53]	α_3 integrin	cdGLG-Hyp-Nc (LXY1)
Ovarian adenocarcinoma (CaOV-3, ES-2, SKOV-3, OVCAR-3), MDA-MB 231 metastatic breast cancer, A172 glioblastoma, and melanoma	α_3 integrin	cd/DGX*GXXc (X* = Cha, Chg, HCit, Cit, F, Y, Nle, M, L, or I) cdG-HCit-GPQc (OA02)
NSCLC	α_3 integrin	cNGXGXXc
DU145 prostate cancer cell line	$\alpha_6\beta_1$ integrin	kikmviswkG, kmviywkaG, kGGrhykfG, yiknrkhhG, LNNIVSVNGRHX, DNRIRLQAKXX
U-87 MG glioblastoma and A375M melanoma [43]	$\alpha_v\beta_3$ integrin	cGRGDdvc (LXW7)
WEHI-279 murine lymphoma cell line	idiotype	RWID, RWFD, xtxGmxkx, xGrfxswx
WEHI-231 murine lymphoma cell line	idiotype	XWYD/T/V, lwxxpewi, kwxGpxw, wGeyixvx
LNCaP prostate cancer cell line [57]	NA	Dimer (QMARIPKRLARH)2KG

Single-letter representation for amino acid according to standard convention, except for those amino acids without single-letter representation: Cha, cyclohexylalanine; Hyp, hydroxyproline; Nle, norleucine; Cit, citrulline.

was screened against LNCaP prostate cancer cells, which were fluorescently tagged through Cell Tracker orange, using an on-bead cell binding assay. A series of dimeric peptides that bound selectively to epithelial cancer cells was identified. One of these peptides, QMARIPKRLARH, in dimeric form, was found to bind to prostate cancer cells, but not the peripheral blood cells.

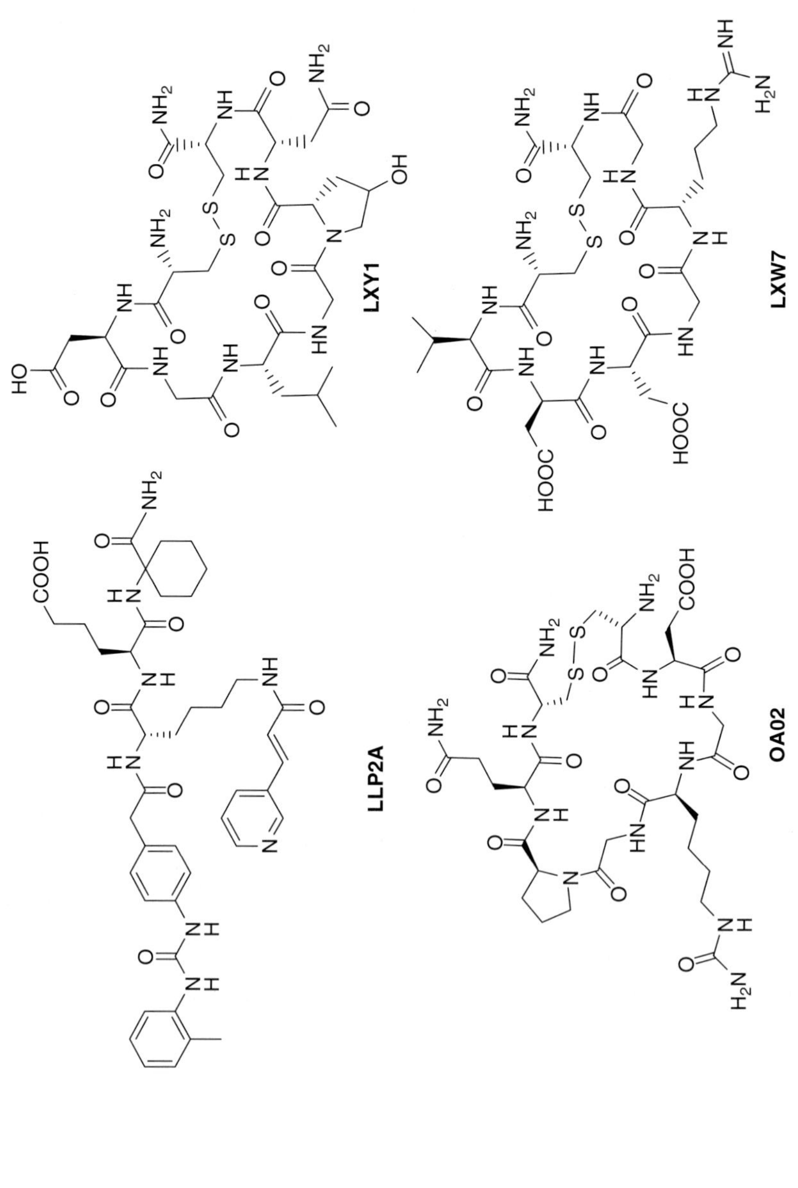

Figure 5.3 Examples of cancer-targeting ligands identified from OBOC libraries.

5.4
Linkers

Targeting ligands can deliver their therapeutic payload to the tumor site efficiently, but the payload needs to be released from the targeting ligands either at the endothelial wall, tumor extracellular matrix, tumor cell surface, endosomes, or lysosomes inside the tumor cells to exert anticancer effects. For linker cleavage, many cancer-targeting ligand–drug conjugate or prodrug designs have exploited the hypoxic and relatively acidic tumor microenvironment, the acidic condition inside the endosomes and lysosomes of the tumor cells, the reductive intracellular microenvironment, and the proteolytic enzymes at the tumor cell extracellular matrix and inside the endosomes or lysosomes. In some instances, cleavage enzymes or cleavage agents can be administered exogenously and delivered to the tumor site (in the case of ADEPT). A summary of linker designs for the cancer-targeting ligand drug–conjugates that take advantages of such physiological alterations in cancer is given in the following. To maximize the therapeutic index of the drug conjugates, premature release of drugs into the circulatory system needs to be minimized.

5.4.1
Acid-Sensitive Linkers

Acid-sensitive linkers are incorporated into the prodrug conjugates such that they can be cleaved under acidic conditions present in tumors, endosomes, and lysosomes [58, 59]. The microenvironment in tumor tissues is often more acidic (0.5–1.0 pH units lower) than normal tissues. A more prominent pH shift takes place during the prodrug conjugate uptake from blood or extracellular spaces (pH 7.2–7.4) into intracellular compartments (pH 4.0–6.5) at endosomes and lysosomes. These changes in pH can be utilized to cleave acid-sensitive linkers extracellularly, particularly when the prodrug stays in the tumor interstitium for a longer duration. Examples of acid-sensitive linkages used in prodrug and conjugate design are imine, hydrazone, acyl hydrazone, ketal, acetal, *cis*-aconityl, and trityl bonds (Figure 5.4).

5.4.2
Enzymatic Cleavage

Linkers have been designed to exploit the presence of hydrolytic enzymes at the tumor site (intracellularly and extracellularly). Enzymatic cleavage of the susceptible linker leads to the release of drugs directly from the drug conjugates. Alternatively, the enzymes may derivatize the linker, which then will degrade spontaneously by elimination. This enzyme-trigger self-immolative linker [59] will be discussed in Section 5.4.3. Figure 5.5 illustrates some of the prodrugs that can be activated by hydrolytic enzymes.

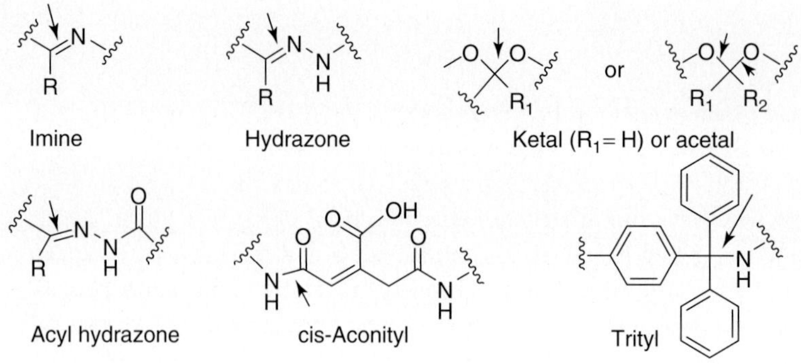

Figure 5.4 Acid-sensitive linkages used in prodrug conjugate design. Cleavage sites are indicated by arrows.

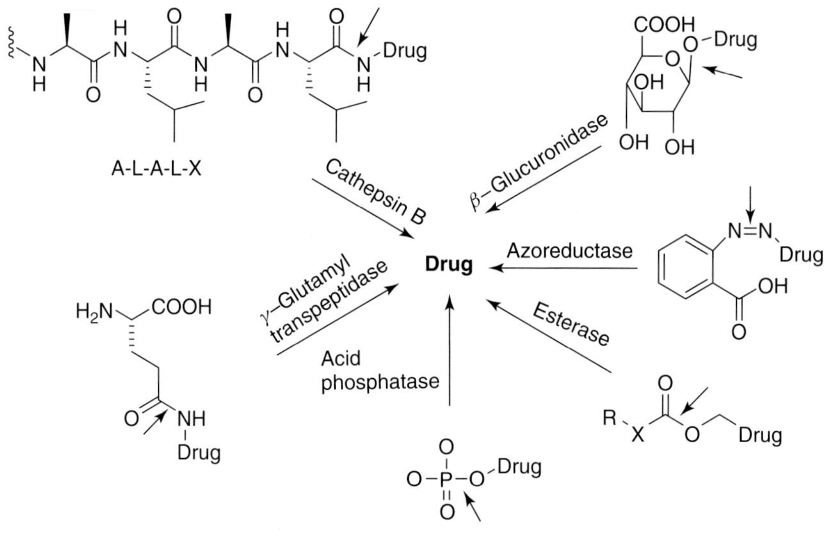

Figure 5.5 Enzymatic cleavage by chemical bonds via tumor-associated enzymes. Enzyme-labile bonds are marked via arrows.

Cathepsins are a family of proteolytic enzymes (cathepsin B, D, H, and L) responsible for the digestion of the basement membrane, as well as activation of enzymes, growth factors, and other proteases involved in the metastatic cascade. Cathepsin B, H, and L are also responsible for the degradation of proteins inside the lysosomes. Peptides with the general structure -RRX-, -ALX-, -GLFGX-, -GFLGX-, and -ALALX- are efficient substrates for these enzymes. Cathepsin D is responsible for the degradation of extracellular matrix, and its substrates include -FAA-F(NO$_2$)-FVL-OM4P-X and Bz-RGFFP-4mβNA. Peptide substrates for other tumor-associated enzymes are: -vLKX-, -aFKX-, or -aWKX- for plasmin, -GGGRRRVX- for urokinase/tissue-type plasminogen activator, morpholinocarbonyl-HSSKLQLX- for prostate-specific antigen, and Ac-PLQLX- and -GPLGIAGQX- for matrix metalloprotease-2 and -9.

Several prodrugs have been approved for cancer treatment. Many of them were developed to overcome formulation problems and designed to be activated by a number of endogenous enzymes (e.g., β-glucuronidase, γ-glutamyl transpeptidase, carboxylesterases, acid phosphatase, and azoreductase) at the tumor sites and/or at the peripheral tissues. For example, irinotecan is an anticancer prodrug and can be converted to SN-38 by endogenous esterase [60]. Estramustine phosphate and fludarabine phosphate are two phosphate-containing prodrugs that can be activated by alkaline phosphatase. Capecitabine (Xeloda®) is another anticancer prodrug that can be converted by three enzymes (carboxylesterase, cytidine deaminase, and thymidine phosphorylase) to 5-fluorouracil. Some of the enzyme-cleavable linkers used in these prodrugs can, in principle, be used for the development of targeting ligand–drug conjugates if cleavage of the linkers at the peripheral sites or during circulating is insignificant.

5.4.3
Self-Immolative Spacers

Self-immolative spacers have three components: drug, linker, and trigger [59]. The tumor-specific cleavage reaction takes place between the trigger and the linker to form a drug–linker derivative, which then degrades spontaneously by elimination or cyclization to release the free drug [61–65]. The general mechanism of action of some of the self-immolative (self-eliminating) spacers is shown in Figure 5.6.

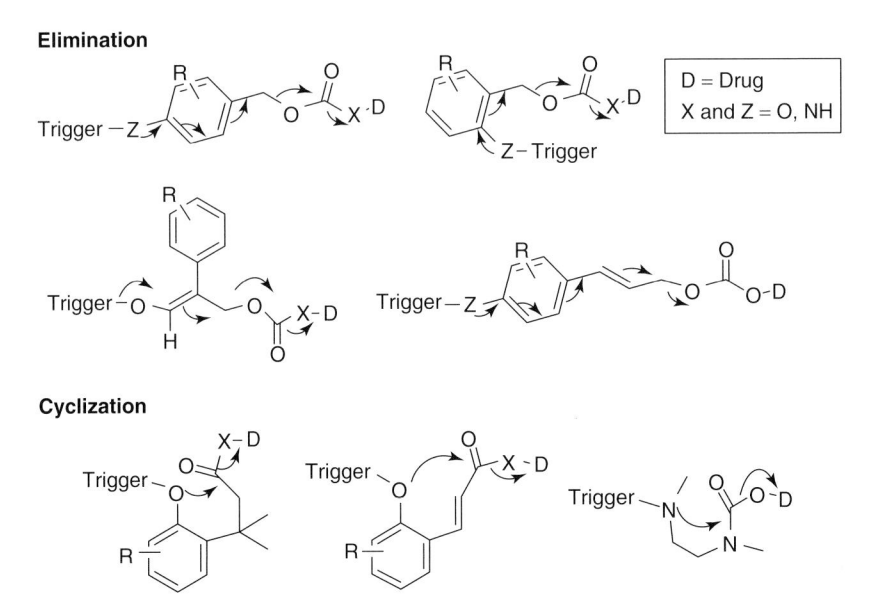

Figure 5.6 Self-immolative spacers in prodrug design.

Dubowchik et al. prepared a series of DOX derivatives with cathepsin B-cleavable dipeptides [66]. They observed that in the presence of the target enzyme, only those derivatives that incorporated the self-immolative moiety could liberate the drug. Self-immolative or cascade-release dendrimers have also been reported [67, 68].

5.4.4
Reductive Cleavage

The presence of hypoxia in human tumors, especially in solid tumors, is well known. Some regions in tumor tissues are poorly vascularized, resulting in low oxygen tension, low pH, low nutrient levels, and overexpression of angiogenic factors and endogenous reductive enzymes [69]. In addition, exogenous reductive enzymes can be delivered to tumor cells through fusion with tumor-specific antibodies or overexpressed in tumor cells through gene delivery approaches. The nontoxic prodrugs targeting hypoxia are substrates for either endogenous reductases enzymes such as diphtheria toxin diaphorase (DTD), β-glucuronidase, or exogenous enzymes, such as carboxypeptidase and nitroreductase [70]. Many reductase-activating anticancer prodrugs have been designed and they often contain functional groups such as quinones, nitroaromatics, N-oxides, and metal complexes [71]. These reducible moieties can be used as linkers to bridge ligand molecules and the anticancer drugs.

The glutathione level is elevated in a number of different human cancer tissues [72] and many chemoresistant cancer biopsy tissues (10-fold higher than before treatment) [73]. The reductively activated disulfide prodrug of paclitaxel, given systemically, has been reported to exhibit significant regressions or cures of cancer in *in vivo* antitumor efficacy studies [74]. A folate receptor targeted camptothecin (CPT) prodrug was synthesized using a hydrophilic peptide spacer linked to folate via a releasable disulfide carbonate linker [75]. The conjugate was found to possess high affinity for folate receptor-expressing cells and inhibited cell proliferation in human KB cells with an IC_{50} of 10 nM.

5.4.5
On-Demand Cleavable Linker

One of the limitations of radioimmunotherapy with radiolabeled mAbs is the long circulating half-life of the radioimmunoconjugates (RICs), resulting in excessive toxicities to normal tissues. One approach to lower such toxicities is to develop RICs with an on-demand cleavable linker that can be cleaved by exogenously administered agents given to the patients after maximal uptake of the RIC in the tumor site has been achieved, so that the radiochelate can be cleared rapidly via the kidneys. The cleavage agent that we chose was TNKase®, a FDA-approved thrombolytic agent (tissue plasminogen activator), and the method we used to identify such linker was the fluorescent-quenched random OBOC combinatorial peptide library approach [44]. D-Amino acid-containing peptides that were specific for TNKase but resistant to cleavage by plasma and tumor-associated proteases were identified. One of these peptide substrates (rqYKYkf) was used to link the DOTA chelate to ChL6, a mAb known to target breast cancer. The addition of TNKase at a clinically achievable plasma level (10 µg/ml) resulted in the release of 28% of the radiometal from the RIC within 72 h. Bernstein et al. [76] reported the development of another on-demand enzyme cleavable linker for their RICs. It is cephalosporin-based and is susceptible to cleavage by β-lactamase, a bacterial enzyme.

5.5 Examples of Cancer-Targeting Ligand–Drug Conjugates

In the above discussion, we have given an overview on cancer-targeting ligand–drug conjugates. We have discussed in detail the development of targeting ligands with a focus on the use of combinational library methods to discover such ligands. We have also briefly discussed the various linker options. Below is an account of selected examples that illustrate how the above concepts were put together for the development of anticancer drug conjugates.

5.5.1 Folic Acid–Drug Conjugates

Folic acid belongs to the vitamin B family and has been widely used as a targeting ligand to develop ligand–drug conjugates. Folic acid can be taken up by epithelial cells through receptor-mediated endocytosis. The binding affinity of folic acid against the two isoforms of membrane-bound folic acid receptors (FR-a and FR-b) is below 1 nM [77]. The FR is an excellent target for tumor-specific drug delivery because: (i) the expression of FR in normal tissues is low, but it is upregulated in many human carcinomas (e.g., cancers of the ovary, brain, kidney, breast, colon, myeloid, and lung) and (ii) FR density appears to increase as the stage/grade of the cancer becomes more advanced [78]. Folic acid has been used as the vehicle for delivery of both low-molecular-weight drugs as well as macromolecular complexes.

Many drugs have been used to prepare low-molecular-weight folate–drug conjugates. These include alkylating agents, platinum complexes, paclitaxel, 5-fluorouracil, CPT, DOX, and mitomycin C (MMC). For example, Lee et al. [79] conjugated paclitaxel to folic acid through an oligoethylene glycol linker. The folate–paclitaxel conjugate exhibited higher cytotoxicity than paclitaxel alone. The IC_{50} values against A-549 (NSCLC), MCF-7 (breast), and HT-29 (colon) cancer cell lines in vitro were up to 10- to 30-fold lower than those of free paclitaxel. However, it was found that the FR-binding affinity of a representative conjugate, C-7-(PEG-3)-folyl-paclitaxel, to the FR-positive KB cells was only a quarter of that of free folic acid. Moreover, these conjugates all failed to demonstrate selective cytotoxicity to FR-expressing KB tumor cells in vitro and in vivo. Another example is the folic acid–MMC conjugate [80]. One such conjugate, called EC72, was synthesized with an intramolecular disulfide bond and it was found to be efficacious against

FR-expressing M109 tumors, but with less toxicity when compared to the free drug.

Folic acid has also been used as a vehicle for the delivery of drug-loaded liposomes, polymeric micelles, proteins, synthetic polymers, and nanoparticles. The use of a macromolecular carrier bearing folic acid molecules as tumor-targeting moieties has an advantage because the FRs in kidneys are expressed in the region where macromolecules cannot reach, thereby avoiding undesired renal toxicity. In vitro studies with folic acid-decorated and rhodamine-labeled liposomes demonstrated binding and subsequent internalization of the liposomes by a high FR-expressing murine lung carcinoma cell line (M109-HiFR cells) [81]. Liposome uptake was shown to be inhibited by free folic acid. The in vitro cytotoxic activity obtained with DOX-loaded folate-targeted liposomes (FTLs) was 10-fold greater than that of the nontargeted liposomes, but was not improved over that of free DOX despite the higher cellular drug levels obtained with the targeted liposomes in M109R-HiFR cells. However, if M109R-HiFR cells were exposed to drugs in vitro and tested in an in vivo adoptive assay for tumor growth in syngeneic mice along a 5-week time span, FTL-DOX was significantly more tumor inhibitory than free DOX. Pinhassi et al. [82] have recently developed a targeted biomacromolecular nanovehicle that can differentially deliver a cytotoxic cargo into FR-overexpressing cells, by tethering both folate and methotrexate (MTX) to arabinogalactan (AG), a highly branched natural polysaccharide with unusual water solubility. Moreover, the target-activated release mechanism was demonstrated by linking MTX via an endosomally cleavable peptide (GFLG). This FA–AG–GFLG–MTX drug conjugate was found to be 6.3-fold more active against FR-overexpressing cells compared to their FR-lacking counterparts.

5.5.2
Peptide Ligand–Drug Conjugates

Peptide-based targeting of tumor-associated receptors is an attractive approach in tumor-specific drug delivery because high-affinity sequences can be discovered through screening of combinatorial libraries. Recently, a number of peptides and their conjugates with cytotoxic agents that target different cancer cell receptors have emerged as potential tumor-specific chemotherapeutic agents. Through screening OBOC combinatorial libraries, we have successfully discovered a few high-specificity and high-affinity peptide or peptidomimetic ligands, including $\alpha_4\beta_1$ integrin targeting LLP2A peptidomimetic ligand against lymphoma cells [51], $\alpha_3\beta_1$ integrin targeting OAO2 peptide against ovarian cancer cells [54], LXY1 peptide against glioblastoma tumor cells [53], and LXY3 peptide against breast cancer cells [83]. We further demonstrated that these peptide ligands can be used to image the corresponding tumor type with high sensitivity and specificity when complexed with streptavidin–near-IR fluorescent dye conjugate in a mouse xenograft model. Application of these novel peptide ligands for tumor-targeted drug or radionuclide delivery is still ongoing.

RGD peptides have been employed as delivery agents for small-molecule drugs, peptides, polymers, liposomes, and radiotracers to $\alpha_v\beta_3$ integrin-expressing tumor endothelial cells. The $\alpha_v\beta_3$ integrin plays a critical role in the adhesion and migration of endothelial cells to extracellular matrix components, and it is overexpressed by proliferating endothelial cells and some tumor cells. Peptides containing the RGD sequence that is present in the extracellular matrix can be used to target integrins and subsequently inhibit angiogenesis. Mukhopadhyay *et al.* [84] designed a series of mono- and bifunctionalized Pt(IV) complexes in which a conjugated peptide containing RGD, (CRGDC)c, (RGDfK)c, or NGR is appended to selectively target tumor endothelial cells. The Pt(IV)–RGD conjugates were demonstrated to be highly and specifically cytotoxic to cell lines containing $\alpha_v\beta_3$ integrin. Huang *et al.* [85] have recently developed a c(RGDyK) targeted SN-38 prodrug with an indolequinone structure for bioreductive drug release (Figure 5.7). There are three moieties in the prodrug design, namely a therapeutic drug SN-38, an indolequinone structure serving as a drug-releasing trigger, and an $\alpha_v\beta_3$ integrin targeting peptide c(RGDyK). Preliminary studies showed that SN-38 was efficiently released from the prodrug in the presence of a recombinant bioreductive enzyme DTD, and the prodrug was found to be essentially noncytotoxic against human cervical carcinoma KB cells at up to 300 nM concentration, whereas there was a 50–70% decrease in cell growth in the presence of DTD.

Figure 5.7 c(RGDyK) targeted SN-38 prodrug incorporating an indolequinone structure for bioreductively triggered drug release.

5.5.3
Peptide Hormone–Drug Conjugates

Many other peptides, such as gastrointestinal peptides, SST, and bombesin, have also been already used for targeting drug delivery. For example, neuropeptide Y (NPY), a 36-amino acid peptide of the pancreatic polypeptide family, which is overexpressed in a number of neuroblastoma tumors, was covalently linked to daunorubicin via two spacers that differ in stability: an acid-sensitive hydrazone bond and a stable amide bond [86]. Both conjugates were able to bind to NPY Y1 receptor-expressing human neuroblastoma cell line SK-N-MC with affinities ranging from 25 to 51 nM, but only the compound containing the acid-sensitive bond ($[^{15}C]$-NPY-Dauno-HYD) showed cytotoxic activity comparable to free daunorubicin. The intracellular distribution study demonstrated that the active conjugate $[^{15}C]$-NPY-Dauno-HYD released daunorubicin, which was localized close to the nucleus, whereas the inactive conjugate $[^{15}C]$-NPY-Dauno-MBS was distributed at a distance from the nucleus and did not seem to release the drug within the cell.

The LHRH receptor can also be utilized for targeted chemotherapy with a cytotoxic agent covalently linked to an LHRH analog. More than 80% of human ovarian and endometrial cancers and about 50% of breast cancers express LHRH receptor. Emons et al. [4] have developed a novel cytotoxic LHRH analog, AN-152 (Figure 5.8), in which DOX is linked to the (D-Lys^6)-LHRH agonist. AN-152 was found to selectively internalize in human ovarian or endometrial cancer cell lines that express LHRH receptors, and DOX was cleaved from LHRH and accumulated in the nucleus after internalization of the ligand–drug conjugate. Furthermore, the antitumor efficacy and toxicity profiles of AN-152 in LHRH receptor-positive endometrial and ovarian tumors *in vivo* were demonstrated to be superior to those of equimolar doses of free DOX. Chandna et al. [87] have recently proposed a multifunctional, multicomponent polymer peptide–drug conjugate (PPDC) that includes one or several molecules of anticancer drug (CPT) conjugated to PEG carrier via citric acid spacers together with a tumor-targeting moiety (LHRH analog)

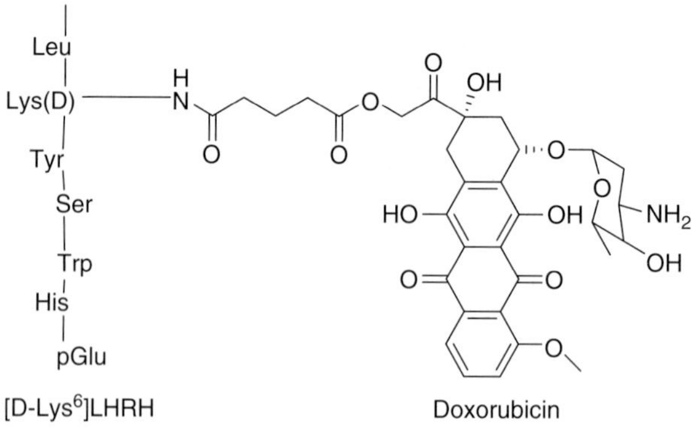

Figure 5.8 LHRH analog AN-152 (cytotoxic agent DOX covalently linked to (D-Lys^6) LHRH).

and a suppressor of cellular antiapoptotic defense (BH3 peptide). The therapeutic efficacy was tested using xenograft models derived from cells isolated from primary tumors of patients with ovarian carcinoma, and it was found that PPDC with multiple copies of drugs and targeting peptides demonstrated significantly higher antitumor activity in primary and metastatic cancers when compared to drug alone or PEG–CPT conjugate without ligand.

5.5.4
Antibody–Drug Conjugates

Early mAb–drug conjugates used mAbs derived from murine hybridomas, which severely impaired their therapeutic efficacy, due to the human antimouse antibody response, resulting in rapid clearance of the immunoconjugates from the bloodstream. To overcome this problem, chimeric and humanized mAbs with decreased immunogenicity have been developed. Five antibodies (naked, no drugs or radionuclides) have been approved by the FDA for the treatment of hematological malignancies and solid tumors [88–90], and many more are currently in clinical trials. These approved antibodies are trastuzumab (Herceptin®), alemtuzumab (Campath®), rituximab (Rituxan®), bevacizumab (Avastin®), and cetuximab (Erbitux®).

Clinical development of antibody–drug conjugates with small-molecule drugs like antifolates [91], vinca alkaloids [92], or anthracyclines [93], however, has been lagging behind, probably because (i) only very small amounts of cytotoxic drug can be conjugated to the antibody (i.e., drug loading) without reducing its affinity to the tumor-associated antigens and (ii) the expression of antigen on tumor cells is also limited. In order to be effective, the therapeutic payload needs to be much more potent than standard chemotherapeutic agents. These payloads include natural product toxin, protein toxin, and radionuclides.

Mylotarg (gemtuzumab; Wyeth) is the only immune toxin conjugate that has been approved by the FDA for the treatment of $CD33^+$ acute myeloid leukemia (AML) [94]. This immunoconjugate consists of humanized anti-CD33 mAb linked to the cytotoxic antibiotic ozogamicin (N-acetyl-γ-calicheamicin). The linker consists of two cleavable bonds. Mylotarg demonstrated clinical efficiency in pediatric patients with advanced $CD33^+$ AML. This drug, however, is never used as front-line therapy in AML because of its severe toxicity. Table 5.5 summarizes many of the immunoconjugates currently undergoing clinical development.

Protein toxins have been used for immunoconjugates. The cell recognition domain of bacterial toxins, such as *Pseudomonas aeruginosa* exotoxin A (PE, 613 amino acids) and diphtheria toxin (DT, 580 amino acids), and plant toxins, such as ricin, is replaced with a new recognition or targeting moiety such as a mAb [97]. Various immunotoxins for the treatment of both hematological malignancies and solid tumors have been evaluated in different stages of clinical trials (Table 5.6). For example, LMB-2 is a single-chain immunotoxin in which the Fv of an antibody to the CD25 subunit of the IL-2 receptor is fused to PE38 (truncated PE). In a phase I trial, clinical responses to LMB-2 were observed in patients with

Table 5.5 Antibody–drug conjugates in clinical trials [95, 96].

Antibody–drug conjugate	Target	Status of clinical trials	Company
SGN-70-MC-VC-MMAF (SGN-75)	CD70/solid tumors	investigational new drug application 2009	Seattle Genetics
1C1-MC-MMAF (MEDI-547)	EphA2/solid tumors	phase I	AstraZeneca MedImmune
MDX-1203-MC-VC-MGBA (duocarmycin)	CD70/renal cell carcinoma	phase I	Medarex
Lintuzumab-MC-VC-MMAE (SGN-35)	CD30/hematologic malignancies, Hodgkin's lymphoma	phase I	Seattle Genetics
BT-062	multiple myeloma	phase I	Biotest/Immunogen
CMC-544 (inotuzumab ozogamicin)	CD22-expressing cells in B-cell Leukemia	phase I	Wyeth
Anti-CD33 mAb–DM4 conjugate (AVE9633)	CD33-expressing cells in acute myeloid leukemia	phase I	Sanofi-Aventis/Immunogen
IMGN388-amide-MCC-DM4	integrin/antivascular/solid tumors	phase I	Centocor (JnJ)/Immunogen
SAR3419-amide-MCC-DM4	CD19/non-Hodgkin's lymphoma	phase I	Sanofi-Aventis/Immunogen
MLN-2704	prostrate-specific membrane antigen-expressing prostate cancer	phase I/II	Millennium Pharmaceuticals
CR011-MC-VC-MMAE	GPNMB/melanoma	phase II	Curagen/Seattle Genetics
HuC242-amide-MCC-DM4	CanAg/gastric cancer	phase II	Immunogen
HuN901-amide-MCC-DM1	CD56/multiple myeloma and small-cell lung cancer	phase II	Immunogen
Trastuzumab-amide-MCC-DM1	HER2/neu/HER2$^+$ breast cancer	phase III	Genentech/Immunogen
Inotuzumab-amide-hydrazonecalicheamicin	CD22/non-Hodgkin's lymphoma	phase II/III	Wyeth
Gentuzumab-amide-hydrazonecalicheamicin (Mylotarg)	CD33/myeloid leukemia	FDA approved 2000	Wyeth

Table 5.6 Examples of antibody–toxin conjugates (immunotoxins) in clinical trials.

Immunotoxins	Toxin	Antigen targeted	Tumor type	Clinical status
DAB389IL2 (IL-2 fused to DT)	DT	IL-2	CTCL, CLL, and NHL	approved by the FDA phase III
IL13-PE38QQR	PE38	IL-13	glioblastomas	phase II ongoing
Anti-tac(scFv)–PE38 (LMB-2; Fv portion of anti-CD25 antibody fused to PE)	PE	CD25 (subunit of IL-2)	HCL, CLL, ATL, CTCL, and NHL	
RFB4(dsFv)–PE38 (BL22; disulfide-linked Fv portion of anti-CD22 antibody fused to PE)	PE38	CD22	HCL, CLL, and NHL	phase II
TP-38 (transforming growth factor-α fused to PE38)	PE38	EGFR	glioblastomas	phase II
SS1(dsFv)–PE38 (SS1P; antimesothelin Fv fused to PE38)	PE38	mesothelin	mesotheliomas, ovarian cancer, and pancreatic cancer	phase II studies in combination with chemotherapy
Anti-B4–bR	bRicin	CD19	NHL	phase II
DT388–GMCSF (granulocyte macrophage-colony stimulating factor fused to DT)	DT	granulocyte macrophage-colony stimulating factor receptor	AML	phase I
RFT5–dgA	dgA	CD25	HD	phase I/II

DT, diphtheria toxin; PE, *Pseudomonas* exotoxin A; PE38, truncated PE; bRicin, blocked ricin; dgA, deglycosylated ricin A chain; CTCL, cutaneous T-cell lymphoma; CLL, chronic lymphocytic leukemia; NHL, non-Hodgkin's lymphoma; HCL, hairy cell leukemia; ATL, adult T-cell leukaemia; AML, acute myelogenous leukemia; HD, Hodgkin's disease.

chemotherapy-resistant hematologic malignancies [98, 99]. Common toxicities were transaminase elevations (liver toxicity) associated with fever (probably mediated by released cytokines). Clinical responses to immunotoxins have mainly been observed in hematological malignancies, where immunotoxins can rapidly reach the tumor cells, and not in solid tumors, where tumor penetration is limited. As immunotoxins contain bacterial or plant proteins, antibody formation prevents retreatment of patients with solid tumors where the immune system is intact. Furthermore, myelosuppression caused by nonspecific binding of the drug conjugates to the reticuloendothelial system is a problem.

5.5.5
ADEPT

In enzyme/prodrug therapy, the prodrug-activating enzyme gene or functional enzyme protein is delivered selectively to tumor tissues, followed by systemic administration of a nontoxic prodrug that can be specifically activated by the exogenous enzyme at the tumor site. There are two enzyme/prodrug strategies: (i) delivery of active enzymes onto tumor tissues, which is also referred as ADEPT, and (ii) delivery of genes that encode prodrug-activating enzymes into tumor tissues, which is also referred to as gene-directed enzyme prodrug therapy (GDEPT). Only ADEPT will be discussed here. ADEPT is a two-step targeted therapy strategy (Figure 5.9) developed independently by Bagshawe [100] and Senter *et al.* [101]. An exogenous enzyme is coupled to a mAb that can specifically target tumor cells. In the first step, this enzyme–mAb conjugate is administered intravenously, and allowed sufficient time to localize on tumor cells and clear from the circulation. In the second step, a prodrug is administered as a selective substrate of the exogenous enzyme, which will be selectively converted into the potent active drug by the antibody-delivered exogenous enzyme in tumor cells or in the tumor microenvironment, thus achieving the selective killing of tumor cells.

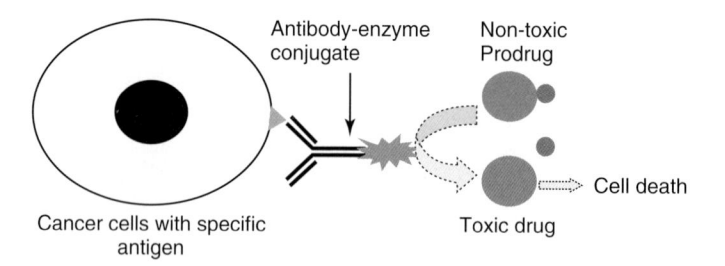

Figure 5.9 Two-step targeted therapy of ADEPT. Antibody–enzyme conjugate is first delivered to the tumor cell surface, followed by administration of nontoxic prodrug, which is activated at the tumor site by the antibody–enzyme conjugate.

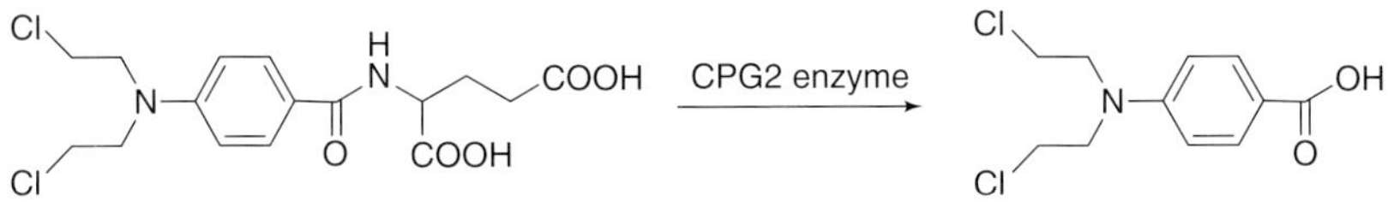

Figure 5.10 The activation of 4-(bis(2-chloroethyl)-amino) benzoyl-L-glutamic acid prodrug to anticancer drug 4-(bis(2-chloroethyl)-amino) benzoic acid by CPG2–mAb conjugate.

An example of ADEPT is to use carboxypeptidases to release the anticancer agent 4-(bis(2-chloroethyl)-amino) benzoic acid. Carboxypeptidase G2 (CPG2)–mAb conjugate has been studied in a human choriocarcinoma cell line and a human colorectal cell line [102]. In the presence of CPG2, the investigated prodrug, 4-(bis(2-chloroethyl)-amino) benzoyl-L-glutamic acid, was converted to an active anticancer agent 4-(bis(2-chloroethyl)-amino) benzoic acid (Figure 5.10). Promising results were obtained in athymic mice with transplanted choriocarcinoma or colorectal xenografts [103].

Although ADEPT has already been demonstrated to be effective in several tumor xenograft studies [104, 105], it still has not yet been translated into clinical practice. A significant obstacle may be the immunogenicity of enzymes used for prodrug activation and the targeting mAb as both were derived from nonhuman sources. This problem can be resolved by the use of human enzymes in conjunction with humanized or human mAbs. A humanized anti-carcinoembryonic antigen (CEA) antibody–human β-glucuronidase fusion protein plus DOX glucuronide prodrug was developed [106]. This ADEPT system exhibited superior antitumor efficacy without any detectable toxicity in tumor xenograft-bearing mice as compared to conventional chemotherapy. These superior therapeutic effects in human tumor xenografts can be explained by the approximately 10-fold higher drug concentrations in tumors of mice treated with this ADEPT system than those treated with free DOX alone. The use of human enzymes, however, poses the potential risk of unwanted activation of prodrugs by endogenous enzymes. Early clinical trials are promising and indicate that ADEPT may become an effective treatment for solid tumors. Examples of ADEPT systems in clinical trials are listed in Table 5.7.

Table 5.7 Examples of ADEPT in clinical trials.

Enzyme	Prodrug	Target	Clinical trial stage
CPG2 linked to F(ab′)$_2$ fragment of murine A5B7 mAb (A5CP)	N-(4-((2-chloroethyl) (2-mesyloxyethyl)amino) benzoyl)-L-glutamic acid	colorectal carcinoma	phase I [103]
A5CP	bis-iodophenol mustard, ZD2767P	advanced colorectal carcinoma	phase I [107]

5.5.6
Polymer–Drug Conjugates

The conjugation of drugs to synthetic and natural macromolecules was initiated more than 50 years ago. For example, Jatzkewitz used a dipeptide spacer to attach a drug (mescaline) to polyvinylpyrrolidone in the early 1950s. When compared to low-molecular-weight drugs, polymer–drug conjugates have several advantages [108]: (i) active uptake by fluid-phase pinocytosis (nontargeted polymer–drug conjugates) or receptor-mediated endocytosis (targeted polymer–drug conjugates), (ii) passive accumulation of the drug at the tumor site by the enhanced permeability and retention (EPR) effect, (iii) prolonged blood circulation time, (iv) reduced nonspecific toxicity of the conjugated drug, and (v) decreased immunogenicity of the targeting moiety. An optimal macromolecule prodrug system would ideally have: (i) a nontoxic and nonimmunogenic polymer, readily excreted or biodegraded by the host, (ii) a linker that is stable in the circulation and degrades at a controlled rate at the site of action, and (iii) a stable formulation that is amenable to commercial production [109]. Table 5.8 lists some of the polymer–drug conjugates currently in different stages of clinical trials.

Duncan and Kopecek developed an N-(2-hydroxypropyl) methacrylamide (HPMA) copolymer-G-F-L-G-DOX conjugate (PK1, FCE28068) currently in clinical trials [109, 112]. PK1 comprises DOX covalently bound to HPMA copolymer by a tetrapeptidyl linker (G-F-L-G), which is stable in the plasma and has been shown

Table 5.8 Polymer–drug conjugates in clinical trials [110, 111].

Conjugates	Target	Status	Company
Cyclodextrin-based polymer–CPT (IT-101)	solid tumors	phase I	Insert Therapeutics
Carboxymethyldextran–exatecan (DE-310)	solid tumors	phase I	Daiichi Pharmaceuticals
PGA–CPT (CT-2106)	colorectal, lung, and ovarian cancers	phase I	Cell Therapeutics
PEG–SN-38 (EZN-2208)	solid tumors	phase I	Enzon
HPMA–platinate	ovarian cancer and melanoma	phase I	Access Pharmaceutical
PEG–CPT (pegamotecan)	solid tumors	phase II	Enzon
HPMA–DOX–galactosamine (PK2, FCE28069)	hepatocellular carcinoma	phase I/II	Pfizer
HPMA–DOX (PK1, FCE28068)	lung and breast cancers	phase II	Pfizer
PGA–paclitaxel (CT-2103, Xyotax)	lung, ovarian, colorectal, breast, and esophageal cancers	phase III	Cell Therapeutics

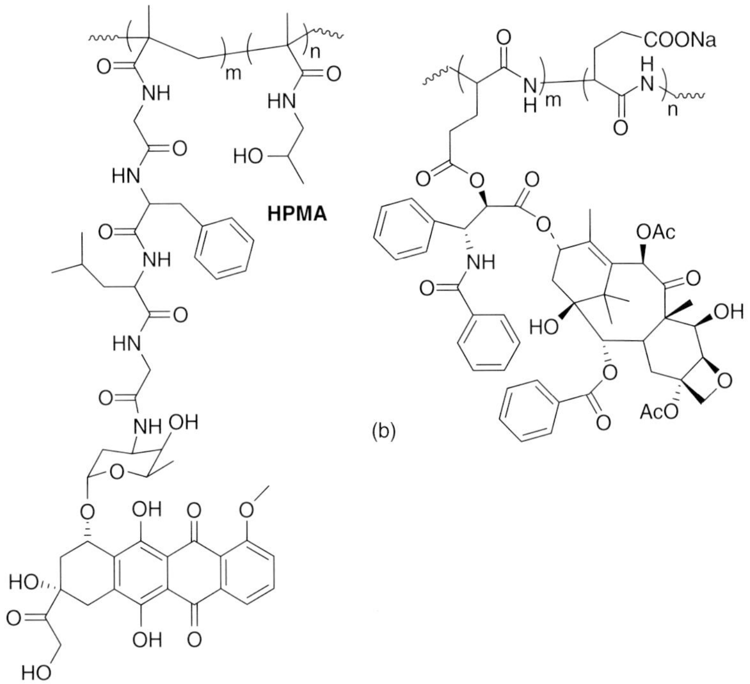

Figure 5.11 Structures of (a) PK1 (HPMA copolymer DOX) and (b) PGA–paclitaxel.

to concentrate within solid tumor models via the EPR effect (Figure 5.11a). It is then cleaved intracellularly by lysosomal cysteine proteinases, thereby allowing intratumoral drug release. The prodrug has a MW of around 30000 Da and a DOX content of around 8.5 wt%. Preclinical work demonstrated that PK1 had dramatically different pharmacokinetics compared with free DOX, with an increased plasma half-life from 5 min to 1 h. The stable peptidyl linker also ensures that little or no free DOX is liberated into the circulation following intravenous administration, thus increasing the therapeutic index of the conjugate. The *in vitro* cytotoxicity against a human ovarian carcinoma cell line indicated that PK1 can overcome the P-glycoprotein cell surface membrane pump associated with the multidrug resistance (MDR) phenotype. *In vivo*, PK1 has been shown to exhibit superior antitumor activity to free DOX after intraperitoneal administration in a large panel of model tumors, including the ascitic tumor model L1210, melanoma B16F10, Walker sarcoma, P388 leukemia, M5076, and the human colon xenograft LS174T. In phase I clinical trials, the maximum tolerated dose was determined to be 320 mg/m^2 after intravenous infusion every 3 weeks to patients with refractory or resistant cancers. No congestive cardiac failure was seen despite individual cumulative doses up to 1680 mg/m^2. Other anthracycline-like toxicities were attenuated. Pharmacokinetic data showed that PK1 had a distribution $t_{1/2}$ of 1.8 h and an elimination $t_{1/2}$ averaging 93 h. ^{131}I-labeled PK1 imaging suggested PK1 was taken up by some tumors. Responses (two partial and two minor responses) were seen in four patients with NSCLC, colorectal cancer, and anthracycline-resistant breast cancer. In the phase II studies [112], up to eight courses of PK1 (280 mg/m² DOX-equivalent) were given intravenously, together with ^{123}I-labeled imaging analog. Of 14 evaluable patients with breast cancer, three had partial responses, all anthracycline-naive patients. In 26 evaluable patients with NSCLC, three chemotherapy-naive patients had partial response. Imaging of 16 patients (five with breast cancer, six with NSCLC, and five with colorectal cancer) showed obvious tumor accumulation in two metastatic breast cancers. These results show six of 62 partial responses with limited side-effects, supporting the concept that polymer–drug conjugate therapeutics can improve anticancer activities with reduced dose-limiting toxicity compared with free drugs.

Several other polymers such as poly(L-glutamic acid) (PGA) and PEG have also been used for conjugation with drugs [111]. PGA–paclitaxel (CT-2103; Xyotax®) has advanced to phase III clinical trials and is positioned to be the first of its class to reach the market. It contains 37 wt% of paclitaxel linked through the 2'-position via an ester bond to the γ-carboxylic of PGA (MW ~ 40 000). PGA is a biodegradable polymer and its backbone is cleaved by cathepsin B to liberate diglutamyl-paclitaxel (Figure 5.11b). The PGA–paclitaxel conjugates were administered intravenously as a single agent for 30 min every 3 weeks (maximum tolerated dose: 266 mg/m²). Compared with conventional paclitaxel-based treatment, PGA–paclitaxel exhibited superior toxicity profiles and antitumor efficacy. A significant number of patients showed partial responses or stable disease (mesothelioma, renal cell carcinoma, NSCLC, and paclitaxel-resistant ovarian cancer patients). Xyotax is currently being evaluated in combination with cisplatin and carboplatin.

5.5.7
Targeting Liposomes and Nanoparticles

There are a variety of nanoparticle systems currently being explored for cancer therapeutics, which include solid nanoparticles, liposomes, dendrimers, polymeric micelles, water-soluble polymers, and protein aggregates. Like the polymeric drug conjugates, nanoparticles target the tumor passively via the EPR effect if their size is smaller than 100 nm [113]. Liposomal DOX (Doxil®) and paclitaxel-loaded human serum albumin nanoaggregates (Abraxane®) are among the first nanotherapeutics approved by the FDA for the treatment of cancers. Nanoparticles can be actively targeted by decorating the particle surface with tumor-targeting ligands [114, 115]. For examples, Farokhzad et al. [114] developed a docetaxel (DTX)-encapsulated poly(D,L-lactic-co-glycolic acid)-b-PEG nanoparticles with surface functionalization of the A10 2'-fluoropyrimidine RNA aptamer (DTX-NP-Apt) that recognizes the extracellular domain of the prostate-specific membrane antigen expressed on the surface of prostate cancer cells. DTX-NP-Apt exhibited significantly enhanced *in vitro* and *in vivo* antitumor efficacy and reduced toxicity when compared to non-targeted nanoparticles that lack the prostate-specific membrane antigen-targeting aptamer (DTX-NP).

Table 5.9 Examples of tumor-targeting nanoparticles.

Targeting nanoparticle	Nanoparticle type	Targeting ligand	Therapeutic agent	Clinical status
FCE28069 (PK2)	polymeric nanoparticle	galactose	DOX	phase I (stopped)
MCC-465	liposome	F(ab')$_2$ fragment of human antibody GAH	DTX	phase I
MBP-426	liposome	transferrin	oxaliplatin	phase I
SGT-53	liposome	antibody fragment to transferrin receptor	plasmid DNA with p53 gene	phase I
CALAA-01	polymeric nanoparticle	transferrin	small interfering RNA	phase I

Although the enhanced therapeutic efficacy of tumor-targeting nanoparticles has been demonstrated in different animal tumor models, the effects of targeting ligands on the biodistribution and pharmacokinetics of nanoparticles are still controversial. Several recent papers have suggested the primary role of tumor-targeting ligands is to enhance intracellular uptake of nanoparticles rather than increasing tumor accumulation [116, 117]. However, other reports indicate that they do play a role in the accumulation in the tumor [118]. Table 5.9 lists some examples of tumor-targeting nanoparticles currently in clinical trials.

5.6
Conclusions and Perspectives

In the last decade, there has been significant progress in our understanding of the molecular basis of cancer. A lot of this knowledge has been applied to the development of target-specific drugs against unique oncogenic aberrations. Unfortunately, many of these new drugs only exhibit modest therapeutic efficacy and often they need to be given together with standard chemotherapy to be clinically useful. Many standard chemotherapeutic agents, when given as free drug, are highly toxic with a very narrow therapeutic index. Targeting ligand–drug conjugates represent a promising approach to allow oncologists to give high doses of toxic but effective drugs to cancer patients while minimizing side-effects in normal tissue. We believe future effective cancer treatment regimens will include a combination of: (i) less-toxic but more specific drugs that can target the molecular defects of cancer (e.g., inhibitors against mitogenic protein kinases, proteasome inhibitors, and mTOR inhibitors), (ii) less-specific but toxic drugs or radionuclides delivered as targeting ligand–drug conjugates, and (iii) adjuvant immunomodulatory agents that can harness the immune response to "mop-up" the residual cancer.

In this chapter, we have reviewed the development of targeting ligand–drug conjugates with an emphasis on the discovery of cancer-targeting ligands and how these ligands can be applied to various drug delivery platforms. Although there has been enormous progress in this field, a lot remains to be worked out. One major challenge of cancer therapy is that tumors are highly heterogeneous, both among patients and within the same patient. For effective drug delivery to all the tumors (big and small, primary site, and metastatic lesions) and to most patients, we may need to use more than one delivery platform to treat a patient. For example, targeted polymeric drugs or nanoparticles may be effective for the treatment of bigger tumors with ample neovasculatures, but totally ineffective for micrometastasis, in which small-molecule ligand–drug conjugates may be more efficacious. To further enhance the therapeutic effects, drugs such as bortizomib, a proteasome inhibitor, that inhibit the antiapoptotic pathway may be added to the therapeutic payload of the drug conjugates. Many drug conjugates tend to cumulate in liver and lung nonspecifically. The challenge will be to optimize the size and surface charge of the drug conjugates such that their uptake into these two vital organs will be minimal. Although many cancer-targeting ligands are available, their utilities in cancer patients remain to be proven. There is great need to develop additional cancer-targeting ligands with high affinity and high specificity against a spectrum of tumor types. These ligands also need to have efficient endocytic activity so that drugs delivered to the tumor site can be rapidly taken up by the tumor cells. Ideally, the remaining unbound drug conjugates will be processed and rendered inactive by metabolism and excretion, perhaps facilitated by the administration of exogenous cleavage agents to cleave the on-demand linkers within the circulating drug conjugates.

Acknowledgments

This work was supported by the National Institutes of Health (R33CA-86364, R21CA135345, R33CA-99136, U19CA113298, R01CA140449, and P50CA097257). We would like to thank Mr. Joel Kugelmass for editorial support.

References

1. Hudson, P.J. and Souriau, C. (2003) Engineered antibodies. *Nat. Med.*, **9**, 129–134.
2. Todorovska, A., Roovers, R.C., Dolezal, O., Kortt, A.A., Hoogenboom, H.R., and Hudson, P.J. (2001) Design and application of diabodies, triabodies and tetrabodies for cancer targeting. *J. Immunol. Methods*, **248**, 47–66.
3. Lopci, E., Nanni, C., Rampin, L., Rubello, D., and Fanti, S. (2008) Clinical applications of ^{68}Ga-DOTANOC in neuroendocrine

tumours. *Minerva Endocrinol.*, **33**, 277–281.

4. Emons, G., Sindermann, H., Engel, J., Schally, A.V., and Grundker, C. (2009) Luteinizing hormone-releasing hormone receptor-targeted chemotherapy using AN-152. *Neuroendocrinology*, **90**, 15–18.

5. Stoltenburg, R., Reinemann, C., and Strehlitz, B. (2007) SELEX – a (r)evolutionary method to generate high-affinity nucleic acid ligands. *Biomol. Eng.*, **24**, 381–403.

6. Davies, A.J. (2007) Radioimmunotherapy for B-cell lymphoma: Y^{90} ibritumomab tiuxetan and I^{131} tositumomab. *Oncogene*, **26**, 3614–3628.

7. DeNardo, S.J., Gumerlock, P.H., Winthrop, M.D., Mack, P.C., Chi, S.G., Lamborn, K.R., Shen, S., Miers, L.A., deVere White, R.W., and DeNardo, G.L. (1995) Yttrium-90 chimeric L6 therapy of human breast cancer in nude mice and apoptosis-related messenger RNA expression. *Cancer Res.*, **55** (23 Suppl.), 5837s–5841s.

8. Aina, O.H., Liu, R., Sutcliffe, J.L., Marik, J., Pan, C.X., and Lam, K.S. (2007) From combinatorial chemistry to cancer-targeting peptides. *Mol. Pharm.*, **4**, 631–651.

9. Smith, G.P. (1985) Filamentous fusion phage: novel expression vectors that display cloned antigens on the virion surface. *Science*, **228**, 1315–1317.

10. Brown, K.C. (2010) Peptidic tumor targeting agents: the road from phage display peptide selections to clinical applications. *Curr. Pharm. Des.*, **16**, 1040–1054.

11. Cai, J., Liu, Z., Wang, F., and Li, F. (2010) Phage display applications for molecular imaging. *Curr. Pharm. Biotechnol.*, **11**, 603–609.

12. Shukla, G.S. and Krag, D.N. (2010) Cancer cell-specific internalizing ligands from phage displayed beta-lactamase-peptide fusion libraries. *Protein Eng. Des. Sel.*, **23**, 431–440.

13. Kay, B.K., Kasanov, J., and Yamabhai, M. (2001) Screening phage-displayed combinatorial peptide libraries. *Methods*, **24**, 240–246.

14. Hoffman, J.A., Giraudo, E., Singh, M., Zhang, L., Inoue, M., Porkka, K., Hanahan, D., and Ruoslahti, E. (2003) Progressive vascular changes in a transgenic mouse model of squamous cell carcinoma. *Cancer Cell.*, **4**, 383–391.

15. Krag, D.N., Shukla, G.S., Shen, G.P., Pero, S., Ashikaga, T., Fuller, S., Weaver, D.L., Burdette-Radoux, S., and Thomas, C. (2006) Selection of tumor-binding ligands in cancer patients with phage display libraries. *Cancer Res.*, **66**, 7724–7733.

16. Wang, R.Z., Zhang, L. H., Wei, X., Yang, Y., Zhang, S., Wu, J., Wu, M., Cao, Y., and Niu, R. (2008) *In vivo* selection of phage sequences and characterization of peptide-specific binding to breast cancer cells. *Chin. J. Clin. Oncol.*, **5**, 128–131.

17. Dong, J, WeiQing, L., Jiang, A., Zhang, K., and Chen, M. (2008) A novel peptide, selected from phage display library of random peptides, can efficiently target into human breast cancer cell. *Chin. Sci. Bull.*, **53**, 860–867.

18. Zang, L., Shi, L., Guo, J., Pan, Q., Wu, W., Pan, X., and Wang, J. (2009) Screening and identification of a peptide specifically targeted to NCI-H1299 from a phage display peptide library. *Cancer Lett.*, **281**, 64–70.

19. Chang, D.K., Lin, C.T., Wu, C.H., and Wu, H.C. (2009) A novel peptide enhances therapeutic efficacy of liposomal anti-cancer drugs in mice models of human lung cancer. *PLoS ONE*, **4**, e4171.

20. Zhang, J., Spring, H., and Schwab, M. (2001) Neuroblastoma tumor cell-binding peptides identified through random peptide phage display. *Cancer Lett.*, **171**, 153–164.

21. Joyce, J.A., Laakkonen, P., Bernasconi, M., Bergers, G., Ruoslahti, E., and Hanahan, D. (2003) Stage-specific vascular markers revealed by phage display in a mouse model of pancreatic islet tumorigenesis. *Cancer Cell.*, **4**, 393–403.

22. Zhu, X., Wu, H., Luo, S., Xianyu, Z., and Zhu, D. (2008) Screening and

identification of a novel hepatocellular carcinoma cell binding peptide by using a phage display library. *J. Huazhong Univ. Sci. Technol. Med. Sci.*, **28**, 299–303.

23. Sun, L., Chu, T., Wang, Y., and Wang, X. (2007) Radiolabeling and biodistribution of a nasopharyngeal carcinoma-targeting peptide identified by in vivo phage display. *Acta Biochim. Biophys. Sin.*, **39**, 624–632.

24. Nothelfer, E.M., Zitzmann-Kolbe, S., Garcia-Boy, R., Kramer, S., Herold-Mende, C., Altmann, A., Eisenhut, M., Mier, W., and Haberkorn, U. (2009) Identification and characterization of a peptide with affinity to head and neck cancer. *J. Nucl. Med.*, **50**, 426–434.

25. Hsiao, J.R., Chang, Y., Chen, Y.L., Hsieh, S.H., Hsu, K.F., Wang, C.F., Tsai, S.T., and Jin, Y.T. (2010) Cyclic alphavbeta6-targeting peptide selected from biopanning with clinical potential for head and neck squamous cell carcinoma. *Head Neck*, **32**, 160–172.

26. Buhl, L., Szecsi, P.B., Gisselo, G.G., and Schafer-Nielsen, C. (2002) Surface immunoglobulin on B lymphocytes as a potential target for specific peptide ligands in chronic lymphocytic leukaemia. *Br. J. Haematol.*, **116**, 549–554.

27. Arap, W., Pasqualini, R., and Ruoslahti, E. (1998) Cancer treatment by targeted drug delivery to tumor vasculature in a mouse model. *Science*, **279**, 377–380.

28. Renschler, M.F., Bhatt, R.R., Dower, W.J., and Levy, R. (1994) Synthetic peptide ligands of the antigen binding receptor induce programmed cell death in a human B-cell lymphoma. *Proc. Natl. Acad. Sci. USA*, **91**, 3623–3627.

29. Qin, X., Wan, Y., Li, M., Xue, X., Wu, S., Zhang, C., You, Y., Wang, W., Jiang, C., Liu, Y., Zhu, W., Ran, Y., Zhang, Z., Han, W., and Zhang, Y. (2007) Identification of a novel peptide ligand of human vascular endothelia growth factor receptor 3 for targeted tumour diagnosis and therapy. *J. Biochem.*, **142**, 79–85.

30. Zou, J., Glinsky, V.V., Landon, L.A., Matthews, L., and Deutscher, S.L. (2005) Peptides specific to the galectin-3 carbohydrate recognition domain inhibit metastasis-associated cancer cell adhesion. *Carcinogenesis*, **26**, 309–318.

31. Fukuda, M.N., Ohyama, C., Lowitz, K., Matsuo, O., Pasqualini, R., Ruoslahti, E., and Fukuda, M. (2000) A peptide mimic of E-selectin ligand inhibits sialyl Lewis X-dependent lung colonization of tumor cells. *Cancer Res.*, **60**, 450–456.

32. Oku, N., Asai, T., Watanabe, K., Kuromi, K., Nagatsuka, M., Kurohane, K., Kikkawa, H., Ogino, K., Tanaka, M., Ishikawa, D., Tsukada, H., Momose, M., Nakayama, J., and Taki, T. (2002) Anti-neovascular therapy using novel peptides homing to angiogenic vessels. *Oncogene*, **21**, 2662–2669.

33. Zhao, X., Hu, J., Huang, R., and Yang, L. (2007) Identification of one vasculature specific phage-displayed peptide in human colon cancer. *J. Exp. Clin. Cancer Res.*, **26**, 509–514.

34. Zhi, M., Wu, K.C., Dong, L., Hao, Z.M., Deng, T.Z., Hong, L., Liang, S.H., Zhao, P.T., Qiao, T.D., Wang, Y., Xu, X., and Fan, D.M. (2004) Characterization of a specific phage-displayed peptide binding to vasculature of human gastric cancer. *Cancer Biol. Ther.*, **3**, 1232–1235.

35. Tu, X., Zang, L., Lan, D., and Liang, W. (2009) Screening and identification of a peptide specifically targeted to NCI-H1299 cells from a phage display peptide library. *Mol. Med. Rep.*, **2**, 1005–1010.

36. Lee, S.M., Lee, E.J., Hong, H.Y., Kwon, M.K., Kwon, T.H., Choi, J.Y., Park, R.W., Kwon, T.G., Yoo, E.S., Yoon, G.S., Kim, I.S., Ruoslahti, E., and Lee, B.H. (2007) Targeting bladder tumor cells *in vivo* and in the urine with a peptide identified by phage display. *Mol. Cancer Res.*, **5**, 11–19.

37. Du, B., Han, H., Wang, Z., Kuang, L., Wang, L., Yu, L., Wu, M., Zhou, Z., and Qian, M. (2010) Targeted drug delivery to hepatocarcinoma *in vivo*

by phage-displayed specific binding peptide. *Mol. Cancer Res.*, **8**, 135–144.

38. Kolonin, M.G., Sun, J., Do, K.A., Vidal, C.I., Ji, Y., Baggerly, K.A., Pasqualini, R., and Arap, W. (2006) Synchronous selection of homing peptides for multiple tissues by *in vivo* phage display. *FASEB J.*, **20**, 979–981.

39. Newton, J.R., Kelly, K.A., Mahmood, U., Weissleder, R., and Deutscher, S.L. (2006) *In vivo* selection of phage for the optical imaging of PC-3 human prostate carcinoma in mice. *Neoplasia*, **8**, 772–780.

40. Zurita, A.J., Troncoso, P., Cardo-Vila, M., Logothetis, C.J., Pasqualini, R., and Arap, W. (2004) Combinatorial screenings in patients: the interleukin-11 receptor alpha as a candidate target in the progression of human prostate cancer. *Cancer Res.*, **64**, 435–439.

41. Maruta, F., Akita, N., Nakayama, J., Miyagawa, S., Ismail, T., Rowlands, D.C., Kerr, D.J., Fisher, K.D., Seymour, L.W., and Parker, A.L. (2007) Bacteriophage biopanning in human tumour biopsies to identify cancer-specific targeting ligands. *J. Drug Target.*, **15**, 311–319.

42. Lam, K.S., Salmon, S.E., Hersh, E.M., Hruby, V.J., Kazmierski, W.M., and Knapp, R.J. (1991) A new type of synthetic peptide library for identifying ligand-binding activity. *Nature*, **354**, 82–84.

43. Xiao, W., Wang, Y., Lau, E.Y., Luo, J., Yao, N., Shi, C., Meza, L., Tseng, H., Maeda, Y., Kumaresan, P., Liu, R., Lightstone, F.C., Takada, Y., and Lam, K.S. (2010) The use of one-bead one-compound combinatorial library technology to discover high-affinity $\alpha_v\beta_3$ integrin and cancer targeting arginine-glycine-aspartic acid ligands with a built-in handle. *Mol. Cancer Ther.*, **9**, 2714–2723.

44. Kumaresan, P.R., Natarajan, A., Song, A., Wang, X., Liu, R., DeNardo, G., DeNardo, S., and Lam, K.S. (2007) Development of tissue plasminogen activator specific "on demand cleavable" (ODC) linkers for radioimmunotherapy by screening one-bead-one-compound combinatorial peptide libraries. *Bioconjug. Chem.*, **18**, 175–182.

45. Meldal, M., Svendsen, I., Breddam, K., and Auzanneau, F.I. (1994) Portion-mixing peptide libraries of quenched fluorogenic substrates for complete subsite mapping of endoprotease specificity. *Proc. Natl. Acad. Sci. USA*, **91**, 3314–3318.

46. Liu, R., Marik, J., and Lam, K.S. (2002) A novel peptide-based encoding system for "one-bead one-compound" peptidomimetic and small molecule combinatorial libraries. *J. Am. Chem. Soc.*, **124**, 7678–7680.

47. Song, A., Zhang, J., Lebrilla, C.B., and Lam, K.S. (2003) A novel and rapid encoding method based on mass spectrometry for "one-bead-one-compound" small molecule combinatorial libraries. *J. Am. Chem. Soc.*, **125**, 6180–6188.

48. Wang, X., Zhang, J., Song, A., Lebrilla, C.B., and Lam, K.S. (2004) Encoding method for OBOC small molecule libraries using a biphasic approach for ladder-synthesis of coding tags. *J. Am. Chem. Soc.*, **126**, 5740–5749.

49. Liu, R. and Lam, K.S. (2001) Automatic Edman microsequencing of peptides containing multiple unnatural amino acids. *Anal. Biochem.*, **295**, 9–16.

50. Amadei, G.A., Cho, C.F., Lewis, J.D., and Luyt, L.G. (2010) A fast, reproducible and low-cost method for sequence deconvolution of "on-bead" peptides via "on-target" maldi-TOF/TOF mass spectrometry. *J. Mass. Spectrom.*, **45**, 241–251.

51. Peng, L., Liu, R., Marik, J., Wang, X., Takada, Y., and Lam, K.S. (2006) Combinatorial chemistry identifies high-affinity peptidomimetics against alpha4beta1 integrin for *in vivo* tumor imaging. *Nat. Chem. Biol.*, **2**, 381–389.

52. Wang, X., Peng, L., Liu, R., Xu, B., and Lam, K.S. (2005) Applications of topologically segregated bilayer beads in "one-bead one-compound" combinatorial libraries. *J. Pept. Res.*, **65**, 130–138.

53. Xiao, W., Yao, N., Peng, L., Liu, R., and Lam, K.S. (2009) Near-infrared optical imaging in glioblastoma xenograft with ligand-targeting alpha 3 integrin. *Eur. J. Nucl. Med. Mol. Imaging*, **36**, 94–103.

54. Aina, O.H., Marik, J., Gandour-Edwards, R., and Lam, K.S. (2005) Near-infrared optical imaging of ovarian cancer xenografts with novel alpha3-integrin binding peptide "OA02". *Mol. Imaging*, **4**, 439–447.

55. Haubner, R., Gratias, R., Diefenbach, B., Goodman, S.L., Jonczyk, A., and Kessler, H. (1996) Structural and functional aspects of RGD-containing cyclic pentapeptides as highly potent and selective integrin $\alpha_v\beta_3$ antagonists. *J. Am. Chem. Soc.*, **118**, 7461–7472.

56. Johansson, E.M., Dubois, J., Darbre, T., and Reymond, J.L. (2010) Glycopeptide dendrimer colchicine conjugates targeting cancer cells. *Bioorg. Med. Chem.*, **18**, 6589–6597.

57. Aggarwal, S., Harden, J.L., and Denmeade, S.R. (2006) Synthesis and screening of a random dimeric peptide library using the one-bead–one-dimer combinatorial approach. *Bioconjug. Chem.*, **17**, 335–340.

58. Dubowchik, G.M. and Walker, M.A. (1999) Receptor-mediated and enzyme-dependent targeting of cytotoxic anticancer drugs. *Pharmacol. Ther.*, **83**, 67–123.

59. Kratz, F., Muller, I.A., Ryppa, C., and Warnecke, A. (2008) Prodrug strategies in anticancer chemotherapy. *ChemMedChem*, **3**, 20–53.

60. Jonsson, E., Dhar, S., Jonsson, B., Nygren, P., Graf, W., and Larsson, R. (2000) Differential activity of topotecan, irinotecan and SN-38 in fresh human tumour cells but not in cell lines. *Eur. J. Cancer*, **36**, 2120–2127.

61. Damen, E.W., Nevalainen, T.J., van den Bergh, T.J., de Groot, F.M., and Scheeren, H.W. (2002) Synthesis of novel paclitaxel prodrugs designed for bioreductive activation in hypoxic tumour tissue. *Bioorg. Med. Chem.*, **10**, 71–77.

62. de Groot, F.M., van Berkom, L.W., and Scheeren, H.W. (2000) Synthesis and biological evaluation of 2′-carbamate-linked and 2′-carbonate-linked prodrugs of paclitaxel: selective activation by the tumor-associated protease plasmin. *J. Med. Chem.*, **43**, 3093–3102.

63. Greenwald, R.B., Choe, Y.H., Conover, C.D., Shum, K., Wu, D., and Royzen, M. (2000) Drug delivery systems based on trimethyl lock lactonization: poly(ethylene glycol) prodrugs of amino-containing compounds. *J. Med. Chem.*, **43**, 475–487.

64. Rivault, F., Tranoy-Opalinski, I., and Gesson, J.P. (2004) A new linker for glucuronylated anticancer prodrugs. *Bioorg. Med. Chem.*, **12**, 675–682.

65. Wang, B., Zhang, H., Zheng, A., and Wang, W. (1998) Coumarin-based prodrugs. Part 3: structural effects on the release kinetics of esterase-sensitive prodrugs of amines. *Bioorg. Med. Chem.*, **6**, 417–426.

66. Dubowchik, G.M., Firestone, R.A., Padilla, L., Willner, D., Hofstead, S.J., Mosure, K., Knipe, J.O., Lasch, S.J., and Trail, P.A. (2002) Cathepsin B-labile dipeptide linkers for lysosomal release of doxorubicin from internalizing immunoconjugates: model studies of enzymatic drug release and antigen-specific *in vitro* anticancer activity. *Bioconjug. Chem.*, **13**, 855–869.

67. Gopin, A., Ebner, S., Attali, B., and Shabat, D. (2006) Enzymatic activation of second-generation dendritic prodrugs: conjugation of self-immolative dendrimers with poly(ethylene glycol) via click chemistry. *Bioconjug. Chem.*, **17**, 1432–1440.

68. McGrath, D.V. (2005) Dendrimer disassembly as a new paradigm for the application of dendritic structures. *Mol. Pharm.*, **2**, 253–263.

69. Brown, J.M. and Wilson, W.R. (2004) Exploiting tumour hypoxia in cancer treatment. *Nat. Rev. Cancer*, **4**, 437–447.

70. McKeown, S.R., Cowen, R.L., and Williams, K.J. (2007) Bioreductive drugs: from concept to clinic. *Clin. Oncol. (R. Coll. Radiol.)*, **19**, 427–442.

71. Chen, Y. and Hu, L. (2009) Design of anticancer prodrugs for reductive activation. *Med. Res. Rev.*, **29**, 29–64.
72. Balendiran, G.K., Dabur, R., and Fraser, D. (2004) The role of glutathione in cancer. *Cell. Biochem. Funct.*, **22**, 343–352.
73. Britten, R.A., Green, J.A., and Warenius, H.M. (1992) Cellular glutathione (GSH) and glutathione S-transferase (GST) activity in human ovarian tumor biopsies following exposure to alkylating agents. *Int. J. Radiat. Oncol. Biol. Phys.*, **24**, 527–531.
74. Vrudhula, V.M., MacMaster, J.F., Li, Z., Kerr, D.E., and Senter, P.D. (2002) Reductively activated disulfide prodrugs of paclitaxel. *Bioorg. Med. Chem. Lett.*, **12**, 3591–3594.
75. Henne, W.A., Doorneweerd, D.D., Hilgenbrink, A.R., Kularatne, S.A., and Low, P.S. (2006) Synthesis and activity of a folate peptide camptothecin prodrug. *Bioorg. Med. Chem. Lett.*, **16**, 5350–5355.
76. Beeson, C., Butrynski, J.E., Hart, M.J., Nourigat, C., Matthews, D.C., Press, O.W., Senter, P.D., and Bernstein, I.D. (2003) Conditionally cleavable radioimmunoconjugates: a novel approach for the release of radioisotopes from radioimmunoconjugates. *Bioconjug. Chem.*, **14**, 927–933.
77. Elnakat, H. and Ratnam, M. (2004) Distribution, functionality and gene regulation of folate receptor isoforms: implications in targeted therapy. *Adv. Drug Deliv. Rev.*, **56**, 1067–1084.
78. Shia, J., Klimstra, D.S., Nitzkorski, J.R., Low, P.S., Gonen, M., Landmann, R., Weiser, M.R., Franklin, W.A., Prendergast, F.G., Murphy, L., Tang, L.H., Temple, L., Guillem, J.G., Wong, W.D., and Paty, P.B. (2008) Immunohistochemical expression of folate receptor alpha in colorectal carcinoma: patterns and biological significance. *Hum. Pathol.*, **39**, 498–505.
79. Lee, J.W., Lu, J.Y., Low, P.S., and Fuchs, P.L. (2002) Synthesis and evaluation of taxol–folic acid conjugates as targeted antineoplastics. *Bioorg. Med. Chem.*, **10**, 2397–2414.
80. Reddy, J.A., Westrick, E., Vlahov, I., Howard, S.J., Santhapuram, H.K., and Leamon, C.P. (2006) Folate receptor specific anti-tumor activity of folate–mitomycin conjugates. *Cancer Chemother. Pharmacol.*, **58**, 229–236.
81. Goren, D., Horowitz, A.T., Tzemach, D., Tarshish, M., Zalipsky, S., and Gabizon, A. (2000) Nuclear delivery of doxorubicin via folate-targeted liposomes with bypass of multidrug-resistance efflux pump. *Clin. Cancer Res.*, **6**, 1949–1957.
82. Pinhassi, R.I., Assaraf, Y.G., Farber, S., Stark, M., Ickowicz, D., Drori, S., Domb, A.J., and Livney, Y.D. (2010) Arabinogalactan–folic acid–drug conjugate for targeted delivery and target-activated release of anticancer drugs to folate receptor-overexpressing cells. *Biomacromolecules*, **11**, 294–303.
83. Yao, N., Xiao, W., Wang, X., Marik, J., Park, S.H., Takada, Y., and Lam, K.S. (2009) Discovery of targeting ligands for breast cancer cells using the one-bead one-compound combinatorial method. *J. Med. Chem.*, **52**, 126–133.
84. Mukhopadhyay, S., Barnes, C.M., Haskel, A., Short, S.M., Barnes, K.R., and Lippard, S.J. (2008) Conjugated platinum(IV)–peptide complexes for targeting angiogenic tumor vasculature. *Bioconjug. Chem.*, **19**, 39–49.
85. Huang, B., Desai, A., Tang, S., Thomas, T.P., and Baker, J.R. Jr. (2010) The synthesis of a c(RGDyK) targeted SN38 prodrug with an indolequinone structure for bioreductive drug release. *Org. Lett.*, **12**, 1384–1387.
86. Langer, M., Kratz, F., Rothen-Rutishauser, B., Wunderli-Allenspach, H., and Beck-Sickinger, A.G. (2001) Novel peptide conjugates for tumor-specific chemotherapy. *J. Med. Chem.*, **44**, 1341–1348.
87. Chandna, P., Khandare, J.J., Ber, E., Rodriguez-Rodriguez, L., and Minko, T. (2010) Multifunctional tumor-targeted polymer–peptide–drug delivery system for treatment of primary and metastatic cancers. *Pharm. Res.*, **11**, 2296–2306.

88. Adams, G.P. and Weiner, L.M. (2005) Monoclonal antibody therapy of cancer. *Nat. Biotechnol.*, **23**, 1147–1157.
89. Fanale, M.A. and Younes, A. (2007) Monoclonal antibodies in the treatment of non-Hodgkin's lymphoma. *Drugs*, **67**, 333–350.
90. Zhang, Q., Chen, G., Liu, X., and Qian, Q. (2007) Monoclonal antibodies as therapeutic agents in oncology and antibody gene therapy. *Cell Res.*, **17**, 89–99.
91. Shen, W.C., Ballou, B., Ryser, H.J., and Hakala, T.R. (1986) Targeting, internalization, and cytotoxicity of methotrexate-monoclonal anti-stage-specific embryonic antigen-1 antibody conjugates in cultured F-9 teratocarcinoma cells. *Cancer Res.*, **46**, 3912–3916.
92. Johnson, D.A. and Laguzza, B.C. (1987) Antitumor xenograft activity with a conjugate of a Vinca derivative and the squamous carcinoma-reactive monoclonal antibody PF1/D. *Cancer Res.*, **47**, 3118–3122.
93. Dillman, R.O., Johnson, D.E., Shawler, D.L., and Koziol, J.A. (1988) Superiority of an acid-labile daunorubicin–monoclonal antibody immunoconjugate compared to free drug. *Cancer Res.*, **48**, 6097–6102.
94. Bross, P.F., Beitz, J., Chen, G., Chen, X.H., Duffy, E., Kieffer, L., Roy, S., Sridhara, R., Rahman, A., Williams, G., and Pazdur, R. (2001) Approval summary: gemtuzumab ozogamicin in relapsed acute myeloid leukemia. *Clin. Cancer Res.*, **7**, 1490–1496.
95. Singh, Y., Palombo, M., and Sinko, P.J. (2008) Recent trends in targeted anticancer prodrug and conjugate design. *Curr. Med. Chem.*, **15**, 1802–1826.
96. Teicher, B.A. (2009) Antibody–drug conjugate targets. *Curr. Cancer Drug Targets*, **9**, 982–1004.
97. Pastan, I., Hassan, R., FitzGerald, D.J., and Kreitman, R.J. (2007) Immunotoxin treatment of cancer. *Annu Rev. Med.*, **58**, 221–237.
98. Kreitman, R.J., Wilson, W.H., Robbins, D., Margulies, I., Stetler-Stevenson, M., Waldmann, T.A., and Pastan, I. (1999) Responses in refractory hairy cell leukemia to a recombinant immunotoxin. *Blood*, **94**, 3340–3348.
99. Kreitman, R.J., Wilson, W.H., White, J.D., Stetler-Stevenson, M., Jaffe, E.S., Giardina, S., Waldmann, T.A., and Pastan, I. (2000) Phase I trial of recombinant immunotoxin anti-Tac(Fv)–PE38 (LMB-2) in patients with hematologic malignancies. *J. Clin. Oncol.*, **18**, 1622–1636.
100. Bagshawe, K.D. (1987) Antibody directed enzymes revive anti-cancer prodrugs concept. *Br. J. Cancer*, **56**, 531–532.
101. Senter, P.D., Saulnier, M.G., Schreiber, G.J., Hirschberg, D.L., Brown, J.P., Hellstrom, I., and Hellstrom, K.E. (1988) Anti-tumor effects of antibody–alkaline phosphatase conjugates in combination with etoposide phosphate. *Proc. Natl. Acad. Sci. USA*, **85**, 4842–4846.
102. Springer, C.J., Antoniw, P., Bagshawe, K.D., Searle, F., Bisset, G.M., and Jarman, M. (1990) Novel prodrugs which are activated to cytotoxic alkylating agents by carboxypeptidase G2. *J. Med. Chem.*, **33**, 677–681.
103. Napier, M.P., Sharma, S.K., Springer, C.J., Bagshawe, K.D., Green, A.J., Martin, J., Stribbling, S.M., Cushen, N., O'Malley, D., and Begent, R.H. (2000) Antibody-directed enzyme prodrug therapy: efficacy and mechanism of action in colorectal carcinoma. *Clin. Cancer Res.*, **6**, 765–772.
104. Alderson, R.F., Toki, B.E., Roberge, M., Geng, W., Basler, J., Chin, R., Liu, A., Ueda, R., Hodges, D., Escandon, E., Chen, T., Kanavarioti, T., Babe, L., Senter, P.D., Fox, J.A., and Schellenberger, V. (2006) Characterization of a CC49-based single-chain fragment–beta-lactamase fusion protein for antibody-directed enzyme prodrug therapy (ADEPT). *Bioconjug. Chem.*, **17**, 410–418.

105. Sharma, S.K., Pedley, R.B., Bhatia, J., Boxer, G.M., El-Emir, E., Qureshi, U., Tolner, B., Lowe, H., Michael, N.P., Minton, N., Begent, R.H., and Chester, K.A. (2005) Sustained tumor regression of human colorectal cancer xenografts using a multifunctional mannosylated fusion protein in antibody-directed enzyme prodrug therapy. *Clin. Cancer Res.*, **11**, 814–825.
106. Bosslet, K., Czech, J., Seemann, G., Monneret, C., and Hoffmann, D. (1994) Fusion protein mediated prodrug activation (FMPA) *in vivo*. *Cell Biophys.*, **24–25**, 51–63.
107. Francis, R.J., Sharma, S.K., Springer, C., Green, A.J., Hope-Stone, L.D., Sena, L., Martin, J., Adamson, K.L., Robbins, A., Gumbrell, L., O'Malley, D., Tsiompanou, E., Shahbakhti, H., Webley, S., Hochhauser, D., Hilson, A.J., Blakey, D., and Begent, R.H. (2002) A phase I trial of antibody directed enzyme prodrug therapy (ADEPT) in patients with advanced colorectal carcinoma or other CEA producing tumours. *Br. J. Cancer*, **87**, 600–607.
108. Kopecek, J. and Kopeckova, P. (2010) HPMA copolymers: origins, early developments, present, and future. *Adv. Drug Deliv. Rev.*, **62**, 122–149.
109. Vasey, P.A., Kaye, S.B., Morrison, R., Twelves, C., Wilson, P., Duncan, R., Thomson, A.H., Murray, L.S., Hilditch, T.E., Murray, T., Burtles, S., Fraier, D., Frigerio, E., and Cassidy, J., Cancer Research Campaign Phase I/II Committee (1999) Phase I clinical and pharmacokinetic study of PK1 [N-(2-hydroxypropyl)methacrylamide copolymer doxorubicin]: first member of a new class of chemotherapeutic agents–drug–polymer conjugates. *Clin. Cancer Res.*, **5**, 83–94.
110. Albain, K.S., Belani, C.P., Bonomi, P., O'Byrne, K.J., Schiller, J.H., and Socinski, M. (2006) PIONEER: a phase III randomized trial of paclitaxel poliglumex versus paclitaxel in chemotherapy-naive women with advanced-stage non-small-cell lung cancer and performance status of 2. *Clin. Lung Cancer*, **7**, 417–419.
111. Li, C. and Wallace, S. (2008) Polymer–drug conjugates: recent development in clinical oncology. *Adv. Drug Deliv. Rev.*, **60**, 886–898.
112. Seymour, L.W., Ferry, D.R., Kerr, D.J., Rea, D., Whitlock, M., Poyner, R., Boivin, C., Hesslewood, S., Twelves, C., Blackie, R., Schatzlein, A., Jodrell, D., Bissett, D., Calvert, H., Lind, M., Robbins, A., Burtles, S., Duncan, R., and Cassidy, J. (2009) Phase II studies of polymer–doxorubicin (PK1, FCE28068) in the treatment of breast, lung and colorectal cancer. *Int. J. Oncol.*, **34**, 1629–1636.
113. Matsumura, Y. and Maeda, H. (1986) A new concept for macromolecular therapeutics in cancer chemotherapy: mechanism of tumoritropic accumulation of proteins and the antitumor agent smancs. *Cancer Res.*, **46**, 6387–6392.
114. Farokhzad, O.C., Cheng, J., Teply, B.A., Sherifi, I., Jon, S., Kantoff, P.W., Richie, J.P., and Langer, R. (2006) Targeted nanoparticle–aptamer bioconjugates for cancer chemotherapy *in vivo*. *Proc. Natl. Acad. Sci. USA*, **103**, 6315–6320.
115. Zhang, X.Y., Chen, J., Zheng, Y.F., Gao, X.L., Kang, Y., Liu, J.C., Cheng, M.J., Sun, H., and Xu, C.J. (2009) Follicle-stimulating hormone peptide can facilitate paclitaxel nanoparticles to target ovarian carcinoma *in vivo*. *Cancer Res.*, **69**, 6506–6514.
116. Bartlett, D.W., Su, H., Hildebrandt, I.J., Weber, W.A., and Davis, M.E. (2007) Impact of tumor-specific targeting on the biodistribution and efficacy of siRNA nanoparticles measured by multimodality *in vivo* imaging. *Proc. Natl. Acad. Sci. USA*, **104**, 15549–15554.
117. Kirpotin, D.B., Drummond, D.C., Shao, Y., Shalaby, M.R., Hong, K., Nielsen, U.B., Marks, J.D., Benz, C.C., and Park, J.W. (2006) Antibody targeting of long-circulating lipidic nanoparticles does not increase tumor localization but does increase internalization in animal models. *Cancer Res.*, **66**, 6732–6740.

118. Wu, A.M., Yazaki, P.J., Tsai, S., Nguyen, K., Anderson, A.L., McCarthy, D.W., Welch, M.J., Shively, J.E., Williams, L.E., Raubitschek, A.A., Wong, J.Y., Toyokuni, T., Phelps, M.E., and Gambhir, S.S. (2000) High-resolution microPET imaging of carcinoembryonic antigen-positive xenografts by using a copper-64-labeled engineered antibody fragment. *Proc. Natl. Acad. Sci. USA*, **97**, 8495–8500.

6
Antibody-Directed Enzyme Prodrug Therapy (ADEPT) – Basic Principles and its Practice So Far

Kenneth D. Bagshawe

6.1
Introduction

In the early years following World War II there was speculation that the aberrant behavior of cancer cells might result from a unique repertoire of enzymes not expressed by normal cells. If such enzymes had been found there was the possibility that they might be used to convert relatively nontoxic prodrugs into potent cytotoxic agents. Evidence for such enzymes has not been found and the prodrug cyclophosphamide proved to be activated, not as hoped, by tumor-located enzymes, but by normal hepatic enzymes [1]. In the 1970s studies were reported using antibody–enzyme conjugates (AECs) [2] Then came the proposal to use an antibody directed at a tumor-related antigen to deliver a unique enzyme to cancer sites and this was combined with the concept of using the enzyme to convert a low-toxicity prodrug to a highly cytotoxic agent [3].

It seemed possible that a differential toxicity between a prodrug and drug of 100-fold, might allow up to a 100 times the dose of cytotoxic agent to be delivered to tumors. Since then prodrug-to-drug toxicity differentials of up to 4000-fold have been reported [4] and more than 100 papers have been published on what has become known as antibody-directed enzyme prodrug therapy (ADEPT).

Despite widespread interest in the approach, after more than 20 years, the only reports of ADEPT in the clinic have, to the best of our knowledge, come from London, UK.

Although the basic concept of ADEPT is simple it clearly requires a multidisciplinary team to achieve all the products required for clinical evaluation. Such a team approach has been applied in London, but it is fair to say that ADEPT has not, so far, achieved its early promise. It is indicated in this chapter that this failure may have resulted from deviation from principles that were apparent at the outset. However, it can be reported that there is a new beginning of ADEPT that is based on those principles. Although some of the ADEPT studies done elsewhere have been summarized here (see Table 6.1), these have been reviewed [5, 6] more extensively elsewhere and the emphasis in this paper will be on the clinical studies in London.

Drug Delivery in Oncology: From Basic Research to Cancer Therapy, First Edition.
Edited by Felix Kratz, Peter Senter, and Henning Steinhagen.
© 2012 Wiley-VCH Verlag GmbH & Co. KGaA. Published 2012 by Wiley-VCH Verlag GmbH & Co. KGaA.

Table 6.1 Examples of enzyme prodrug systems.

Enzyme	Prodrug	Drug	References
Alkaline phosphatase	etoposide phosphate	etoposide	[7]
	mitomycin C phosphate	mitomycin	[8]
	doxorubicin phosphate	doxorubicin	[9]
	phenol mustard phosphate	phenol mustard	[10]
Alcohol dehydrogenase	alcohol	–	[11]
β-Lactamase	cephalosporin mustards	nitrogen mustards	[12, 13]
β-Glucoronidase	phenol mustard glucuronidase	phenol mustard	[14, 15]
	daunorubicin glucuronidase	daunorubicin	[16, 17]
Carboxyesterases	CPT-11 and irinotecan	SN38	[18]
Carboxypeptidase A	methotrexate peptide	methotrexate	[19]
	methotrexate alanine	methotrexate	[20]
Carboxypeptidase G2	benzoic mustard glutamates	–	–
	CMDA	benzoic acid mustard	[21]
	bis-iodophenol mustard	phenol mustard	[22]
Glycosidases	glycosides	duocarmycin	[23]
Nitroreductase	CB1954	5-(aziridin-1-yl)-4-hydroxy-amino-2-nitro benzamide	[24]
Penicillin amidase	palytoxin	palytoxin	[25]

6.2
Principles and the Components of ADEPT

Before the ADEPT proposal was published [3] the logistics of the system, the *in vivo* behavior of its components, and preliminary animal studies provided evidence for the feasibility of a form of ADEPT (Figure 6.1) that translated into the clinic. To understand ADEPT it is essential to consider both its individual components and their behavior *in vivo*. The term "AEC" will be used in this chapter to cover both chemical conjugates and, where appropriate, fusion proteins.

6.2.1
Target

Ideally, the target antigen would be unique to the target cells, but more often it may be necessary to accept that the distinction between cancer and normal tissue is one of overexpression of the target antigen by cancer cells. In the case of carcinoembryonic antigen (CEA) as a target in gastrointestinal tumors, there is the redeeming feature that the low-level expression of CEA by normal

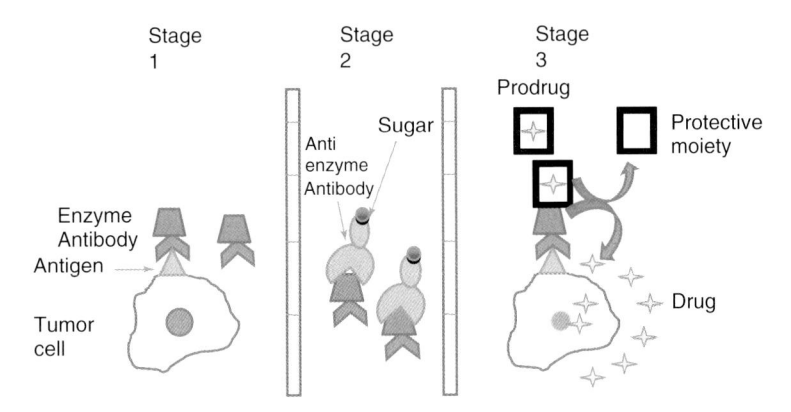

Figure 6.1 ADEPT. Stage 1: antibody binding to antigen delivers enzyme to tumor cells. Stage 2: antienzyme antibody inactivates and clears enzyme from blood. Stage 3: enzyme converts prodrug to cell killing drug within the tumor.

cells is restricted to intracellular sites not normally accessible to intravenously administered antibodies [26].

An early consideration was that the target antigen should be expressed on the surface of the cancer cell. This would allow the enzyme to have access to prodrug molecules in tumor extracellular fluid (ECF). Internalization of the AEC by target-expressing cells would result in its degradation and would deny that access, and was therefore undesirable. The target antigen should be expressed on a high proportion of the cancer cells, but heterogeneity in expression of antigens is a well-known feature of epithelial cancers [27]. Since the conversion of prodrug to drug is anticipated to occur in tumor ECF, the generated drug should be free to enter cells that fail to express the target antigen as well as those that do express it. This so-called "bystander effect" is one of the potential advantages of the ADEPT system that has been demonstrated with *in vitro* models [28].

Secretion of the targeted antigen into the ECF and into the blood may result in binding of AEC to the secreted antigens and it may be supposed that the presence of antigen in blood would negate delivery of AEC to tumors through immune complex formation in blood. This did not prove to be the case in imaging studies, with the freely secreted choriocarcinoma antigen, human chorionic gonadotropin (hCG), when it was present in blood at very high concentrations (above 200 000 IU/ml) [29].

6.2.2
Antibody

It is clear that the AEC must be a stable complex and the antibodies used in ADEPT studies have been IgG monoclonals of class 1 or 2. Conjugation of antibody to enzyme by heterobifunctional agents had to be such that the binding site of the antibody and the active site of the enzyme were not sterically obstructed.

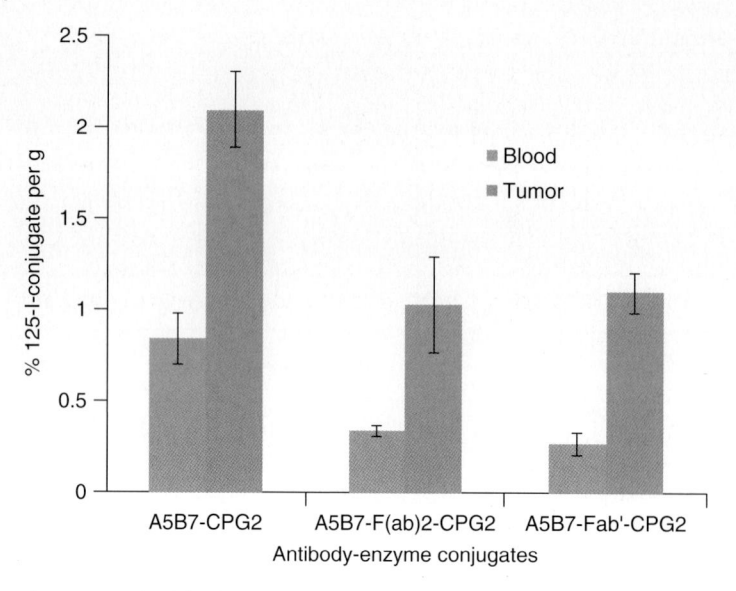

Figure 6.2 Blood level and tumor localization at 72 h after injection of ^{125}I-labeled AEC (25 units per mouse) in LS174T xenografted mice.

Experience with the use of radiolabeled antibodies for imaging purposes showed it was advantageous to use Fab$_2$ fragments, which cleared from blood more quickly than intact IgG molecules. This resulted in the use of Fab$_2$ molecules in the AEC used in the early London studies. This was probably mistaken since we had already shown that the Fc component prolonged antibody retention at tumor sites [30] (Figure 6.2) and for therapy, prolonged retention of the AEC at tumor sites was desirable. Prolonged retention of AEC in tumors would allow more time for prodrug administration. As mentioned in the previous section, internalization of the AEC is likely to be counterproductive. The use of single-chain Fv (scFv) antibody fragments in fusion proteins will be discussed in the context of later developments.

Although it is likely that small molecules penetrate better into tumors it is undesirable that they should be small enough to be subject to renal clearance or any form of rapid clearance from the circulation since this could result in reduction of enzyme concentration in tumors.

6.2.3
Enzyme

The need for an enzyme that was not expressed in any normal human tissue was paramount to avoid activation of prodrug at unwanted sites. This excluded virtually all human enzymes and all mammalian enzymes with analogous human forms, and pointed to bacterial enzymes that have no human equivalents, such as carboxypeptidase G2 (CPG2) and β-lactamase. The downside of bacterial enzymes is their potent immunogenicity that limits their repeated use. Techniques now exist for replacing amino acid sequences that are immunogenic in man [31, 32], but these have yet to be fully exploited in ADEPT. Other techniques for avoiding immunogenicity will be summarized later. It remains to be seen whether tolerance to such potent immunogens as bacterial enzymes can be induced within the time constraints imposed by the progression of cancers. The possible use of mutated human enzymes now exists. This requires that prodrug activation results from the mutated enzyme, but not from the native form. It requires modification of the prodrug as well as that of the enzyme and, of course, the mutated enzyme must remain nonimmunogenic.

6.2.4
Prodrug and Drug

It is self-evident that the prodrug should be a substrate for the selected enzyme and only for the selected enzyme. The enzyme and the prodrug have to be designed as an entity.

The advantage of the ADEPT system results from its potential to deliver a much higher concentration of cytotoxic agent to cancers than is possible with conventional chemotherapy. It follows that the action of the generated drug should be concentration-dependent over a wide range of concentrations. The action of many conventional cytotoxic agents is dose-dependent over only a limited range of concentrations and many are limited by well-known resistance mechanisms. These considerations pointed to the use of alkylating agents, the cytotoxicity of which appears to be dose-dependent over a wide range of concentrations [33, 34].

Another fundamental requirement of the prodrug is one that has been frequently ignored in ADEPT studies. If a high concentration of a drug is generated at one (or many) cancer site(s) the drug will inevitably diffuse back from the site(s) into the blood and access normal vulnerable tissues. This can only be avoided by ensuring that the drug has a short half-life so that it has decayed by the time it enters the blood. As was pointed out in the first ADEPT paper [3], this probably requires the drug to have a half-life measured in seconds rather than minutes.

Several ADEPT studies have ignored these considerations and have started from the premise that making a prodrug from an already licensed drug (see Table 6.1), however inappropriate for ADEPT, would facilitate its route to the clinic.

6.3
Third Essential

It is clear that the driving force by which molecules enter and exit from a tumor mass is the concentration gradient – the difference between plasma concentration and tumor ECF concentration. Antibody binding to cell-bound antigens modifies this process, but is subject to on/off rates.

It was evident from studies using radiolabeled antibodies directed at tumor-associated antigens that only a comparatively small proportion of any administered dose of AEC localized at cancer sites [29]. Most of it remained in the circulation until cleared by hepatic or renal routes. It was obvious that to give prodrug when there is still enzyme in blood was equivalent to giving a potentially large dose of a conventional cytotoxic agent. Even a very low concentration of enzyme in the presence of a high concentration of substrate could generate a lot of drug. It is perhaps not immediately evident that clearing enzyme from blood is a two-phase process.

So long as the plasma concentration is higher than that in the tumor ECF, the AEC will enter tumor extracellular space. Its retention there depends on the availability of binding sites and the antibody's affinity for them. Thus, the first phase of ensuring the absence of enzyme in plasma before prodrug is given is clearing the substantial amount of AEC in blood that has not localized at tumor sites. As the plasma concentration falls, antibody off rates result in slow release of AEC back into the tumor ECF and the reversed concentration gradient takes it back into the circulation. The second and more prolonged phase is that of clearing enzyme that leaks back from tumor sites into blood. It can be assumed that AEC in nontumor tissues where antigen binding has not occurred quickly returns to the blood as the plasma concentration falls.

These points were confirmed in the early preclinical studies. Nude mice bearing drug-resistant choriocarcinoma had a high concentration of the target antigen, hCG, in blood. Complete eradication of 1-cm^3 tumors was achieved with an antibody directed at hCG and conjugated to CPG2; this was followed after 72 h by the prodrug 4-((2-chloroethyl)(2-methoxy)ethyl)amino benzoyl-L-glutamic acid (CMDA) [35]. The same protocol, but with an anti-CEA antibody given to colon cancer (LS174T)-bearing nude mice, in which the target antigen was not detectable in blood, resulted in toxicity, but little tumor regression. With prolongation of the interval between administration of AEC and prodrug there was neither toxicity nor tumor regression. It was concluded that the success with the choriocarcinoma model resulted from accelerated clearance of AEC from blood by hCG in blood. In the colon model there was enzyme in blood when prodrug was given in the first case, resulting in toxicity, and in the second case, enzyme had cleared both from tumor and blood, resulting in neither tumor inhibition nor toxicity. It was clear that an agent was necessary to accelerate removal of enzyme from blood before prodrug could be given [36].

Antienzyme antibodies were made that would accelerate clearance of the AEC from blood, but one of them inactivated the enzyme (Figure 6.3). It was evident that enzyme inactivation was an almost instantaneous event and therefore more controllable than accelerated clearance. It was concluded that an enzyme-inactivating antibody would be appropriate both for inactivating enzyme that failed to localize at tumor sites and for the slow leak back of enzyme from tumor sites. The question arose whether the enzyme-inactivating antibody would inactivate enzyme in tumors and this was demonstrated to be possible. By galactosylating the antibody its rapid elimination from blood via hepatic galactose receptors was ensured and it

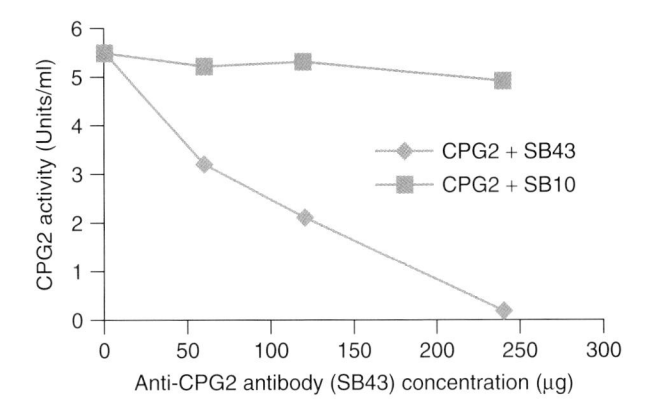

Figure 6.3 Incubation of CPG2 with SB43 *in vitro* results in inactivation of CPG2 activity in a dose-dependent manner, whereas an irrelevant antibody has no effect on CPG2 activity.

was confirmed that administration of the galactosylated SB43gal had no detectable effect on tumor enzyme levels [37].

With the three-component ADEPT system, growth delay was obtained in LS174T tumors and in ovarian tumor xenografts [38, 39].

6.4
ADEPT Studies Elsewhere

Some of the studies by other groups are summarized in Table 6.1, which illustrates the variety of enzymes and prodrug systems that have been reported. It is surprising that in many cases the issue of prodrug activation by residual plasma enzyme has not been addressed. It is also noted that many studies employed prodrugs based on existing licensed drugs. As already mentioned, the half-lives of most conventional drugs are such that they would inevitably escape from tumors and access normal cell renewal systems. The half-lives of some conventional drugs are summarized for convenience in Table 6.2.

An interesting study [41] used a nonglycosylated fusion protein that combined an antibody directed at the antigen Tag72 with the bacterial enzyme β-lactamase. Retention of enzyme activity at tumor sites showed a $t_{1/2}$ of 36.9 h in the LS174T xenografts, indicating marked dissociation between clearance from tumor and that from blood. The drug liberated from the novel prodrug was melphalan which, as shown in Table 6.2, has a $t_{1/2}$ of 1.8 h. This would allow plenty of time for the drug to escape from the tumor and cause the observed toxicity.

The advantage of using intact IgG as the targeting molecule was illustrated by a study in breast cancer xenografts [42]. A second antibody was not used, but prodrug was delayed until 12 days post-AEC and good therapeutic results obtained, demonstrating prolonged retention of the AEC in the tumors.

Table 6.2 Examples of half-lives of some conventional cytotoxic drugs (modified from [40]).

Drugs	$t_{1/2}$
Anthracyclines	22–48 h
Cyclophosphamide	1.0–6.0 h
Etoposide	4.0–8.0 h
5-Fluorouracil	10–20 min
Melphalan	1.8 h
Nitrosoureas	68 min
Procarbazine	7 min
Taxol	5.0 h
Vinblastine	2.27 h

Another interesting study reported a thermostable human endopeptidase engineered to achieve greater stability at 37 °C that has been chemically conjugated to antibody. It is argued that the low level of normal enzyme in normal tissues should not activate the prodrug [43], but results are awaited.

The important process of reducing or eliminating the antigenicity of bacterial enzymes has begun with β-lactamase [44]. The options for overcoming this problem are several, but the substitution of human amino acid sequences for response-provoking epitopes, if it can be achieved without functional loss, seems likely to be the most secure route. The fact that this has not been done so far with CPG2 may have resulted from the thorny issue of intellectual property rights. Alternatives include the masking of epitopes with poly(ethylene glycol) (PEG) or PEG-like molecules. There is also the possibility of inducing immune tolerance with heavy PEGylation [45, 46]. The use of modern immunosuppressants has not yet been reported in this context. Humanized antibodies with catalytic function, so-called abzymes, have been a long time in the wings, but may yet emerge [47–49].

6.5
Reagents for First Clinical Trials in London (1990–1995)

A consideration of the expression of CEA by colorectal carcinomas suggested this frequently fatal human cancer as a suitable target for clinical trial.

A murine anti-CEA monoclonal antibody (A5B7) was produced in our laboratory and prepared in Fab$_2$ form [50]. CPG2, which cleaves the terminal glutamate from folate-type molecules, was produced in Government Laboratories, PHLS at Porton Down, Salisbury, UK [51]. A5B7 in Fab$_2$ form was conjugated to CPG2 by a heterobifunctional agent [52] and formed the AEC. Colleagues from the Institute of Cancer Research, London, suggested a benzoic acid mustard that would be relatively easy to make in the laboratory and that would be inactivated by a terminal glutamate. A series of prodrugs was made and one, CMDA, was selected for further studies [21]. Scale-up of CMDA for clinical use was performed in a Cancer Research Campaign facility at the University of Strathclyde. CMDA had the disadvantage of being soluble only in dimethyl sulfoxide. The galactosylated murine monoclonal antibody (SB43) that inactivated CPG2 [53] and the A5B7 anti-CEA antibody were produced on a scale for a pilot clinical trial by Cell Tech Laboratories, Slough, UK.

6.5.1
First ADEPT Clinical Trial

Nineteen patients were aged 28–75 years, with advanced carcinomas of the colon, rectum, or appendix with multisite metastatic disease, that expressed CEA on histological examination. All had undergone initial surgery and available chemotherapy, but now had progressive, drug-resistant disease. Expected survival times were not more than 8 weeks.

As the prodrug had not been used clinically it was necessary to perform a dose-escalation study as a preliminary part of the study. The scale of the dose-escalation and the main study was limited by the amount of available agents.

The prodrug dose-escalation study showed that CMDA was well tolerated over the dose range covered (0.2–2.4 g/m^2) [54].

In the main study a variety of protocols were explored. The doses of AEC ranged from 20 000 to 30 000 enzyme units/m^2. The dosage of SB43gal ranged from 90 to 240 mg/m^2. The total dosage of prodrug ranged from 1.4 to 10 g/m^2. The other important variables were the time interval between administration of AEC and prodrug, and the duration of SB43gal administration. In an attempt to delay the host antibody response to the murine antibodies and the bacterial enzyme six patients received cyclosporine. Cyclosporine delayed the antibody response allowing up to three cycles of therapy to be given in some cases, but it increased toxicity significantly and was judged to have contributed to the two deaths that occurred during treatment.

Most patients had grade 3 or 4 reversible myelosuppression, which was attributable to the half-life of the drug that proved to be about 30 min. Of eight patients who received the highest doses of prodrug, four achieved partial responses and one had a mixed response in which all but one mass shrank by more than 50%.

Seven patients survived 6 months or more, including three who died at 18 months, at 25 months, and at 3 years [55].

The first conclusion from the study was that the drug generated from CMDA had a half-life that was much too long and was the probable cause of the myelosuppression.

The second conclusion was that the AEC and the SB43 were well tolerated, and that the SB43 quickly reduced blood enzyme levels to the limit of detection (Figure 6.4).

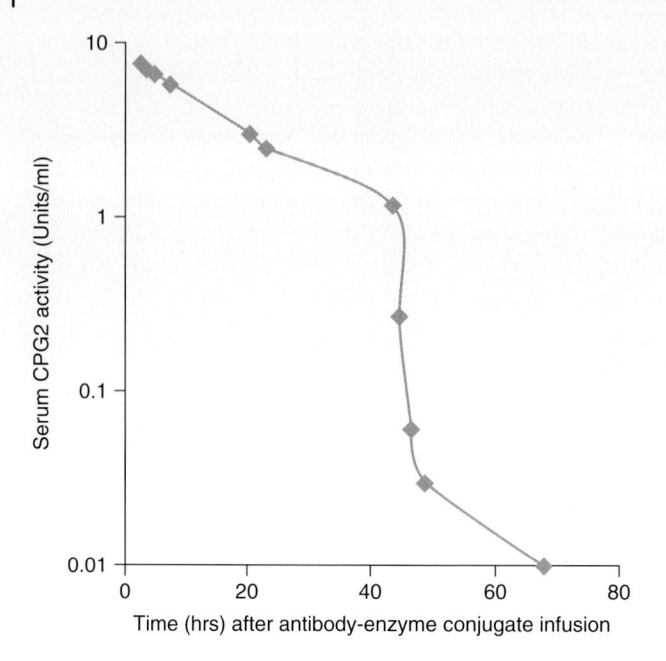

Figure 6.4 ADEPT patient given AEC followed at 48 h later by SB43gal infusion. SB43gal reduced serum CPG2 activity to below the level of detection so that prodrug was given at 72 h after the conjugate.

It became clear that the amount of SB43 given needed to be proportionate to the dose of AEC for the first few hours of administration, but it could then be infused at a greatly reduced rate to inactivate enzyme leaking back from tumor sites.

Given the limitations of the agents used it was an encouraging start.

6.5.2
Subsequent ADEPT Clinical Studies in London

A second, even smaller-scale clinical trial (10 patients) took place at another center in London using the same agents as used in the first clinical trial, but using substantially reduced doses of AEC. In this study biopsies of tumors were obtained from some patients after the SB43gal enzyme-inactivating antibody had been given. In all cases, the tumor/blood enzyme ratio was greater than 10 000 : 1. One patient in this study, who had tumor growing through the abdominal wall around a colostomy site, had near-complete resolution of the growth [56].

The challenge for the chemists at this time was to produce a potent drug with a very short half-life. This resulted in the production of what is described as a bis-iodophenol; it also is inactivated by a terminal glutamate that is cleaved by CPG2 [22]. The $t_{1/2}$ of the drug proved too short to measure, but is believed to be of the order of 1 min. It had been designated ZD2767P.

6.5.3
Two-Phase ADEPT Clinical Studies in London

At this time a major pharmaceutical company took control of ADEPT developments. Using more amenable xenograft targets than the LS174T model used in the previous studies, it was found that good responses were obtained with the ZD2767p prodrug, without the use of the enzyme-inactivating antibody [57]. Xenograft models in nude mice have been invaluable in the development of ADEPT, but what works in the nude mouse does not always translate into the human. Nevertheless, on the basis of the new animal data it was decided to proceed to a further clinical trial omitting the enzyme-inactivating antibody SB43.

The agents used in the next trial therefore consisted only of the original AEC and the prodrug ZD2767P. Twenty seven patients entered this trial. It was necessary to wait several days after the AEC was given before plasma enzyme fell to a value below 0.05 U/ml when it was judged safe for prodrug administration. Three doses of the prodrug were then given. As predicted from the earlier mouse studies, there were no responses, not even minor ones [58].

6.6
Technology Advances

It was true that chemical conjugates of antibody and enzyme had limitations, particularly with respect to batch variation. New techniques based on combinatorial libraries of scFv genes began to be used in conjunction with filamentous phage technology to produce antibody fragments with superior binding characteristics to those produced by hybridoma technology [59]. Chester *et al.* generated a library of antibodies from murine spleen cells after the mice had been immunized with CEA. Antibodies were selected for high affinity by selection in decreasing antigen concentrations. One of these scFv antibodies (MFE-23) was stable, and showed efficient localization in human colon cancers both *in vitro* and *in vivo*.

Recombinant DNA technology offered the means to generate a single molecule with antibody and enzymic function. Fusion proteins had been described by Neuberger and Bosslet [60, 61]. A genetic construct consisting of the gene encoding MFE-23 linked to the gene for CPG2 was developed [62, 63]. CPG2 is a noncovalently bound dimer and the resulting fusion protein (MFECP) has two scFv antibodies attached to the enzyme. An incidental benefit from the fusion protein was the attachment of a His tag for purification purposes, which masked the dominant epitope [64] so that some patients did not have an immune response to a single exposure to the fusion protein.

It has been argued that small antibody fragments are superior to larger ones in terms of tumor penetration, but they have not been shown to be advantageous in the case of AECs. The issue of residence time at tumor sites, possibly dependent on the Fc component, may be more important.

The yield of the fusion protein MFECP in bacterial expression systems proved to be rather poor, but it was very good when expressed in the yeast *Pichia pastoris* [65]. This new expression system, necessary for production purposes, resulted in the clinical studies in London deviating away from the original ADEPT principles for more than 12 years. Why did this happen? Proteins expressed by *P. pastoris* are mannosylated [66]. The presence of this sugar on MFECP modified its circulatory characteristics in the body fundamentally [67].

Big Pharma had opined that a three-component therapy system was one component too many. So would this sugared fusion protein replace both the original, chemically conjugated AEC and the enzyme-inactivating agent SB43, and make ADEPT a simpler two-component system (i.e., fusion protein and prodrug)? The idea that MFECP would clear quickly from blood was thought to be advantageous in the light of the previous trial where waiting for the enzyme to clear from blood delayed prodrug administration until a time when there was little or no enzyme remaining at tumor sites.

The presence of the mannose on MFECP ensured that its clearance, via hepatic mannose receptors, would begin as soon as its administration by intravenous infusion was started [67]. Its plasma concentration therefore would fail to reach the high concentration achieved by the original AEC. The blood/tumor gradient would be reduced. So, for a given amount of administered enzyme, the amount delivered to tumors would be less.

In addition, the rapid fall in the enzyme concentration after completion of the AEC infusion would be accompanied by a leak back of enzyme into the blood. The glycosylated fusion protein would not be able to eliminate the leak back of enzyme from tumors into blood: it was part of the problem. So how long was it appropriate to wait before giving the prodrug?

If the prodrug was delayed until there was no detectable enzyme in blood, the probability was that there would be too little enzyme in tumors to activate much prodrug. Thus, was there a concentration of enzyme in plasma that would not activate enough prodrug to result in toxicity?

Encouragement came from studies in the mouse [68]. It was found that in nude mice bearing xenografts of LS174T or SW1222 human colon cancers, tumor/blood ratios of 1400 : 1 and 344 : 1 were obtained respectively. Plasma enzyme activity fell to 0.001 and 0.0038 units in these models by 6 h after administration. A single ADEPT cycle with prodrug (ZD2767P) given at 6, 7, and 8 h after MFECP produced reproducible growth delay in both xenograft models. Multiple ADEPT cycles (9–10 cycles over 21 days) produced complete regressions in the SW1222 xenografts. These mouse data suggested that there would be a short time interval in the human when there was still sufficient enzyme at tumor sites, but a very low concentration of enzyme in blood. Would this prove to be the case?

Introducing a new fusion protein into the clinic in the twenty-first century encounters regulatory restrictions that require the production of materials intended for the clinic to Good Manufacturing Practice standards [69]. As in previous trials, the patients all had advanced disease and had become resistant to all available conventional chemotherapy. In patients it was found that it took much longer to give a single cycle of therapy and was much more variable between patients than had been the case in the mouse models. Initially, prodrug was not given until the plasma enzyme concentration was less than 0.02 units, but this was later lowered to 0.005 units. The best response in the study was a 10% reduction in tumor diameter in one patient. A single cycle of therapy did not achieve significant responses in any other patient although 11 of 28 patients were judged to have stable disease at 8 weeks post-therapy [70].

A subsequent analysis of the same patient data together with data from additional patients who received two or more cycles of ADEPT during a period of up to 12 days has been published to date, only in an abstract by Wilkins *et al.* [7]. This analysis focused on the total dosage of prodrug given. The total dose of prodrug ranged from 37 to 3226 mg/m^2 on one or more cycles. The maximum tolerated dose was 1200 mg/m^2 in two complete ADEPT cycles. Human anti-CPG2 antibodies were found in 40% of patients after one cycle of ADEPT. Sixty-nine percent of the patients who received a total prodrug dose of 0.900 mg/m^2, had stable disease at 8 weeks post-therapy and 44% of these had "clinically significant" responses. Of the nine patients studied by ^{18}F-fluorodeoxyglucose positron emission tomography, four had partial responses predictive of prolonged survival by the criteria introduced by Green *et al.* [8]. Further treatment could not be given because patients developed antibodies to CPG2, but they were also limited by myelosuppression. It seems likely that the myelosuppression results from the low concentration of enzyme in plasma when prodrug was given.

Whilst it can be claimed that these results are superior to those achieved in such patients by any conventional drug, they still fall far short of those achieved in the first clinical trial and the results potentially achievable by adherence to the original principles as set out in this chapter.

6.7
ADEPT Future

Currently, the process of rebuilding ADEPT has begun. The new ADEPT team accepts the need to adhere to the original principles outlined earlier in this chapter as well as make use of the technological advances that have occurred in the past 20 years.

References

1. Chang, T.K., Weber, G.F., Crespi, C.L., and Waxman, D.J. (1993) Differential activation of cyclophosphamide and ifosphamide by cytochromes P-450 2B and 3A in human liver microsomes. *Cancer Res.*, **53**, 5629–5637.
2. Philpott, G.W., Shearer, W.T., Bower, R.J., and Parker, C.W. (1973) Selective cytotoxicity of hapten-substituted cells with an antibody–enzyme conjugate. *J. Immunol.*, **111**, 921–929.
3. Bagshawe, K.D. (1987) Antibody directed enzymes revive anti-cancer prodrugs concept. *Br. J. Cancer*, **56**, 531–532.
4. Tietze, L.F., Major, F., Schuberth, I., Spiegl, D.A., Krewer, B.,

Maksimenka, K., Bringmann, G., and Magull, J. (2007) Selective treatment of cancer: synthesis, biological evaluation and structural elucidation of novel analogues of the antibiotic CC-1065 and the duocarmycins. *Chemistry*, **13**, 4396–4409.

5. Senter, P.D. and Springer, C.J. (2001) Selective activation of anticancer prodrugs by monoclonal antibody–enzyme conjugates. *Adv. Drug Deliv. Rev.*, **53**, 247–264.

6. Bagshawe, K.D. (2006) Antibody-directed enzyme prodrug therapy (ADEPT) for cancer. *Expert Rev. Anticancer Ther.*, **6**, 1421–1431.

7. Senter, P.D., Saulnier, M.G., Schreiber, G.J., Hirschberg, D.L., Brown, J.P., Hellstrom, I., and Hellstrom, K.E. (1988) Anti-tumor effects of antibody–alkaline phosphatase conjugates in combination with etoposide phosphate. *Proc. Natl. Acad. Sci. USA*, **85**, 4842–4846.

8. Senter, P.D., Schreiber, G.J., Hirschberg, D.L., Ashe, S.A., Hellstrom, K.E., and Hellstrom, I. (1989) Enhancement of the *in vitro* and *in vivo* antitumor activities of phosphorylated mitomycin C and etoposide derivatives by monoclonal antibody–alkaline phosphatase conjugates. *Cancer Res.*, **49**, 5789–5792.

9. Senter, P.D. (1990) Antitumor effects of antibody enzyme conjugates in combination with prodrugs. *Front. Radiat. Ther. Oncol.*, **24**, 132–141.

10. Wallace, P.M. and Senter, P.D. (1991) *In vitro* and *in vivo* activities of monoclonal antibody–alkaline phosphatase conjugates in combination with phenol mustard phosphate. *Bioconjug. Chem.*, **2**, 349–352.

11. Savage, P., Cowburn, P., Clemens, D., Hurley, T., Laguda, B., Martin-Duque, P., Vassaux, G., and Lemoine, N.R. (2004) Suicide gene therapy: conversion of ethanol to acetaldehyde mediated by human beta 2 alcohol dehydrogenase. *Cancer Gene Ther.*, **11**, 774–781.

12. Svensson, H.P., Kadow, J.F., Vrudhula, V.M., Wallace, P.M., and Senter, P.D. (1992) Monoclonal antibody–beta-lactamase conjugates for the activation of a cephalosporin mustard prodrug. *Bioconjug. Chem.*, **3**, 176–181.

13. Kerr, D.E., Vrudhula, V.M., Svensson, H.P., Siemers, N.O., and Senter, P.D. (1999) Comparison of recombinant and synthetically formed monoclonal antibody–beta-lactamase conjugates for anticancer prodrug activation. *Bioconjug. Chem.*, **10**, 1084–1089.

14. Bosslet, K., Czech, J., Seemann, G., Monneret, C., and Hoffmann, D. (1994) Fusion protein mediated prodrug activation (FMPA) *in vivo*. *Cell Biophys.*, **24-25**, 51–63.

15. Roffler, S.R., Wang, S.M., Chern, J.W., Yeh, M.Y., and Tung, E. (1991) Anti-neoplastic glucuronide prodrug treatment of human tumor cells targeted with a monoclonal antibody–enzyme conjugate. *Biochem. Pharmacol.*, **42**, 2062–2065.

16. Chen, B.M., Chan, L.Y., Wang, S.M., Wu, M.F., Chern, J.W., and Roffler, S.R. (1997) Cure of malignant ascites and generation of protective immunity by monoclonal antibody-targeted activation of a glucuronide prodrug in rats. *Int. J. Cancer*, **73**, 392–402.

17. Bakina, E. and Farquhar, D. (1999) Intensely cytotoxic anthracycline prodrugs: galactosides. *Anticancer Drug Des.*, **14**, 507–515.

18. Senter, P.D., Beam, K.S., Mixan, B., and Wahl, A.F. (2001) Identification and activities of human carboxylesterases for the activation of CPT-11, a clinically approved anticancer drug. *Bioconjug. Chem.*, **12**, 1074–1080.

19. Kuefner, U., Lohrmann, U., Montejano, Y.D., Vitols, K.S., and Huennekens, F.M. (1989) Carboxypeptidase-mediated release of methotrexate from methotrexate alpha-peptides. *Biochemistry*, **28**, 2288–2297.

20. Haenseler, E., Esswein, A., Vitols, K.S., Montejano, Y., Mueller, B.M., Reisfeld, R.A., and Huennekens, F.M. (1992) Activation of methotrexate-alpha-alanine by carboxypeptidase A–monoclonal antibody conjugate. *Biochemistry*, **31**, 891–897.

21. Springer, C.J., Antoniw, P., Bagshawe, K.D., Searle, F., Bisset, G.M., and Jarman, M. (1990) Novel prodrugs

which are activated to cytotoxic alkylating agents by carboxypeptidase G2. *J. Med. Chem.*, **33**, 677–681.

22. Springer, C.J., Dowell, R., Burke, P.J., Hadley, E., Davis, D.H., Blakey, D.C., Melton, R.G., and Niculescu-Duvaz, I. (1995) Optimization of alkylating agent prodrugs derived from phenol and aniline mustards: a new clinical candidate prodrug (ZD2767) for antibody-directed enzyme prodrug therapy (ADEPT). *J. Med. Chem.*, **38**, 5051–5065.

23. Tietze, L.F., Lieb, M., Herzig, T., Haunert, F., and Schuberth, I. (2001) A strategy for tumor-selective chemotherapy by enzymatic liberation of seco-duocarmycin SA-derivatives from nontoxic prodrugs. *Bioorg. Med. Chem.*, **9**, 1929–1939.

24. Knox, R.J., Friedlos, F., Sherwood, R.F., Melton, R.G., and Anlezark, G.M. (1992) The bioactivation of 5-(aziridin-1-yl)-2,4-dinitrobenzamide (CB1954) – II. A comparison of an *Escherichia coli* nitroreductase and Walker DT diaphorase. *Biochem. Pharmacol.*, **44**, 2297–2301.

25. Bignami, G.S., Senter, P.D., Grothaus, P.G., Fischer, K.J., Humphreys, T., and Wallace, P.M. (1992) N-(4′-hydroxyphenylacetyl)palytoxin: a palytoxin prodrug that can be activated by a monoclonal antibody–penicillin G amidase conjugate. *Cancer Res.*, **52**, 5759–5764.

26. Boxer, G., Stuart-Smith, S., Flynn, A., Green, A., and Begent, R. (1999) Radioimmunoluminography: a tool for relating tissue antigen concentration to clinical outcome. *Br. J. Cancer*, **80**, 922–926.

27. Edwards, P.A. (1985) Heterogeneous expression of cell-surface antigens in normal epithelia and their tumours, revealed by monoclonal antibodies. *Br. J. Cancer*, **51**, 149–160.

28. Cheng, T.L., Wei, S.L., Chen, B.M., Chern, J.W., Wu, M.F., Liu, P.W., and Roffler, S.R. (1999) Bystander killing of tumour cells by antibody-targeted enzymatic activation of a glucuronide prodrug. *Br. J. Cancer*, **79**, 1378–1385.

29. Begent, R.H., Searle, F., Stanway, G., Jewkes, R.F., Jones, B.E., Vernon, P., and Bagshawe, K.D. (1980) Radioimmunolocalization of tumours by external scintigraphy after administration of ^{131}I antibody to human chorionic gonadotrophin: preliminary communication. *J. R. Soc. Med.*, **73**, 624–630.

30. Harwood, P.J., Pedley, R.B., Boden, J., Rawlins, G., Pentycross, C.R., Rogers, G.T., and Bagshawe, K.D. (1985) Prolonged localisation of a monoclonal antibody against CEA in a human colon tumour xenograft. *Br. J. Cancer*, **52**, 797–799.

31. Holgate, R.G. and Baker, M.P. (2009) Circumventing immunogenicity in the development of therapeutic antibodies. *IDrugs*, **12**, 233–237.

32. Baker, M.P. and Carr, F.J. (2010) Pre-clinical considerations in the assessment of immunogenicity for protein therapeutics. *Curr. Drug Saf.*, **5**, 308–313.

33. Frei, E., III, Teicher, B.A., Holden, S.A., Cathcart, K.N., and Wang, Y.Y. (1988) Preclinical studies and clinical correlation of the effect of alkylating dose. *Cancer Res.*, **48**, 6417–6423.

34. Teicher, B.A. and Frei, E. III (1988) Development of alkylating agent-resistant human tumor cell lines. *Cancer Chemother. Pharmacol.*, **21**, 292–298.

35. Springer, C.J., Bagshawe, K.D., Sharma, S.K., Searle, F., Boden, J.A., Antoniw, P., Burke, P.J., Rogers, G.T., Sherwood, R.F., and Melton, R.G. (1991) Ablation of human choriocarcinoma xenografts in nude mice by antibody-directed enzyme prodrug therapy (ADEPT) with three novel compounds. *Eur. J. Cancer*, **27**, 1361–1366.

36. Bagshawe, K.D. (1989) The First Bagshawe Lecture. Towards generating cytotoxic agents at cancer sites. *Br. J. Cancer*, **60**, 275–281.

37. Sharma, S.K., Bagshawe, K.D., Burke, P.J., Boden, J.A., Rogers, G.T., Springer, C.J., Melton, R.G., and Sherwood, R.F. (1994) Galactosylated antibodies and antibody–enzyme conjugates in antibody-directed enzyme prodrug therapy. *Cancer*, **73**, 1114–1120.

38. Sharma, S.K., Bagshawe, K.D., Springer, C.J., Burke, P.J., Rogers, G.T., Boden, J.A., Antoniw, P., Melton, R.G., and

Sherwood, R.F. (1991) Antibody directed enzyme prodrug therapy (ADEPT): a three phase system. *Dis. Markers*, **9**, 225–231.

39. Sharma, S.K., Boden, J.A., Springer, C.J., Burke, P.J., and Bagshawe, K.D. (1994) Antibody-directed enzyme prodrug therapy (ADEPT). A three-phase study in ovarian tumor xenografts. *Cell Biophys.*, **24–25**, 219–228.
40. Holland, J.F., Frei, E., Bast, R.C., Kufe, D.W., Morton, D.L.,and Weichselbaum, R.R., (eds) (1997) *Cancer Medicine*, 4th edn, Williams & Wilkins Baltimore, MD,
41. Alderson, R.F., Toki, B.E., Roberge, M., Geng, W., Basler, J., Chin, R., Liu, A., Ueda, R., Hodges, D., Escandon, E., Chen, T., Kanavarioti, T., Babe, L., Senter, P.D., Fox, J.A., and Schellenberger, V. (2006) Characterization of a CC49-based single-chain fragment–beta-lactamase fusion protein for antibody-directed enzyme prodrug therapy (ADEPT). *Bioconjug. Chem.*, **17**, 410–418.
42. Eccles, S.A., Court, W.J., Box, G.A., Dean, C.J., Melton, R.G., and Springer, C.J. (1994) Regression of established breast carcinoma xenografts with antibody-directed enzyme prodrug therapy against c-erbB2 p185. *Cancer Res.*, **54**, 5171–5177.
43. Heinis, C., Alessi, P., and Neri, D. (2004) Engineering a thermostable human prolyl endopeptidase for antibody-directed enzyme prodrug therapy. *Biochemistry*, **43**, 6293–6303.
44. Harding, F.A., Liu, A.D., Stickler, M., Razo, O.J., Chin, R., Faravashi, N., Viola, W., Graycar, T., Yeung, V.P., Aehle, W., Meijer, D., Wong, S., Rashid, M.H., Valdes, A.M., and Schellenberger, V. (2005) A beta-lactamase with reduced immunogenicity for the targeted delivery of chemotherapeutics using antibody-directed enzyme prodrug therapy. *Mol. Cancer Ther.*, **4**, 1791–1800.
45. Abuchowski, A., McCoy, J.R., Palczuk, N.C., van Es, T., and Davis, F.F. (1977) Effect of covalent attachment of polyethylene glycol on immunogenicity and circulating life of bovine liver catalase. *J. Biol. Chem.*, **252**, 3582–3586.
46. Novikov, B.N., Grimsley, J.K., Kern, R.J., Wild, J.R., and Wales, M.E. (2010) Improved pharmacokinetics and immunogenicity profile of organophosphorus hydrolase by chemical modification with polyethylene glycol. *J. Control. Release*, **146**, 318–325.
47. Wentworth, P., Datta, A., Blakey, D., Boyle, T., Partridge, L.J., and Blackburn, G.M. (1996) Toward antibody-directed "abzyme" prodrug therapy, ADAPT: carbamate prodrug activation by a catalytic antibody and its *in vitro* application to human tumor cell killing. *Proc. Natl. Acad. Sci. USA*, **93**, 799–803.
48. Kakinuma, H., Fujii, I., and Nishi, Y. (2002) Selective chemotherapeutic strategies using catalytic antibodies: a common pro-moiety for antibody-directed abzyme prodrug therapy. *J. Immunol. Methods*, **269**, 269–281.
49. Abraham, S., Guo, F., Li, L.S., Rader, C., Liu, C., Barbas, C.F. III, Lerner, R.A., and Sinha, S.C. (2007) Synthesis of the next-generation therapeutic antibodies that combine cell targeting and antibody-catalyzed prodrug activation. *Proc. Natl. Acad. Sci. USA*, **104**, 5584–5589.
50. Pedley, R.B., Begent, R.H., Boden, J.A., Boden, R., Adam, T., and Bagshawe, K.D. (1991) The effect of radiosensitizers on radio-immunotherapy, using ^{131}I-labelled anti-CEA antibodies in a human colonic xenograft model. *Int. J. Cancer*, **47**, 597–602.
51. Sherwood, R.F., Melton, R.G., Alwan, S.M., and Hughes, P. (1985) Purification and properties of carboxypeptidase G2 from *Pseudomonas* sp. strain RS-16. Use of a novel triazine dye affinity method. *Eur. J. Biochem.*, **148**, 447–453.
52. Melton, R.G., Boyle, J.M., Rogers, G.T., Burke, P.J., Bagshawe, K.D., and Sherwood, R.F. (1993) Optimisation of small-scale coupling of A5B7 monoclonal antibody to carboxypeptidase G2. *J. Immunol. Methods*, **158**, 49–56.
53. Sharma, S.K., Bagshawe, K.D., Burke, P.J., Boden, R.W., and Rogers, G.T. (1990) Inactivation and clearance of an anti-CEA carboxypeptidase G2 conjugate in blood after localisation in a xenograft model. *Br. J. Cancer*, **61**, 659–662.

54. Bagshawe, K.D., Sharma, S.K., Springer, C.J., Antoniw, P., Boden, J.A., Rogers, G.T., Burke, P.J., Melton, R.G., and Sherwood, R.F. (1991) Antibody directed enzyme prodrug therapy (ADEPT): clinical report. *Dis. Markers*, **9**, 233–238.
55. Bagshawe, K.D. (1994) Antibody-directed enzyme prodrug therapy. *Clin. Pharmacokinet.*, **27**, 368–376.
56. Napier, M.P., Sharma, S.K., Springer, C.J., Bagshawe, K.D., Green, A.J., Martin, J., Stribbling, S.M., Cushen, N., O'Malley, D., and Begent, R.H. (2000) Antibody-directed enzyme prodrug therapy: efficacy and mechanism of action in colorectal carcinoma. *Clin. Cancer Res.*, **6**, 765–772.
57. Blakey, D.C., Burke, P.J., Davies, D.H., Dowell, R.I., East, S.J., Eckersley, K.P., Fitton, J.E., McDaid, J., Melton, R.G., Niculescu-Duvaz, I.A., Pinder, P.E., Sharma, S.K., Wright, A.F., and Springer, C.J. (1996) ZD2767, an improved system for antibody-directed enzyme prodrug therapy that results in tumor regressions in colorectal tumor xenografts. *Cancer Res.*, **56**, 3287–3292.
58. Francis, R.J., Sharma, S.K., Springer, C., Green, A.J., Hope-Stone, L.D., Sena, L., Martin, J., Adamson, K.L., Robbins, A., Gumbrell, L., O'Malley, D., Tsiompanou, E., Shahbakhti, H., Webley, S., Hochhauser, D., Hilson, A.J., Blakey, D., and Begent, R.H. (2002) A phase I trial of antibody directed enzyme prodrug therapy (ADEPT) in patients with advanced colorectal carcinoma or other CEA producing tumours. *Br. J. Cancer*, **87**, 600–607.
59. Chester, K.A., Begent, R.H., Robson, L., Keep, P., Pedley, R.B., Boden, J.A., Boxer, G., Green, A., Winter, G., and Cochet, O. (1994) Phage libraries for generation of clinically useful antibodies. *Lancet*, **343**, 455–456.
60. Neuberger, M.S., Williams, G.T., and Fox, R.O. (1984) Recombinant antibodies possessing novel effector functions. *Nature*, **312**, 604–608.
61. Bosslet, K., Czech, J., and Hoffmann, D. (1994) Tumor-selective prodrug activation by fusion protein-mediated catalysis. *Cancer Res.*, **54**, 2151–2159.
62. Michael, N.P., Chester, K.A., Melton, R.G., Robson, L., Nicholas, W., Boden, J.A., Pedley, R.B., Begent, R.H., Sherwood, R.F., and Minton, N.P. (1996) In vitro and in vivo characterisation of a recombinant carboxypeptidase G2::anti-CEA scFv fusion protein. *Immunotechnology*, **2**, 47–57.
63. Bhatia, J., Sharma, S.K., Chester, K.A., Pedley, R.B., Boden, R.W., Read, D.A., Boxer, G.M., Michael, N.P., and Begent, R.H. (2000) Catalytic activity of an *in vivo* tumor targeted anti-CEA scFv::carboxypeptidase G2 fusion protein. *Int. J. Cancer*, **85**, 571–577.
64. Mayer, A., Sharma, S.K., Tolner, B., Minton, N.P., Purdy, D., Amlot, P., Tharakan, G., Begent, R.H., and Chester, K.A. (2004) Modifying an immunogenic epitope on a therapeutic protein: a step towards an improved system for antibody-directed enzyme prodrug therapy (ADEPT). *Br. J. Cancer*, **90**, 2402–2410.
65. Chester, K.A., Bhatia, J., Boxer, G., Cooke, S.P., Flynn, A.A., Huhalov, A., Mayer, A., Pedley, R.B., Robson, L., Sharma, S.K., Spencer, D.I., and Begent, R.H. (2000) Clinical applications of phage-derived sFvs and sFv fusion proteins. *Dis. Markers*, **16**, 53–62.
66. Medzihradszky, K.F., Spencer, D.I., Sharma, S.K., Bhatia, J., Pedley, R.B., Read, D.A., Begent, R.H., and Chester, K.A. (2004) Glycoforms obtained by expression in *Pichia pastoris* improve cancer targeting potential of a recombinant antibody–enzyme fusion protein. *Glycobiology*, **14**, 27–37.
67. Kogelberg, H., Tolner, B., Sharma, S.K., Lowdell, M.W., Qureshi, U., Robson, M., Hillyer, T., Pedley, R.B., Vervecken, W., Contreras, R., Begent, R.H., and Chester, K.A. (2007) Clearance mechanism of a mannosylated antibody–enzyme fusion protein used in experimental cancer therapy. *Glycobiology*, **17**, 36–45.

68. Sharma, S.K., Pedley, R.B., Bhatia, J., Boxer, G.M., El-Emir, E., Qureshi, U., Tolner, B., Lowe, H., Michael, N.P., Minton, N., Begent, R.H., and Chester, K.A. (2005) Sustained tumor regression of human colorectal cancer xenografts using a multifunctional mannosylated fusion protein in antibody-directed enzyme prodrug therapy. *Clin. Cancer Res.*, **11**, 814–825.

69. Tolner, B., Smith, L., Hillyer, T., Bhatia, J., Beckett, P., Robson, L., Sharma, S.K., Griffin, N., Vervecken, W., Contreras, R., Pedley, R.B., Begent, R.H., and Chester, K.A. (2007) From laboratory to phase I/II cancer trials with recombinant biotherapeutics. *Eur. J. Cancer*, **43**, 2515–2522.

70. Mayer, A., Francis, R.J., Sharma, S.K., Tolner, B., Springer, C.J., Martin, J., Boxer, G.M., Bell, J., Green, A.J., Hartley, J.A., Cruickshank, C., Wren, J., Chester, K.A., and Begent, R.H. (2006) A phase I study of single administration of antibody-directed enzyme prodrug therapy with the recombinant anti-carcinoembryonic antigen antibody–enzyme fusion protein MFECP1 and a bis-iodo phenol mustard prodrug. *Clin. Cancer Res.*, **12**, 6509–6516.

Part II
Tumor Imaging

7
Imaging Techniques in Drug Development and Clinical Practice
John C. Chang, Sanjiv S. Gambhir, and Jürgen K. Willmann

7.1
Introduction

Recent advances in cancer research have led to a better understanding of signaling networks that drive the unlimited proliferation of cancer cells, resulting in new therapeutic approaches that target these signaling chains. The total research and development costs through phase III of clinical trials for novel drugs range from US$ 800 to 900 million as of 2001, with the costs expected to double by 2013 [1].

Given such substantial research and developmental costs, it is critical that the appropriate targets, delivery routes, and efficacies of novel drug candidates are determined at an early stage [1, 2]. Once a selected target and compound have been assessed *in vitro*, preclinical studies need to be obtained in animals to assess *in vivo* delivery, potency, and efficacy prior to actual clinical trials to assess the safety and general effectiveness of the medication. Given this extended process, early elimination of ineffective compounds can dramatically decrease development costs (Figure 7.1). With cancer being a heterogeneous process in terms of angiogenesis, growth factor and receptor expression, as well as genotypes [3–5], the response to chemotherapy can be heterogeneous as well. Thus, it is important to have effective monitoring tools to aid the elimination of ineffective drugs early on in the drug development pipeline.

Monitoring of tumor response can be performed with different techniques, including direct tissue sampling, assessing circulating blood biomarkers or tumor cells in the blood, or by noninvasive imaging techniques [6–9]. Tissue sampling involves either image-guided needle biopsy or open surgical biopsy, both of which carry substantial associated risks such as infection, bleeding, and hypersensitivity reactions to anesthetics. However, the greatest disadvantage of using direct tissue sampling is often incomplete evaluation of tumor response since only a fraction of the tumors can usually be sampled by biopsies [10]. While assessing circulating biomarkers or tumor cells in the blood has shown promise in predicting tumor response, progression-free survival, and overall survival [7, 11, 12], this requires that the tumor cells have invaded vessels and migrated into the blood to be detected or that they have shed biomolecules (e.g., proteins, microRNA)

Drug Delivery in Oncology: From Basic Research to Cancer Therapy, First Edition.
Edited by Felix Kratz, Peter Senter, and Henning Steinhagen.
© 2012 Wiley-VCH Verlag GmbH & Co. KGaA. Published 2012 by Wiley-VCH Verlag GmbH & Co. KGaA.

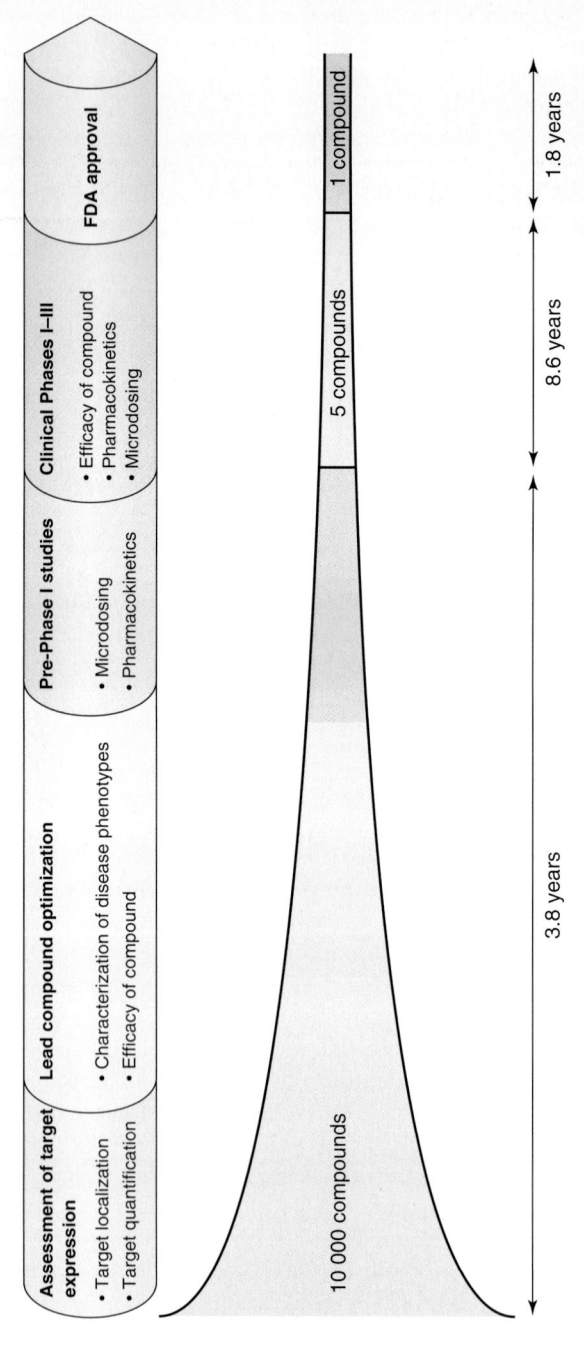

Figure 7.1 Process of drug development from target identification to drug approval. The process of drug development begins with identifying an appropriate target for treatment that leads to development of an inhibiting or activating molecule that is tested in clinical trials before US Food and Drug Administration (FDA) approval. The whole process of drug development and validation takes an average of 14.6 years with overall costs of up to US$1 billion. It is estimated that out of 10 000 initial compounds only one makes it to FDA approval. (Reproduced with permission from [1].)

into the blood at high enough concentrations to be detected through current detection tools such as enzyme-linked immunosorbent assays (ELISAs) or reverse transcription-polymerase chain reaction (RT-PCR) [6–9]. In addition, the results can be confounded by normal cells expressing the same biomarkers also shed into the blood [13]. Noninvasive imaging is probably the most promising approach for obtaining rapid evaluation of tumor response [1, 2, 10]. Currently already clinically available imaging modalities such as positron emission tomography-computed tomography (PET-CT), magnetic resonance imaging (MRI), ultrasound, and CT, allow accurate noninvasive assessment of several characteristics of cancer, such as metabolic activity, tumor perfusion, and tumor size to mention just a few.

In order to appropriately assess drug delivery, drug activity, and tumor response, one must understand the physiologic changes that accompany the neoplastic process, the properties of the drug delivered, and the imaging techniques that attempt to integrate these three processes. In this chapter, biological changes of neoplastic processes will be summarized to cover the relevant genetic, signaling, metabolic, and vascular changes, which will be followed by a discussion on potentially relevant oncological imaging biomarkers. A short summary on the fundamentals of various imaging techniques will be followed by examples that demonstrate how these techniques can accelerate drug development and improve patient care.

7.2
Cancer Biology

7.2.1
Tumor Genetic Heterogeneity

It has been hypothesized that tumors acquire and accumulate genetic mutations on their progression to metastasis. This process is initiated when an initial mutation leads to increased proliferation and acquired ability to escape apoptosis [14], which allows neoplastic cells to maintain and preserve their survival advantage (Figure 7.2). Once this has been achieved, angiogenesis is required to supply the metabolic needs of the growing mass. Hypoxic conditions created by the growing mass then induce expression of large sets of genes (e.g., hypoxia inducible factor (HIF) and its downstream effectors) that allows the tumor to revert to a more primitive phenotype and acquire aerobic glycolysis to lower local pH and disrupt the surrounding stromal tissues [15]. This primitive phenotype also accelerates genetic mutations to reach dysregulated proliferation and leads to tumor genetic heterogeneity [3, 4].

7.2.2
Altered Tumor Metabolism

In becoming cancerous, neoplastic cells develop altered metabolism of glucose for energy, amino acids for protein synthesis, lipids for membrane synthesis, and

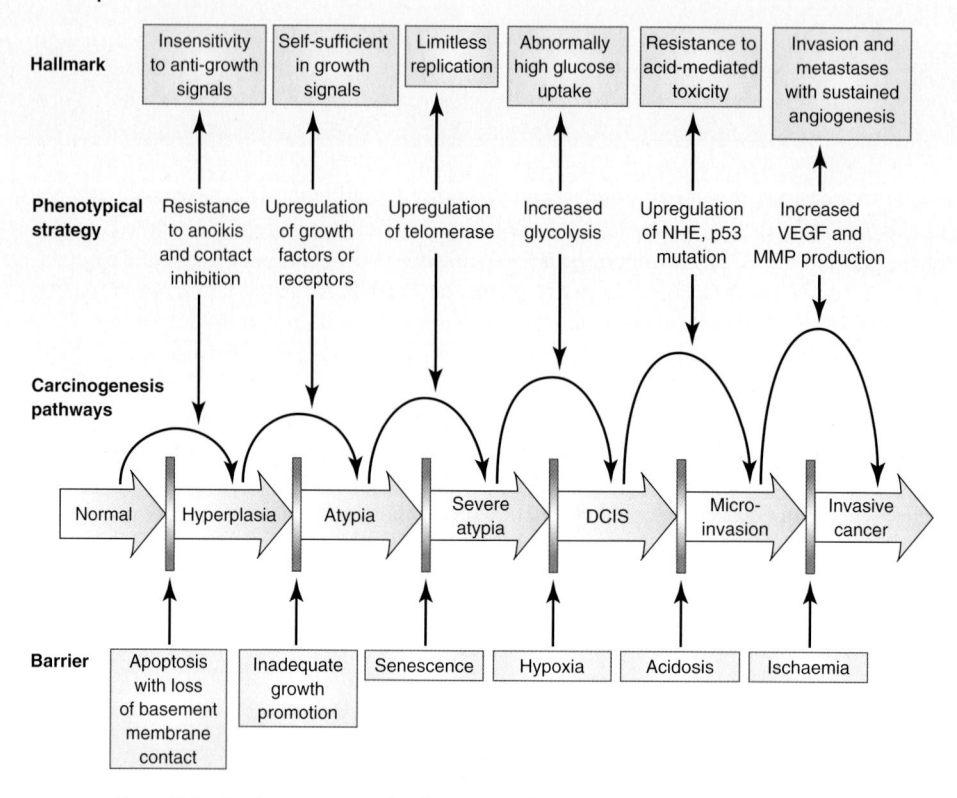

Figure 7.2 Barriers to cancer development as proposed by Gatenby et al. In the process of becoming malignant, each cell needs to overcome six proposed barriers with the potential strategies listed. The sequence of barriers and strategies are not necessarily sequential. NHE, Na$^+$/H$^+$ exchanger; MMP, matrix metalloproteinase; DCIS, ductal carcinoma in situ. (Reproduced with permission from [14].)

nucleic acids for chromosomal replication [16, 17] (Figure 7.3). Regarding glucose metabolism, malignant cells increase expression of glucose-uptake transporter 1 (GLUT-1) that facilitates glucose transport in response to aerobic glycolysis (Warburg effect) [18]. Fatty acid synthase (FAS) and choline kinase (ChoK) expression is elevated as a downstream effect of oncogene activation (*erbB2*, *ras*, *src*, and *raf*) and loss of tumor suppression (PTEN) [17, 19]. Increased amino acid metabolism is reflected through increased uptake of glutamine, which can be shunted for synthesis of other amino acids and of nucleic acids [17, 20]. Although neoplastic cells retain the ability to synthesize nucleic acids *de novo*, nucleic acids are typically recycled to conserve energy, thus allowing imaging with thymidine analogs [16, 21].

7.2.3
Tumor Angiogenesis

In response to the retention of HIF secondary to underlying genetic mutations (such as von Hippel-Lindau protein in renal cell carcinoma [22]), numerous

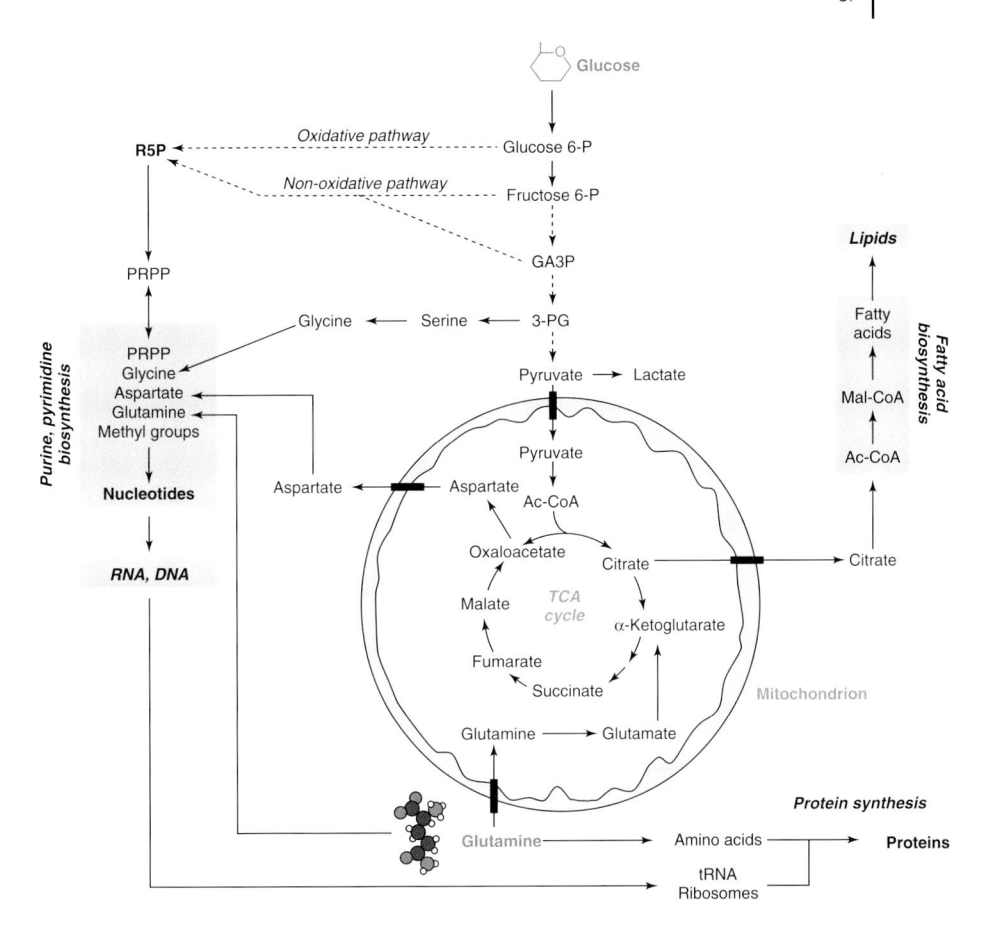

Figure 7.3 Simplified depiction of tumor cell metabolic pathways. Glucose and fatty acid pathways can be assessed with both PET and MRS, although at different points. In the glucose pathway, PET detects the glucose uptake while MRS detects the resulting lactate. In the fatty acid pathway, ^{11}C-choline/acetate uptake reflects lipid synthesis while MRS detects the end-product in lipids. Amino acid can only be assessed with PET as MRS has insufficient peak for delineation. P, phosphate; GA3P, glyceraldehyde 3-phosphate; Ac-CoA, acetyl coenzyme A; Mal-CoA, malonyl coenzyme A; 3-PG, 3-phosphoglycerate; PRPP, phosphoribosyl pyrophosphate. (Reproduced with permission from [20].)

primitive genes are activated that alter energy and iron metabolism, cell signaling through hormonal expression, and vascular growth through vascular endothelial growth factor (VEGF) secretion. VEGF has seven members in the VEGF homology domain (VEGF-A, VEGF-B, VEGF-C, VEGF-D, VEGF-E, VEGF-F, and placenta growth factor [23]). These growth factors act through two types of receptors, VEGFR1 and VEGFR2. VEGFR1 governs the physiologic and developmental angiogenesis, while VEGFR2 is responsible for the mitogenic, angiogenic, and permeability-enhancing effects of VEGF (typically overexpressed in malignancies).

When VEGF/VEGFR overexpression is present in tumors, the prognosis tends to be poorer due to the increased probability of vascular invasion through increased interaction between tumor and vessels. Despite the increased vessel density, tumor oxygenation remains heterogeneous and suboptimal reflecting inefficient vasculature [15, 23–25].

7.2.4 Receptor Pathologies

In addition to genetic heterogeneity, metabolic switch, and tumoral angiogenesis, tumor cells can upregulate receptors that can drive tumor proliferation. For example, breast cancer can overexpress estrogen receptor (ER) or progesterone receptor (PR), which leads to response to hormonal therapy. Human epidermal growth factor receptor 2 (HER2) expression confers a more aggressive phenotype but which responds to trastuzumab (Herceptin®) therapy [6–9]. Similarly, upregulation of epidermal growth factor receptor (EGFR) in solid tumors such as colon, lung, and renal cancers can contribute to tumor proliferation which leads to greater sensitivity to anti-EGFR therapy such as gefitinib (Iressa®), sorafenib (Nexavar®), and axitinib [26–28].

7.3 Cancer Biomarkers

The expense and time associated with traditional clinical trials using, for example, overall and progression-free survival as trial endpoints have spurred on research to seek biomarkers (biological markers) that can be used to provide objective, rapid evaluation, or predict response to therapy at early stages of therapy [1, 9, 29, 30]. Classically, these markers have been hematological or histological in nature [6–9, 29]. Recently, various imaging techniques have been proposed as producing data for surrogate biomarkers to assess tumor response to therapy [29, 30]. The origins for the discovery and development of many of these biomarkers are based on the tumor pathophysiology described above.

7.3.1 Histological Biomarkers

Histological biomarkers are typically overexpressed receptors of growth factors or hormones that can be measured through staining techniques such as immunohistochemistry [6–9]. Examples of these molecules include KIT, ER/PR, EGFR, and HER2/neu (Table 7.1). Overexpression of KIT (platelet-derived growth factor receptor α) in gastrointestinal stromal tumor (GIST) can predict tumor response to imatinib mesylate (Gleevec®) [6]. ER/PR positivity in breast cancer is associated with response to antiestrogenic therapy such as tamoxifen, raloxifen (Evista®), and anastrazole (Arimidex®), which block estrogenic action either at the receptor

Table 7.1 Common biomarkers in clinical use.

Predictive biomarkers			Surveillance biomarkers		Imaging biomarkers		
Marker	Cancer	Prediction	Marker	Cancer	Marker	Modality	Physiology
KIT	GIST	response to imatinib (Gleevec)	CA 125	ovarian cancer	^{18}F-FDG	PET	glucose uptake, glycolysis
ER/PR	breast	response to antiestrogen therapy	CA 19-9	pancreatic cancer	lactate	MRS	glycolysis
HER2/*neu*	breast	response to trastuzumab (Herceptin)	α-fetoprotein	hepatocellular carcinoma, germ cell tumor	^{18}F-FLT	PET	thymidine uptake, proliferation
EGFR	lung, renal	response to EGFR blockers	CEA	colon cancer	^{11}C-MET	PET	protein synthesis
			thyroglobulin	thyroid cancer	tumor perfusion	CT/MRS/ultrasound	restricted diffusion tumor vascularity
			PSA	prostate cancer	antibody-targeted agent	PET/ultrasound MRS	specific protein expression
			5-HIAA/VMA (urinary metabolites of serotonin and catecholamine)	pheochromocytoma			
			β-human chorionic gonadotropin	germ cell tumor			

[a]Three types of biomarkers are currently in clinical use. Predictive biomarkers tend to detect signaling protein expression that can predict a patient's response to therapy. Surveillance markers are related to proteins expressed by the native tissue, although no intracellular signaling property is known to exist. Although these markers cannot predict a patient's response, they have been used to monitor recurrence. Imaging biomarkers are currently available predominantly for research studies, except for ^{18}F-FDG, which is used to predict patient response to chemotherapy [1, 2, 6].

site or at the production site [6]. EGFR positivity in non-small-cell lung cancer (NSCLC) has been shown to predict response to EGFR blocker such as gefitinib [28, 31]. HER2/*neu* is unique in that it not only predicts response of breast cancer to trastuzumab therapy, but also its prognosis in terms of patient survival [31, 32].

7.3.2
Hematological Biomarkers

Hematological biomarkers are typically nonspecific proteins expressed by the tumor and secreted into the blood. Unfortunately, they often have minimal predictive values in terms of response to therapy or patient survival. However, clinically they are very useful as surveillance markers in patients with certain tumors (Table 7.1) [6]. For example, cancer antigens 19-9 and 125 (CA 19-9 and CA 125) have been used to follow recurrence of pancreatic and ovarian malignancies, respectively. Similarly, carcinoembryonic antigen (CEA), thyroglobulin, and prostate-specific antigen (PSA) have been used to detect recurrences of colon, thyroid, and prostate cancers, respectively [6].

More recently, significant research on circulating tumor cells and nucleic acids has shown their promise as biomarkers [7, 8, 31]. Pre- and post-therapy circulating tumor cells have been shown to predict a patient's response to therapy and prognosis in breast and gastrointestinal tumors [7, 8]. In addition, circulating HER2 DNA has been shown to predict response to trastuzumab therapy [12]. Additional research and technological development is needed to further assess the use of hematological biomarkers for both early detection and treatment monitoring of diseases.

7.3.3
Imaging Biomarkers

Due to the subjective nature of clinical symptoms, the time-intensive nature of traditional clinical endpoints such as overall survival and progression-free survival, and the aforementioned shortcomings of other current markers such as hematological biomarkers [9, 30, 31], imaging has been proposed as a promising, noninvasive alternative approach. Depending on the assessed parameters, the detection of response can occur as early as hours instead of days or months following treatment initiation [30, 33]. Traditionally, on imaging exams, response to cytotoxic therapy has been determined using tumor size as the main criterion according to the Response Evaluation Criteria In Solid Tumors (RECIST) criteria (measuring up to 10 measurable lesions with a maximum of five lesions per organ) [34]. According to the RECIST criteria, complete response is defined as complete resolution of all lesions; partial response is defined as greater than 30% decrease in the sum of the longest dimensions of all measured lesions; and progression of disease is defined as presence of any new lesions or greater than 20% increase in the sum of the longest dimensions of all measured pre-existing lesions [34]. However, it has be shown that RECIST criteria alone may not be sufficient to monitor treatment response in patients treated with modern molecularly targeted drugs as size criteria often lag behind therapeutic effects by several weeks or months, making rapid adjustment to therapy/clinical trials impossible [35].

Recently, the widespread use of PET has allowed rapid noninvasive evaluation of tumor response at the molecular level [1, 36]. This has allowed metabolic response (i.e., using 2-^{18}F-fluoro-2-deoxyglucose (FDG)) as well as tumor response to be assessed within a few weeks post-therapy [37–44]. Glucose uptake has been applied to assess tumor response to adjuvant and neoadjuvant chemotherapy from multiple organs such as breast, lung, and lymphoid tissue [36, 45]. Detection of decreased proliferation (i.e., nucleic acid uptake) has been shown to be possible within 2 days of therapy [2, 46] in breast, lung, and lymphoid tumors [2, 28, 47, 48].

With the success of PET, several other imaging modalities have been developed to assess tumor physiological parameters [36], and to aid in quantitative and objective tumor response assessment (see below).

7.4
Imaging Techniques

The most commonly used imaging techniques in both patient care and preclinical drug development in oncology are reviewed in this section. These include single-photon emission computed tomography (SPECT), PET, MRI, CT, ultrasound, and optical imaging. For more details, please refer to other review articles [1, 49–54].

7.4.1
SPECT

SPECT is perhaps the most traditional molecular imaging technique with probes that have been developed to assess physiological/biochemical processes. The radiotracers used to tag the probes are typically high-energy γ-emitters ranging from 100 to 300 keV with half-lives of the tracers lasting from 6 h to several days (^{99m}Tc, 6 h; ^{123}I, 13 h; ^{111}In, 67 h; ^{201}Tl, 73 h; ^{67}Ga, 78 h; ^{131}I, 8 days) [53]. Scintillation crystals with associated photomultiplier tubes are used as detector to measure the high-energy photons from the disintegration process [53].

The interrogation of physiologic processes is achieved through radiolabeling of analogs/ligands of physiological enzymes/receptors. Many of these probes have been developed and applied in clinical practice including $^{123/131}$I for evaluating thyroid carcinoma, ^{99m}Tc diphosphonates for evaluating bone remodeling (e.g., from metastases), ^{111}In-pentetreotide for evaluating tumors with somatostatin receptors (SSTRs) such as neuroendocrine tumors, and $^{123/131}$I-metaiodobenzylguanidine for evaluating pheochromocytoma, neuroblastoma, and paraganglioma [53]. Other nonspecific radiotracers including ^{67}Ga, ^{201}Th chloride, and ^{99m}Tc-sestamibi label malignancies due to nonspecific (lipophilicity for sestamibi) and metabolic uptake mechanisms (transferrin receptor for gallium and sodium/potassium pump for thallium) [53]. More targeted molecular probes have recently been developed to interrogate apoptosis, angiogenesis, as well as HER2 [1, 2, 55].

7.4.2
PET/PET-CT

PET employs positron-emitting radioisotopes for localization of the radiotracer. Commonly used radioisotopes include ^{11}C ($t_{1/2}$ = 20 min), ^{13}N ($t_{1/2}$ = 10 min), ^{15}O ($t_{1/2}$ = 2 min), ^{64}Cu ($t_{1/2}$ = 12 h), ^{124}I ($t_{1/2}$ = 4 days), and ^{18}F ($t_{1/2}$ = 110 min) [53]. These decaying isotopes emit a positron from the unstable nucleus, which is captured by an electron from the same atom, neighboring atom, or neighboring molecule, giving it an inherent resolution limit on the scale of millimeters. This annihilation process produces two 511-keV photons (from conservation of mass with $E = mc^2$, c being the speed of light and m the mass of two electrons) that traverse in opposite directions in order to conserve momentum [53]. The two photons are then detected by a ring detector consisting of scintillation detectors whose signals are amplified by photomultiplier tubes [53]. The images are reconstructed by collecting each volume for several minutes to minimize noise. As the high-energy photons traverse through the body, they are absorbed by the soft tissue whose attenuation is corrected for to produce a more accurate value of the radiotracer concentration [53].

Radiotracers can be targeted to specific receptors or metabolic processes through appropriate conjugation to small molecules. This has been accomplished for detecting glucose metabolism using ^{18}F-FDG [53], nucleic acid uptake using 3′-deoxy-3′-fluorothymidine [46], and amino acid uptake with L-methyl-^{11}C-methionine (^{11}C-MET) and ^{18}F-fluorophyenylalanine [46]. In addition, hormonal receptor and angiogenesis imaging have been achieved using 16-α-^{18}F-fluoro-17β-estradiol (^{18}F-FES), ^{18}F-galacto-RGD, and ^{64}Cu-DOTA-labeled VEGF121 mutants, respectively, to mention only a few (DOTA = 1,4,7,10-tetraazacyclododecane-N,N',N'',N'''-tetraacetic acid) [2, 46, 56].

7.4.3
MRI

MRI creates images of aligned resonating nuclei by employing a strong, static magnetic field with superimposed, transverse perturbation field. Typical nuclei are hydrogen atoms, although other nuclei such as ^{13}C, ^{31}P, and ^{19}F can also be detected with appropriate receiver coils [50]. The contrast of MRI depends on the rate of recovery and dephasing of longitudinal (T_1) and transverse (T_2) polarization [50]. In general, the signal is weak due to a very low percentage of nuclei able to generate a magnetic resonance signal. Modulation of the resonance signal can be achieved by dephasing the resonating nuclei through applied gradient fields, through which the diffusion of nuclei can be inferred to generate a diffusion-weighted sequence to detect pathology [57]. The frequency of the nuclear spins can be mapped onto a spectrum to infer the chemical species within a voxel, allowing assessment of metabolic process and the underlying pathology [50].

Image contrast on MRI can be enhanced with administration with agents that shorten longitudinal recovery time, alter the local magnetic field, or through hyperpolarization of administered contrast agents typically containing ^{13}C, ^{15}N, or ^{31}P (which can increase signal intensity by up to six orders of magnitude) [50]. Contrast agents observed in the first-pass can interrogate tissue vascularity and vessel permeability [57]. This is performed with contrast agents that shorten longitudinal magnetization recovery time. Those agents can also be attached to antibodies or nanoparticles that target specific proteins, thus allowing molecular imaging using MRI [58]. However, depending on the type of agent, the necessary concentration to produce detectable signal may reach micro- to millimolar levels.

7.4.4
CT

CT images are generated by irradiating the subject with X-rays emitted from a rotating source paired with a set of detectors on the opposite end of the gantry (i.e., the frame around which the source and detector rotate) [51]. By detecting the absorption of the in-line tissue from at least 180° of irradiation, net absorption at a specific radial projection can be measured to derive a specific CT absorption value (Hounsfield Unit (HU)) for each pixel by using a back-projection algorithm [51]. During the back-projection calculation, filters are used to either sharpen or smooth the edges to increase/decrease the transition at the interface of tissues [51]. With CT, the resolution is submillimeter, allowing excellent evaluation of tumor size and location.

Radiation absorption between different tissues, however, does not differ significantly to cause a clearly visible boundary between different soft tissues if they abut each other. This difference can be enhanced with intravenous contrast administration, with best results being obtained when there is significant difference in vascular density or permeability between the adjacent tissue [49]. Recently, contrast agents consisting of nanoparticles have been able to image expression of targeted proteins – a field research that is still in its infancy [59–61]. Another technique that has used to assess underlying cancer physiology is CT perfusion, similar to MRI perfusion studies. By using CT perfusion, neoplastic vascular density and microvasculature permeability can be assessed during the first pass of contrast agents. This technique has been used successfully for stroke prognostication and is currently being evaluated for applicability in body tumor prognostication [62]. A limitation, however, of CT perfusion is the substantial irradiation exposure of patients due to repetitive CT scans obtained over a region of interest.

7.4.5
Ultrasound

Ultrasound imaging is based on differences in sound wave propagation. Modern solid-state transducers emit and detect sound waves that are reflected proportional to the mismatch between media at an interface [54]. The intensity of reflection determines the brightness of the interface on the image. If there is a complete mismatch (such as that of tissue and bone or tissue and air), near complete reflection of the incident wave occurs [54]. The spatial resolution depends on the frequency of the waves, with a higher frequency yielding higher-resolution images.

However, high-frequency waves also have short attenuation distances, limiting imaging to superficial structures [54].

The contrast between tissues can be enhanced with contrast agents such as contrast microbubbles (gas-filled microspheres that stay within the vascular compartment). These contrast agents have been used predominantly for interrogating vascularity of lesions [63]. However, recent work (described in more detail below) has shown the great potential of ultrasound to become a molecular imaging tool to image and quantify expression levels of molecular targets expressed on vascular endothelial cells [64–67]. Recent work on clinical-grade contrast agents [66] suggests that molecular ultrasound imaging will also enter the clinical arena in the near future.

7.4.6
Fluorescence/Bioluminescence

Optical imaging has traditionally been a research tool rather than true clinical modality because of extensive tissue absorption that limits tissue penetration to a few millimeter [52]. Tissue penetration of up to several centimeters is possible with near-IR wavelengths where protein and hemoglobin absorption of light is at a minimum [52]. Although this spectrum would be desirable for clinical imaging, most current fluorophores used for optical imaging emit light in the visible range, limiting their use in the clinical realm due to limited tissue penetration.

Fluorophores are critical to the success of optical imaging as these probes are usually conjugated to probes for the detection and quantification of specific molecules. Traditional fluorophores consist of complex small molecules with numerous double bonds that are unstable under prolonged excitation [68]. Recently, semiconducting nanoparticles have provided long-lasting fluorescence with emission wavelength adjusted by particle size [69]. Lastly, luciferase has been used as active fluorophore to minimize absorption [70]. Combinations of quantum dots and either traditional fluorophore or luciferase have been used to successfully assess molecular interactions and enzyme functions [70]. Further details of the rapidly expanding field of optical imaging are reviewed elsewhere [55, 71–73].

7.5
Examples of Imaging Assessment of Tumor Response

In this section, applications of various imaging techniques for drug development and cancer treatment monitoring using different imaging techniques are reviewed.

7.5.1
SPECT

In clinical oncology, SPECT imaging has been used primarily to locate specific tumors and their metastasis to bones. Neuroendocrine tumors as well as pheochromocytoma and paraganglioma can be identified using ^{111}In-pentetreotide and $^{123/131}$I-MIBG [53]. For thyroid cancer, treatment, diagnosis, and surveillance can be accomplished with iodine probes (^{123}I for diagnosis/surveillance and ^{131}I for treatment) [53]. ^{99m}Tc-sestamibi, ^{67}Ga, and ^{201}Th chloride have been used to diagnose various other tumors, including lymphoma, parathyroid adenoma, breast cancer, lung cancer, seminoma, and osteosarcoma [53].

Recent advances in radiochemistry have made molecular imaging with SPECT possible. Angiogenesis has been assessed by labeling VEGF with ^{99m}Tc or ^{123}I. Following labeling with ^{99m}Tc, VEGF121 has been used to assess tumor vasculature in a mouse mammary adenocarcinoma model before and after cyclophosphamide therapy [74]. ^{123}I-labeled VEGF165 has been administered intravenously to pancreatic adenocarcinoma patients to reveal the sites of the primary lesion as well as metastatic sites; however, the metabolically unstable ^{123}I labeling led to significant uptake in the thyroid gland [75]. HER2 has also been imaged with indium-labeled trastuzumab showing metastatic lesions not demonstrable by routine staging studies [76]. ^{99m}Tc-labeled Annexin-V has been used to assess apoptosis in solid tumors following therapy, but the relatively low signal-to-background ratio has prevented this technique from being clinically useful so far [77].

7.5.2
PET/PET-CT

7.5.2.1 Microdosing

Pharmacokinetics, drug distribution, and achievable concentration are important parameters that relate to patient safety and drug efficacy, and are typically studied prior to initiation of a phase I clinical trial. Evaluation of these parameters is important because suboptimal pharmacokinetics and distribution can cause up to 40% of the candidates to fail in a phase I clinical trial [1]. The evaluation of these parameters is done during a phase 0 study when few patients are involved in this process, typically using microdosing studies during which small amounts of radiotracer-labeled drug candidates are administered to monitor their pharmacokinetics and biodistribution in human subjects. Owing to the low level of administered radiotracer-labeled drug, PET is particularly suited for this evaluation because of the sensitive (picomolar) and quantitative nature of the imaging technology [33].

Microdosing studies have been used to evaluate the pharmacokinetics and distribution data for several drug candidates. These include N-(2-(dimethylamino)ethyl)acridine-4-carboxamide (DACA, a topoisomerase I and II inhibitor) and temozolomide. These studies identified the distribution of the candidate drugs as well as their local activation within the neoplastic tissue [78–80]. Myocardial toxicity of DACA was also evaluated during the microdosing study [80].

As very low levels of the drug candidate are used in microdosing studies, questions have been raised regarding the relevance of the acquired pharmacokinetic data to human clinical trials. The CREAM (Consortium for Resourcing and Evaluating AMS Microdosing) trial was conducted to answer this question by simultaneously evaluating microdose and full-dose of the candidate [81]. This study showed that the pharmacokinetic data acquired from the microdosing study can mimic that of the regular dose. However, first-pass metabolism, gastrointestinal transporter mechanisms, plasma protein binding, and efficacy and safety data cannot be fully evaluated due to such low levels of the drug candidates administered.

7.5.2.2 Cancer Metabolism and Proliferation

Evaluating the metabolic response of cancers has become increasingly important, particularly with more cytostatic agents in clinical trials that lengthen progression-free and overall survival with only partial or no size response as judged by traditional RECIST criterion [82]. Radiotracers targeting the metabolic pathways have been synthesized, with the glucose analog (^{18}F-FDG) being currently the most popular agent. Others include ^{11}C- and ^{18}F-labeled amino acids as well as ^{11}C-labeled choline as described in the following section. Labeled DNA analogs have also been used to assess the proliferation rate of the malignant disease, including 3'-deoxy-3'-fluorothymidine (FLT) and 2'-fluoro-5-(^{11}C-methyl)-1-β-D-arabinofuranosyluracil (FMAU).

FDG imaging has provided important and prompt assessment of tumor metabolism and viability in various trials. In clinical practice, FDG imaging has shown that changes of tumor metabolism from therapy can be detected as early as 1–21 days in patients with GIST treated with imatinib mesylate as well as in

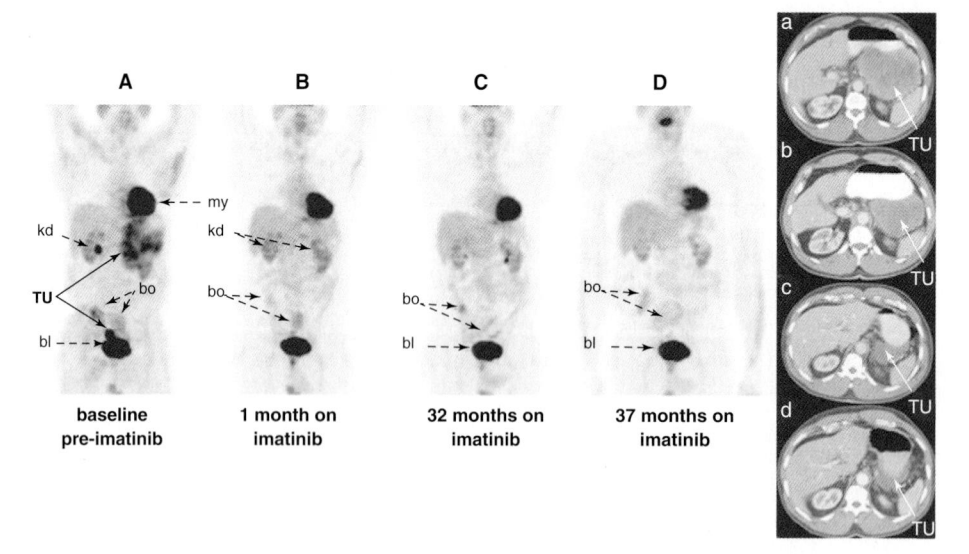

Figure 7.4 FDG-PET images of the response of GIST to imatinib shows complete metabolic response at 1 month. PET scan allows early detection of response to therapy that on the corresponding CT shows a gradual decrease in size (which would be classified as partial response at best during the early time period). A/a, pretherapy images; B/b, 1 month on imatinib; C/c, 32 months on imatinib; D/d, 37 months on imatinib. (Reproduced with permission from [83].)

lung cancer after platinum-based combination chemotherapies [37, 38]. Decrease in metabolic activity has also correlated with improved survival in lymphoma [40, 43], lung cancer [38, 42], esophageal cancer [39, 44], sarcoma [41], cervical cancer [83], and breast cancer [84]. In drug development, FDG imaging allowed better response prediction with cytostatic agents than CT, as these agents prolong survival without any change in tumor size [82, 85]. This was also the case in clinical trials of patients with GIST tumors treated with imatinib mesylate where response to therapy actually led to an increase in tumor size from internal hemorrhage despite a significant decrease in metabolic activity (Figure 7.4) [86]. In lung, esophageal, and lymphoid cancers, changes in tumor size significantly lagged behind metabolic response (Figure 7.5) [45], making tumor metabolism a better marker for assessment than for tumor size.

Changed amino acid metabolism in tumors has also been assessed by PET imaging [46]. The radiotracer that is closest to clinical use is ^{11}C-MET, while several others are in development, including ^{18}F-fluorophenylalanine, L-2-^{18}F-fluorotyrosine, O-(2-^{18}F-fluoroethyl)-L-tyrosine (^{18}F-FET), and ^{18}F-1-amino-3-fluoro-cyclobutane carboxylic acid (^{18}F-FACBC). Decrease in ^{11}C-MET activity following temozolomide therapy for astrocytomas correlated with longer survival (Figure 7.6) [87] and could distinguish radiation necrosis from recurrence or residual tumor [88]. However, because of the short half-life of ^{11}C-MET, its current use is limited clinically. Other tracers that have been tested clinically include ^{18}F-FET [89] and ^{18}F-FACBC [90], which showed clinical potential, though further evaluation is required.

Cellular proliferation has been assessed with PET using ^{18}F-FLT and ^{18}F-FMAU which target thymidine kinase-1 and -2, respectively. These molecules are phosphorylated intracellularly by the thymidine kinase such that they become too

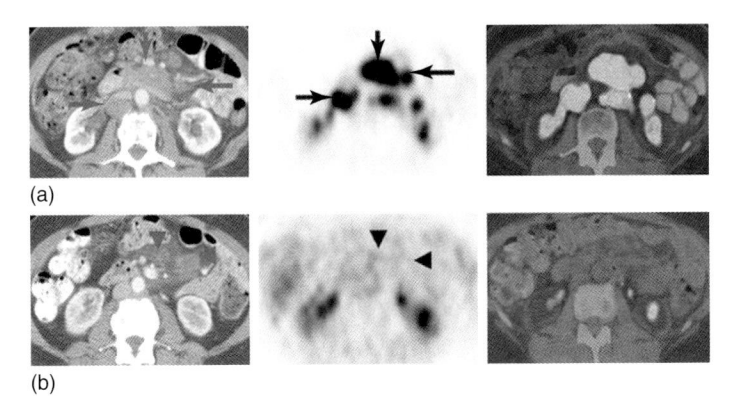

Figure 7.5 Complete metabolic response of non-Hodgkin's lymphoma. (a) FDG-PET and CT images demonstrate significant metabolic activity prior to initiating chemotherapy. (b) After two cycles of R-CHOP therapy, the metabolically active lymph nodes have decreased, with a number without metabolism. (Reproduced with permission from [43].)

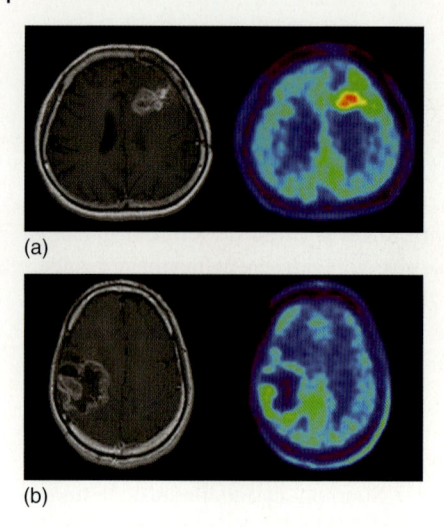

Figure 7.6 ^{11}C-MET PET scan can help differentiate tumor recurrence from gliosis. (a) Rim-enhancing lesion on T$_1$-weighted MRI of the brain correlates with increased uptake on PET scan, which was shown to be a recurrent tumor. (b) Rim-enhancing lesion demonstrates near cortical uptake and was shown on biopsy to represent gliosis. (Reproduced with permission from [84].)

hydrophilic to diffuse across the cellular membrane. It is known that thymidine kinase-1 is expressed predominantly when the cell is proliferating while thymidine kinase-2 is mitochondrial and associated with mitochondrial mass. As nucleic acid sources can be synthesized *de novo* by the cells or through salvage pathways, the level of radiotracer uptake can vary depending on the therapeutic means. For example, inhibition of DNA synthesis by 5-fluorouracil leads to increased FLT uptake secondary to increased salvage of nucleic acid, which can be misinterpreted as progressive disease despite tumor response [46]. On the other hand, therapies that do not lead to increased salvage uptake such as paclitaxel lead to more straightforward interpretation of the results [91].

In clinical trials, predominantly FLT has been used so far to assess efficacy of therapies while FMAU is used much less often [46]. FLT has been shown to detect early response to therapy at 2 days post-treatment [2, 46] with a decrease in radiotracer uptake in lymphoma [47], breast cancer (Figure 7.7) [48], and lung cancer [28]. Despite its ability to detect early response, no clinical trials have so far shown how that response translates to patient progression-free survival or overall survival.

7.5.2.3 Hypoxia

Tumor hypoxia imaging has been researched since the 1930s with recent findings showing hypoxia to be associated with worse outcome. This has led to the development of noninvasive imaging resulting in multiple radiotracers. $^{60/62/64}$Cu-labeled diacetyl-bis(N^4-methylthiosemicarbazone) ($^{60/62/64}$Cu-ATSM) and ^{18}F-fluoromisonidazole (^{18}F-FMISO) have been developed to reach hypoxic

[^{18}F]FLT uptake
100%

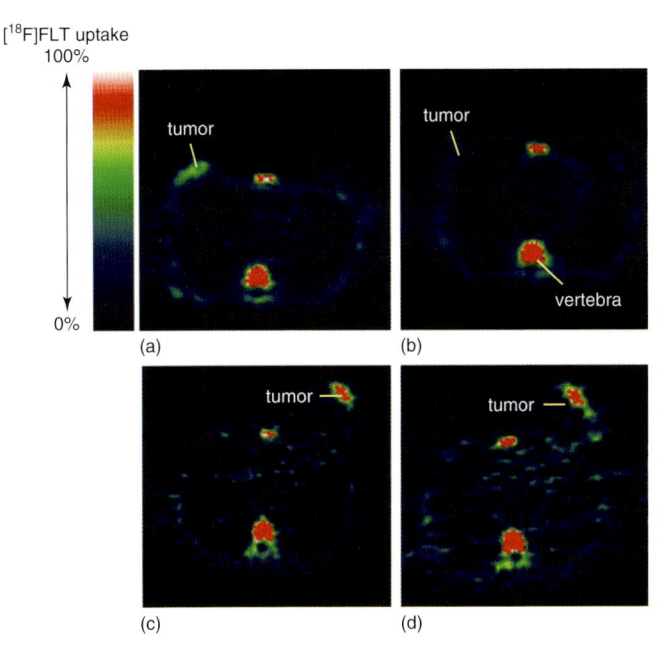

0%

(a) (b)

(c) (d)

Figure 7.7 FLT-PET showing responders and nonresponders for breast cancer patients. Responding patients as judged by tumor size based on RECIST criterion at 60 days post-therapy showed a decrease in nucleotide uptake (a, pretreatment and b, post-treatment) while nonresponders did not demonstrate any decrease in tumor activity (c, pretreatment and d, post-treatment). (Reproduced with permission from [48].)

zones by diffusion with subsequent reduction and entrapment in the hypoxic microenvironment [46]. When used to image tumors, $^{60/62/64}$Cu-ATSM has shown that pretreatment uptake is associated with shortened progression-free survival in lung, cervical, and rectal cancers (Figure 7.8) [92–94]. ^{18}F-FMISO has been tested since the 1990s for assessing tumor hypoxia [95], the results of which demonstrated shorter survival for patients with hypoxic tumors involving NSCLC, head and neck cancer, as well as prostate cancer. However, ^{18}F-FMISO does not have a great imaging profile as the washout of tracer from normal tissue is slow, leading to a low tumor-to-background ratio (approximately 1.2 : 1) [96, 97].

7.5.2.4 Biomarker Imaging

As described previously, biomarkers reflect a biochemical or physiological process relevant to tumor existence that, for example, can represent either a receptor or a secreted protein [9, 29, 30]. Either antibodies or ligand peptides to these biomolecules can be conjugated with, for example, a radiotracer to assess the level of expression by the target tumor. Traditionally, biomarkers have been assessed with lower-energy radiotracers including ^{111}In and ^{99m}Tc (Table 7.2). However, with the discovery of $^{60/62/64}$Cu and ^{124}I, PET agents are increasingly used to assess tumor expression of receptors or growth factors, including steroid receptors, EGFRs, and SSTRs [2]. Sex

(a) (b)

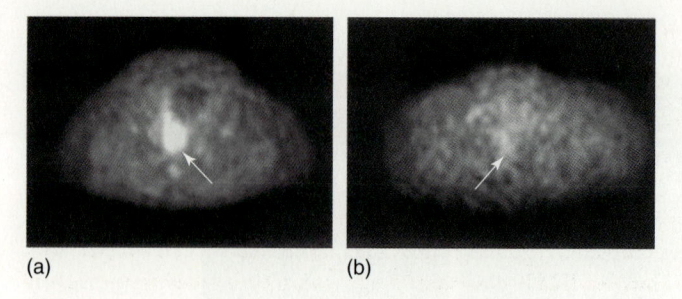

Figure 7.8 ^{60}Cu-ATSM PET images showing uptake predicts worse outcome. Patient (a) shows cervical tumor hypoxia with tumor recurrence following radiation therapy, while the lack of uptake in patient (b) yielded a recurrence-free period of at least 23 months. (Reproduced with permission from [89].)

Table 7.2 Common molecular imaging probes and their targets [2, 23, 53, 97, 100].

Molecular probes	Imaging target
Angiogenesis	
^{99m}Tc-VEGF121	VEGFR
^{123}I-VEGF165	VEGFR
^{64}Cu-DOTA-VEGF121	VEGFR
^{124}I-HuMV833	VEGFR
^{18}F-galacto-RGD	$\alpha_V\beta_3$ integrin
^{64}Cu-DOTA-etaracizumab	$\alpha_V\beta_3$ integrin
anti-VEGFR2/$\alpha_V\beta_3$ microbubble	VEGFR/$\alpha_V\beta_3$ integrin
Hypoxia	
^{18}F-FMISO	tumor hypoxia
^{64}Cu-ATSM	tumor hypoxia
Hormonal receptors	
^{18}F-FES	ER
^{18}F-FDHT	testosterone receptor
^{111}In-octreotide	SSTR
^{68}Ga-octreotide	SSTR
^{68}Ga-DOTA-F(ab')$_2$-trastuzumab	HER2
^{111}In-DTPA-trastuzumab	HER2
Proliferation/metabolism	
^{18}F-FLT	nucleic acid analog
^{18}F-FMAU	nucleic acid analog
^{11}C-MET	amino acid analog
^{18}F-FDG	glucose analog
Hepatobiliary agent	
gadoxetate disodium (Eovist)	liver uptake and biliary excretion
^{99m}Tc-iminodiacetic acid	liver uptake and biliary excretion

hormone receptors for estrogen and dihydrotestosterone have been targeted for PET imaging with ^{18}F-FES and 16β-^{18}F-fluoro-5α-dihydrotestosterone (^{18}F-FDHT). In breast cancer, ^{18}F-FES has been shown to image ER levels within the tumor [46]. Increased radiotracer activity predicted response to antiestrogen therapy in patients [98]. The subsequent decrease in radiotracer activity after initiation of therapy occurred within 7 days and likely reflected receptor downregulation as necrosis secondary to tamoxifen reached steady state around 3–5 weeks post-therapy [46, 99].

Other signaling receptors such as EGFRs and SSTRs have been imaged with radiolabeled PET probes. EGFR has been imaged with both small-molecule and antibody agents. These include reversible agents such as ^{11}C-erlotinib; irreversible agents such as ^{18}F-ML04 and ^{124}I-IPQA; and labeled monoclonal antibodies (mAbs) such as DTPA–cetuximab, DTPA–poly(ethylene glycol)–cetuximab, and DOTA–cetuximab using ^{64}Cu, ^{88}Y, ^{111}In, and ^{125}I (DTPA = diethylenetriamine pentaacetic acid) [2].

7.5.2.5 Angiogenesis

Tumor angiogenesis leads to a worse prognosis and is related to overexpression of VEGFR2. Probes have been developed to target VEGFR2 for assessing the level of expression, although these probes are not specific to type 2 receptors. These include ^{64}Cu-DOTA-VEGF121 and ^{124}I-HuMV833 (mouse monoclonal anti-VEGF antibody). Recently, mutant ^{64}Cu-DOTA-labeled VEGF121 with mutations located at sites 63, 64, and 67 has led to more specific VEGFR2 imaging [101]. In addition, because tumor neovasculature has been shown to overexpress $\alpha_V\beta_3$ integrin, agents targeting this receptor have also been developed. These include ^{64}Cu- and ^{18}F-labeled RGD peptides, including dimeric RGD labeled with ^{18}F, ^{18}F-galacto-RGD (Figure 7.9) [56], and ^{64}Cu-labeled humanized mAb ^{64}Cu-DOTA–etaracizumab [2]. All these agents have been imaged in preclinical *in vivo* studies, but their efficacy and prognostication will need to be further characterized with additional clinical trials.

7.5.2.6 Apoptosis

Following treatment, malignant cells typically respond with apoptosis, which is organized death of the cell [102, 103]. These have been imaged with both SPECT as described previously using Tc-Annexin-V or with PET using predominantly small molecules. These include molecules that image caspase-3 (^{18}F-ICMT 11, ^{18}F-WC-IV-3), membrane potential collapse (^{18}F-FBnTP), or membrane disruption (Aposense® compounds such as ML-10, DDC, or NST-732). Of these, the Aposense compounds, particularly ^{18}F-ML-10, have been tested in humans to evaluate response to therapy, while others have been primarily tested in animals [102, 103].

7.5.3
MRI

Currently, MRI technology does not have well-developed molecular probes that are in routine clinical practice. The closest probes had been reticuloendothelial

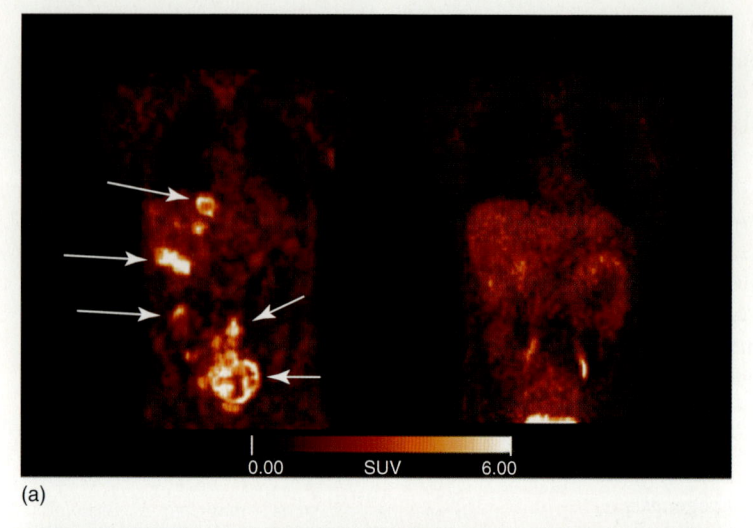

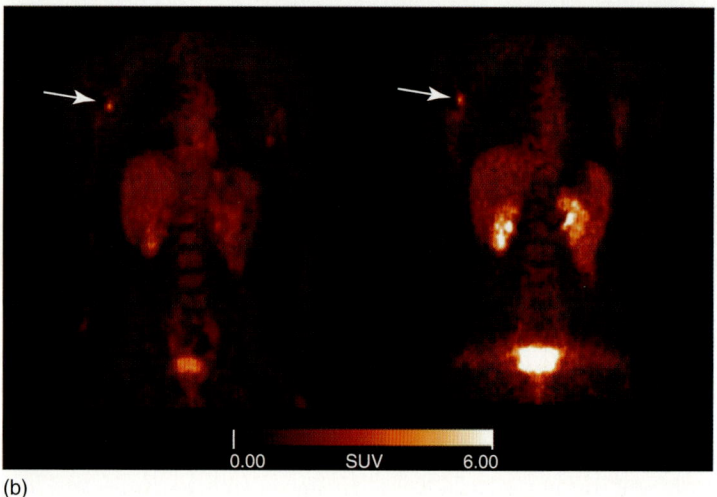

Figure 7.9 $\alpha_v\beta_3$ Imaging (^{18}F-galacto-RGD tracer) of melanoma metastasis. Patient (a) demonstrates metastasis (arrows) to liver on FDG study (left), which does not demonstrate angiogenesis as there is lack of anti-$\alpha_v\beta_3$ activity. In patient (b), there is both FDG and anti-$\alpha_v\beta_3$ activity, showing angiogenesis in the nodal metastasis (arrow). (Reproduced with permission from [56].)

cell-specific superparamagnetic iron oxide nanoparticles. However, recently those products have been withdrawn by the manufacturers owing to lack of demand. Another cell-specific nontargeted MRI contrast agent, Eovist® (also called Primovist®, gadoxetate disodium; Bayer) has received FDA approval for clinical use in liver imaging, particularly for characterizing focal liver lesions such as hepatocellular carcinoma or focal nodular hyperplasia, and is currently undergoing clinical testing. Although molecularly targeted contrast agents have been tested in preclinical trials in various animal models, none of them has been tested in humans or is close to clinical practice. These typically consist of either micellar, dendrimers, or nanoaggregates of gadolinium-based agents to increase T_1 relaxivity [104].

However, because MRI can develop high contrast images based on spin phases and local microenvironmental influences on hydrogen spins, noncontrast and vascular contrast administration images can be obtained to assess tumor physiology of malignant processes. These techniques include the diffusion-weighted sequence to interrogate free diffusion of water, magnetic resonance spectroscopy (MRS) to interrogate local metabolites, as well as dynamic contrast enhanced (DCE)-MRI to evaluate tumor perfusion and vascular permeability.

7.5.3.1 Cellular Structure

With magnetic resonance, water diffusion can be assessed with diffusion-weighted imaging (DWI). In malignant processes, increased cellularity restricts the diffusion of water leading to an abnormally increased signal on DWI images and is reflected in decreased signal intensity on the apparent diffusion coefficient (ADC) map. This technique has been tested for predicting patient response with brain, breast, rectal, and liver cancers to therapy consisting of either radiotherapy, chemotherapy, or hormonal therapy with measurements obtained both before and after therapy [36].

In pretherapy studies, the DWI study has shown potential predictive value regarding tumor response to therapy when correlated to either tumor size change or histopathological evaluation. In rectal cancer, pretherapy studies typically showed correlation of response with the ADC map of the cancer [105–107], with low pretherapy ADC correlating with tumor response, while high ADC correlated with less-predictable response [106, 108].

In studies conducted after initiation of therapy, ADC maps of tumors also changed with the therapy when correlated with the gold standard of tumor volume/size and histopathological analysis. This technique has been applied to brain [109, 110], rectal [111], breast (Figure 7.10) [112], bone [113], as well as prostate bony metastasis [114]. These studies have been conducted from 4 to 28 days after initiation of therapy, demonstrating histological evidence of cellular death or tumor shrinkage. However, data correlating ADC to progression-free and overall survival is still lacking.

7.5.3.2 Metabolic Response

MRS has predominantly been used as a diagnostic tool to characterize a mass as malignant or not. In particular, this technique has been used extensively in neurosurgery to evaluate post-therapy tumor recurrence. However, recent work has applied MRS to both preclinical and clinical evaluation of tumor response to drug therapies, as described in the following paragraphs.

In preclinical evaluation of therapies to inhibit metabolic processes, tumors have shown alterations of levels of phospholipids and lactate using MRS [115]. Contrary to expectations of decreased proliferation, treatment with inhibitors of phospholipid synthesis and histone deacetylase has led to increased phospholipid levels, suggesting the pathways to be significantly more complex than realized

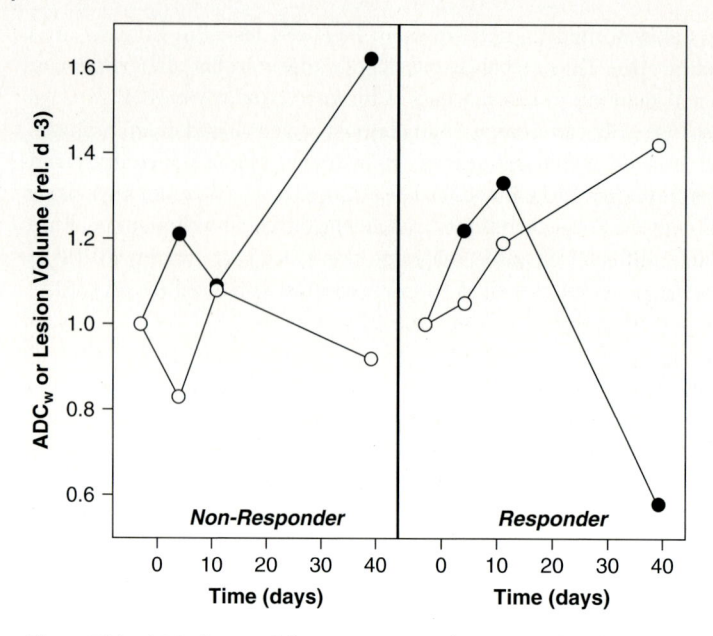

Figure 7.10 ADC changes following initiation of chemotherapy in breast cancer patients with liver metastasis. In responders, the ADC values (open circles) demonstrated a gradual increase, whereas nonresponders demonstrated stable ADC values. These ADC changes correspond to tumor volume (filled circles) decrease and increase, respectively. (Reproduced with permission from [107].)

[115, 116]. Increased aerobic glycolysis due to HIF-1α overexpression leads to overproduction of lactate whose level has been shown to decrease following response to imatinib mesylate therapy in chronic myeloid leukemia [115]. However, direct data regarding progression-free and overall survival have not been obtained.

Clinically, MRS has also been used to assess tumor response to chemotherapy for breast, liver, head, and neck, as well as lymphoid tumors [36]. Studies involving breast cancer have shown that water/fat ratio as well as choline peak alteration correlate with tumor response to chemotherapy that can be seen within the first day postchemotherapy [117, 118]. Similar findings were seen in hepatocellular carcinoma, lymphoma, and glioma [119–121], which demonstrated a post-therapy decrease in choline peak. In head and neck cancers, response to chemotherapy has been assessed by monitoring the phosphomonoester peak that, when measured pretherapy, can correlate with tumor response [122].

7.5.3.3 Tumor Perfusion

With dynamic imaging following intravenous contrast administration, tumor vascularity and vessel permeability can be measured by MRI techniques to infer the level of tumor hypoxia and response to therapy. In addition, tumor vascularity and vessel permeability can serve as imaging biomarkers of tumor response to angiogenesis inhibitors such as bevacizumab (Avastin®) and tyrosine kinase inhibitors such as sorafenib, sunitinib (Sutent®), axitinib, and erlotinib (Tarceva®).

DCE-MRI research has demonstrated potential prognostication of patient response to therapy from changes in vascularity and permeability. Rectal cancer that demonstrates high permeability pretherapy has shown better response than those with lower permeability [123]. Cervical cancer that demonstrated increased permeability 2 weeks after initiation of therapy showed significantly better therapeutic response than those with lower permeability [124]. For all studied cancers, including head and neck cancer, NSCLC, and cervical cancer, a high level of enhancement after completion of therapy was associated with increased recurrence rate and shorter survival [125–127]. DCE-MRI has also been applied to evaluate early-phase clinical trials that assessed the safety of antiangiogenic agents such as axitinib and bevacizumab [128, 129]. In assessing tumor response to axitinib, DCE-MRI showed that greater plasma concentration of axitinib correlated with significant decrease in K_{trans} (which measures the permeability of the vessels, typically requiring complex calculations) and initial area under curve (a practical measure of K_{trans}) at day 2 postinitiation of therapy [128]. In breast cancer treated with bevacizumab, all perfusion parameters decreased following one cycle of therapy, although both responders and nonresponders demonstrated such decrease [129]. Although these findings show that DCE-MRI can serve as a specific biomarker of tumor response to antiangiogenic therapy, they also raise questions regarding their applicability in predicting overall survival, particularly when both responders and nonresponders demonstrate a decrease in perfusion parameters. Further research and likely large-scale trials will be needed to determine DCE-MRI's predictive value for survival benefits from cytostatic therapy.

7.5.4
CT Imaging

CT has traditionally been used for anatomic evaluation of tumor location and response to therapy by the RECIST criteria [34]. This has served well in the evaluation of response in clinical practice and drug trials when cytotoxic drugs were used. With increasing use of cytostatic drugs that inhibit growth factor receptors, such evaluation may be limited, as described above. Fortunately, many of the cytostatic drugs ultimately influence angiogenesis, as seen with anti-VEGF and anti-EGF therapies, as mentioned previously. Changes in tumor vascularity as a response to therapy can be assessed with CT perfusion [62].

Clinical research has shown that CT perfusion has potential for evaluating tumor vascularity as a diagnostic tool and assessment for response to therapy. In evaluating pulmonary nodules, CT perfusion appears to have more than 90% sensitivity and 60% specificity for detecting malignancy in the pulmonary nodule [130] and for evaluating its metabolic response as perfusion values have been correlated with FDG uptake [131]. In clinical trials, CT perfusion has been applied to evaluate response of lymphoma [132], rectal cancer [133], prostate cancer [134, 135], and head and neck cancer [136]. However, additional research is needed to understand and gain control over the internal variability of this technique, which typically varies from 10 to 30% in data-derived perfusion variables [62]. Given that most oncology patients will obtain CT-based follow-up body scans for surveillance, CT perfusion can be easily included as part of the surveillance/monitoring study. However, the radiation exposure from perfusion CT scans is formidable [137], with radiation dose nearly doubling that of regular CT to approximately 30–40 mSv total dose [135]. The increased radiation dose also raises concern for increasing future cancer risk for these patients [135].

Owing to the lack of highly attenuating contrast agents, CT has not typically been thought of as a molecular imaging modality [60, 138]. However, recent research has found that gold nanoparticles can be modified on the surface with antibodies to target cancer with specific protein expression [61]. Gold is desirable because of its significant radiation attenuation and its biochemical inertness. In addition, poly(ethylene glycol)-coated gold nanoparticles can stay within the vasculature for up to 6 h [59], making it suitable as a vascular contrast agent. Although metallic nanoparticles can serve as a CT contrast agent, a significant amount of research is still needed to make it a clinically viable technique.

7.5.5
Ultrasound

Although ultrasound has traditionally been considered primarily an anatomical/morphological and functional imaging tool, the introduction of nontargeted contrast microbubbles allowed the quantitative assessment of tumor vascularity and perfusion at the capillary level. These contrast agents are currently approved for clinical use in Europe, Asia, and parts of Canada, with an ongoing phase III clinical trial in the US for characterization of focal liver lesions [139]. Owing to the angiogenic tendencies of aggressive tumors, many antiangiogenic therapies have been developed to "normalize" the tumor vasculature and to sensitize tumors to traditional chemotherapeutic agents [140]. Contrast enhanced ultrasound (CEUS) can assess native tumor vascularity and perfusion in the setting of breast, melanoma, colon, GIST, renal, ovarian, and primary hepatocellular carcinomas [140, 141]. CEUS also demonstrated the ability to assess tumor response in GIST treated with imatinib mesylate [100] and renal cell carcinoma treated with sorafenib [142]. Initial increases in vascularity can occur following therapy with subsequent vessel normalization – a finding that has been observed with CEUS as well [143, 144].

Recent advances in microbubble modification have made molecular imaging possible with ultrasound (Figure 7.11) [145]. Targeted microbubble sonography has been used to follow tumor response to anti-VEGF therapy, which showed a significant decrease in ultrasound signal intensity following therapy [64, 66]. Mouse models of xenograft ovarian tumor cells have demonstrated improved visualization with dual-targeted contrast microbubbles that can attach simultaneously to two tumor angiogenic markers, $\alpha_v\beta_3$ integrin and VEGFR2 [146]. In a mouse model of colonic tumor xenograft, using novel clinical-grade targeted microbubbles to human KDR (VEGFR2), a decrease in tumor vascularity has been shown as early as 24 h after treatment initiation, whereas tumor size did not change in the same time [66]. These results suggested that molecular ultrasound may become a quantitative

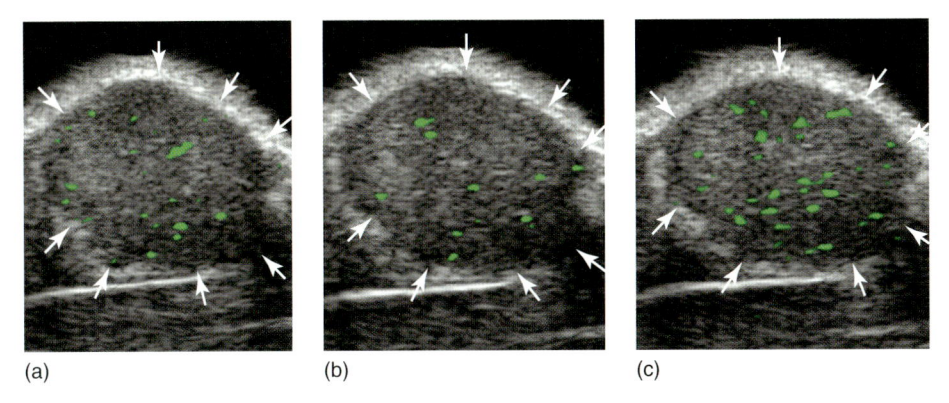

Figure 7.11 Dual-targeted microbubbles allow evaluation of tumor angiogenesis with higher sensitivity than single-targeted microbubbles. (a) Molecular signal from microbubbles targeted to VEGFR2. (b) Molecular signal from microbubbles targeted to $\alpha_v\beta_3$ integrin. (c) Microbubbles conjugated with antibodies to both receptors demonstrate greater signal in the same subcutaneous human ovarian adenocarcinoma xenograft compared to single-targeted microbubbles. (Reproduced with permission from [100].)

high-throughput modality to screen for tumor response at the molecular level following antiangiogenic therapy. Owing to its real-time capabilities, low cost, lack of irradiation, and wide availability, molecular ultrasound is a promising technique not only for drug development, but also for clinical practice, and through the development of novel clinical-grade targeted ultrasound contrast agents, clinical translation of molecular ultrasound in the near future is expected.

7.5.6
Fluorescence/Bioluminescence

Optical imaging currently has a minimal role in clinical imaging as the imaging depth is limited to a couple centimeters at most, depending on the chosen wavelength. However, it has tremendous value in basic research and drug development because of its real-time capability and inexpensive equipment. In addition, numerous probes have also been conjugated to optical emitters for assessing tumor biomarker expression [147, 148].

In drug development, identification of tumor biomarkers for assessing tumor targets and validation of response is one of the important first steps. These have been evaluated optically with fluorescent probes both *in vitro* and *in vivo* using mouse models of xenograft human tumors [147]. In assessing tumor response to mAb therapies, near-IR probes were linked to anti-EGFR antibodies that appropriately identified the cells bearing EGFR *in vitro*. When injected into tumor-bearing mice, these probes also appropriately identified these markers [149]. After treatment with antibody therapy, the apoptotic response of EGFR-bearing tumor cells was validated with Annexin-V-conjugated fluorescent probes [149]. Activatable probes for assessing tumor cells have been tested using cross-linked donor–receptor pairs

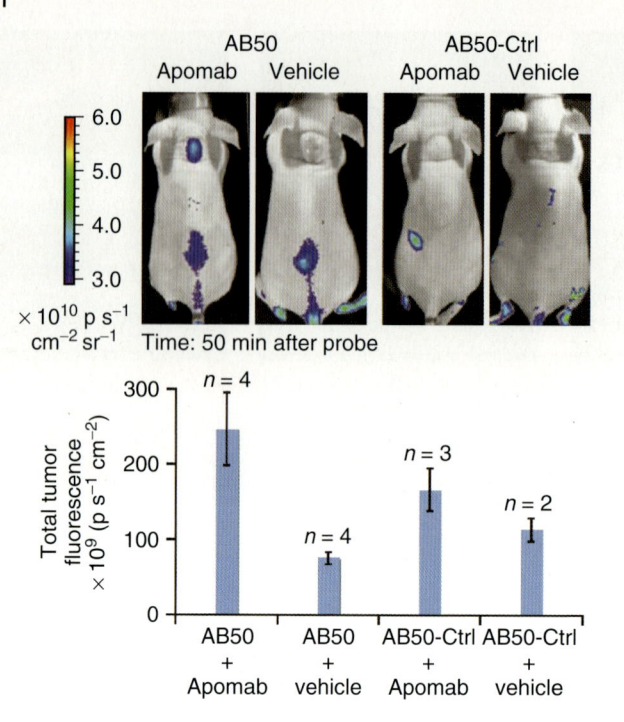

Figure 7.12 Near-IR imaging of activatable apoptosis probe. Peptide-based near-IR probes with a caspase-activatable group images early apoptosis after treatment with apoptosis inducing mAb (Apomab®; Genentech). Activatable probes (AB50) demonstrate differential uptake between Apomab-treated and untreated mice while no difference is seen in control probes without the active acyloxymethyl group (AB50-Ctrl). (Reproduced with permission from [146].)

with the quencher being degraded in the endosomal environment [150]. More complex optical probes have also been developed to interrogate the activation of caspase through an optimized peptide sequence that labeled the caspase with high specificity (Figure 7.12) [151]; HIF and von Hippel-Lindau protein interaction in reconstituting luciferase activity using DNA transfection technique [152]; EGFR labeling *in vivo* for detection of head and neck cancers in mice [153, 154] as well as demonstrating activation of EGFR through split luciferase components [155]; and NF-κB [156] and protein kinase A [156, 157] expression by gene transfer. Other activatable probes include endosomal degradation of indocyanine green quencher [158] and matrix metalloproteinase-cleavable Cy5.5-conjugated peptide [159].

7.6
Challenges of Imaging in Drug Development and Validation

Several challenges need to be resolved to make imaging an integral part of the process of drug development and validation [1]. Most often imaging, in particular molecular imaging, is regarded as useful in the prephase I studies of drug development only. However, molecular imaging may be incorporated into the whole drug development process starting as early as assessment of target expression and lead compound optimization as well as during testing of drugs in clinical trials [1]. This allows integration of molecular imaging into the whole process of drug development and helps to exclude a possible drug candidate early in the testing process if needed. Once a particular imaging technique or combinations of different imaging techniques have been proven useful for following a drug during development, these imaging techniques may be used as a valuable biomarker or even surrogate endpoint for each particular drug in the whole preclinical and clinical process of drug development. It is particularly important that the preclinical and clinical groups within pharmaceutical and biotechnology companies are actively cooperating and working with imaging subgroups to plan for incorporation of imaging into the entire pipeline of drug development [1]. Far too often, this does not occur and leads to the suboptimal use of imaging.

Furthermore, imaging techniques need to continue being sufficiently validated to be useful for all different phases of the drug development process [1]. The decision by a pharmaceutical company to use an imaging modality for drug development strongly depends on the accuracy and reliability of the imaging test. Further improvement is needed regarding the robustness of the imaging techniques, the ease of operation, and the tools for quantitative data analysis of molecular imaging assays, such as determination of concentrations, activities, and flux rates [1].

Finally, even if a drug fails to make it further in the drug development process, a close partnership between pharmaceutical and imaging communities may also enhance the development of new imaging tracers for diagnostics only [1]. Since many components of drug and imaging probe development are near identical, it is highly likely that future companies will be able to exploit joint development strategies. In fact, even if a given agent fails as a drug it may lead to the development of a useful imaging agent. If libraries of failed drugs could become available for mining for imaging probe development this would likely be highly useful. It is also quite possible that an imaging agent initially intended for diagnostics, when optimized for administration dose, could itself be useful as a pharmaceutical. Hopefully, companies in the near future will evolve so that imaging and therapeutics are fully integrated.

7.7
Conclusions and Future Perspectives

Owing to high drug development costs, there is a need to prevent late-phase trial failures through early detection of ineffective drug candidates. By eliminating ineffective candidates early, hundreds of millions of dollars of developmental costs can potentially be saved. The process begins with target and pathway identification with *in vitro* assessment that progresses to small animal testing, both of which are well served with optical or ultrasound imaging due to the rapid turnaround

216 | *7 Imaging Techniques in Drug Development and Clinical Practice*

Optical imaging

Advantages:
- High-throughput screening for target confirmation and compound optimization
- High sensitivity

Disadvantages:
- Limited clinical translation
- Low depth penetration

Magnetic resonance imaging

Advantages:
- Clinical translation
- High resolution and soft-tissue contrast

Disadvantages:
- Costs
- Imaging time

Ultrasound imaging

Advantages:
- Clinical translation
- High spatial and temporal resolution
- Low costs

Disadvantages:
- Operator dependency
- Targeted imaging limited to vascular compartment

PET imaging

Advantages:
- Clinical translation
- High sensitivity with unlimited depth penetration

Disadvantages:
- Cost

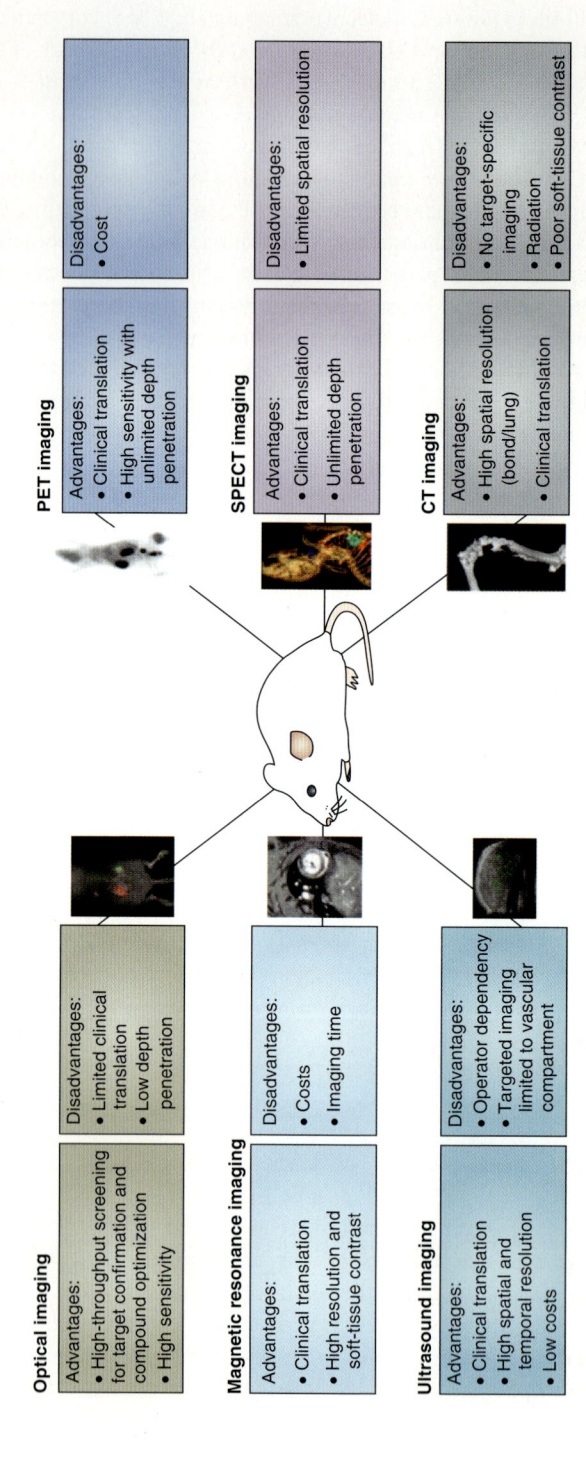

SPECT imaging

Advantages:
- Clinical translation
- Unlimited depth penetration

Disadvantages:
- Limited spatial resolution

CT imaging

Advantages:
- High spatial resolution (bond/lung)
- Clinical translation

Disadvantages:
- No target-specific imaging
- Radiation
- Poor soft-tissue contrast

Figure 7.13 Summary of the key advantages and disadvantages of currently used imaging modalities for oncological drug development and clinical practice. (Reproduced with permission from [1].)

time and the low cost of the equipment. Once the pathway and concept have been proven, phase I and II clinical trials can begin, during which time toxicity, dosing, biodistribution, and early efficacy can be assessed both clinically as well as with PET (particularly for dosing, biodistribution, and tumor metabolic response), MRI (for assessing tumor metabolic state, vascularity, size, and cellularity), CT (for assessing size and vascularity), and ultrasound (assessment of size and vascularity). Finally, large-scale, phase III clinical trials can then be obtained if the drug candidate survives the early clinical testing. In phase III clinical trials, at this time, proven techniques (predominantly PET) can be used to demonstrate early tumor response to candidate therapy that will lead to overall survival or progression-free survival benefit from the candidate drug (Figure 7.13).

Throughout the drug development process, imaging plays a crucial role for target identification and early failure detection. Additional imaging techniques are also being investigated to allow different multimodality evaluation of *in vivo* molecular interactions, which may be translated into the clinic in the near future to aid patient care [160]. With advances in molecular imaging, it is expected that the focus of forthcoming development will be on further integration of imaging in drug development and response monitoring as well as in molecular probe development for a greater number of modalities. By increasing the available probes for a greater number of modalities, more physiologically important targets can be evaluated for their efficacy in cancer treatment. In turn, these probes can be applied to monitor patient response to make treatment more personalized. By increasing the number of molecular imaging modalities, more options are available to improve the resolution, timing, and cost of monitoring response in various research and clinical circumstances. Thus, future of imaging is likely to become significantly more functional as well as molecularly based, providing relevant physiological information for clinicians and scientists to guide patient treatment.

References

1. Willmann, J.K. *et al.* (2008) Molecular imaging in drug development. *Nat. Rev. Drug Discov.*, **7**, 591–607.
2. Josephs, D., Spicer, J., and O'Doherty, M. (2009) Molecular imaging in clinical trials. *Target. Oncol.*, **4**, 151–168.
3. Khalique, L. *et al.* (2007) Genetic intra-tumour heterogeneity in epithelial ovarian cancer and its implications for molecular diagnosis of tumours. *J. Pathol.*, **211**, 286–295.
4. Losi, L. *et al.* (2005) Evolution of intra-tumoral genetic heterogeneity during colorectal cancer progression. *Carcinogenesis*, **25**, 916–922.
5. Pan, H. *et al.* (2005) Loss of heterozygosity patterns provide fingerprints for genetic heterogeneity in multi-step cancer progression of tobacco smoke-induced non-small cell lung cancer. *Cancer Res.*, **65**, 1664–1669.
6. Lenhard, R.E. Jr., Osteen, R.T., and Gansler, T. (2001) *Clinical Oncology*, American Cancer Society, Atlanta, GA.
7. Matsusaka, S. *et al.* (2010) Circulating tumor cells as a surrogate marker for determining response to chemotherapy in patients with advanced gastric cancer. *Cancer Sci.*, **101**, 1067–1071.
8. Nakamura, S. *et al.* (2009) Multi-center study evaluating circulating tumor cells as a surrogate for response

to treatment and overall survival in metastatic breast cancer. *Breast Cancer*, **17**, 199–204.

9. Smith, J.J., Sorensen, A.G., and Thrall, J.H. (2003) Biomarkers in imaging: realizing radiology's future. *Radiology*, **227**, 633–638.

10. Padhani, A.R. and Miles, K.A. (2010) Multiparametric imaging of tumor response to therapy. *Radiology*, **256**, 348–364.

11. Dawood, S. and Cristofanilli, M. (2007) Integrating circulating tumor cell assays into the management of breast cancer. *Curr. Treat. Options Oncol.*, **8**, 89–95.

12. Sorensen, B.S. et al. (2010) Circulating HER2 DNA after trastuzumab treatment predicts survival and response in breast cancer. *Anticancer Res.*, **30**, 2463–2468.

13. Dotan, E. et al. (2009) Circulating tumor cells: evolving evidence and future challenges. *Oncologist*, **14**, 1070–1082.

14. Gatenby, R.A. and Gillies, R.J. (2008) A microenvironmental model of carcinogenesis. *Nat. Rev. Cancer*, **8**, 56–62.

15. Gillies, R.J. et al. (2002) MRI of the tumor microenvironment. *J. Magn. Res. Imaging*, **16**, 430–450.

16. Barwick, T. et al. (2009) Molecular PET and PET/CT imaging of tumour cell proliferation using F-18 fluoro-L-thymidine: a comprehensive evaluation. *Nucl. Med. Commun.*, **30**, 908–917.

17. Plathow, C. and Weber, W.A. (2008) Tumor cell metabolism imaging. *J. Nucl. Med.*, **49** (Suppl. 6), 43S–63S.

18. Gillies, R.J., Robey, I., and Gatenby, R.A. (2008) Causes and consequences of increased glucose metabolism of cancers. *J. Nucl. Med.*, **49**, 24S–42S.

19. Aboagye, E.O. and Bhujwalla, Z.M. (1999) Malignant transformation alters membrane choline phospholipid metabolism of human mammary epithelial cells. *Cancer Res.*, **59**, 80–84.

20. DeBerardinis, R.J. et al. (2008) Brick by brick: metabolism and tumor cell growth. *Curr. Opin. Genet. Dev.*, **18**, 54–61.

21. Berg, J.M., Tymoczko, J.L., and Stryer, L. (2002) *Biochemistry*, 5th edn, Freeman, New York.

22. Suarez, C., Morales, R., and Munoz, E. (2010) Molecular basis for the treatment of renal cell carcinoma. *Clin. Transl. Oncol.*, **12**, 15–21.

23. Cai, W. and Chen, X. (2008) Multimodality molecular imaging of tumor angiogenesis. *J. Nucl. Med.*, **49**, 113S–128S.

24. Bhujwalla, Z. et al. (2001) Vascular differences detected by MRI for metastatic versus nonmetastatic breast and prostate cancer xenografts. *Neoplasia*, **3**, 143–153.

25. Ferrara, N. (2004) Vascular endothelial growth factor: basic science and clinical progress. *Endocr. Rev.*, **25**, 581–611.

26. Choueiri, T.K. (2008) Axitinib, a novel anti-angiogenic drug with promising activity in various solid tumors. *Curr. Opin. Investig. Drugs*, **9**, 658–671.

27. Ratain, M.J. et al. (2006) Phase II placebo-controlled randomized discontinuation trial of sorafenib in patients with metastatic renal cell carcinoma. *J. Clin. Oncol.*, **24**, 2505–2512.

28. Sohn, H.J. et al. (2008) [^{18}F]Fluorothymidine positron emission tomography before and 7 days after gefitinib treatment predicts response in patients with advanced adenocarcinoma of the lung. *Clin. Cancer Res.*, **14**, 7423–7429.

29. Ilyin, S.E., Belkowski, S.M., and Plata-Salaman, C.R. (2004) Biomarker discovery and validation: technologies and integrative approaches. *Trends Biotech.*, **22**, 411–416.

30. Pien, H.H. et al. (2005) Using imaging biomarkers to accelerate drug development and clinical trials. *Drug Discov. Today*, **10**, 259–266.

31. Ludwig, J.A. and Weinstein, J.N. (2005) Biomarkers in cancer staging, prognosis, and treatment selection. *Nat. Rev. Cancer*, **5**, 845–856.

32. Slamon, D.J. et al. (2001) Use of chemotherapy plus a monoclonal antibody against HER2 for metastatic breast cancer that overexpresses HER2. *N. Engl. J. Med.*, **344**, 783–792.

33. Rudin, M. and Weissleder, R. (2003) Molecular imaging in drug discovery and development. *Nat. Rev. Drug Discov.*, **2**, 123–131.
34. Padhani, A.R. and Ollivier, L. (2001) The RECIST criteria: implications for diagnostic radiologists. *Br. J. Radiol.*, **74**, 983–986.
35. Wahl, R.L. et al. (2009) From RECIST to PERCIST: evolving considerations for PET response criteria in solid tumors. *J. Nucl. Med.*, **50** (Suppl. 1), 122S–150S.
36. Harry, V.N. et al. (2010) Use of new imaging techniques to predict tumor response to therapy. *Lancet Oncol.*, **11**, 92–102.
37. Van den Abbeele, A.D. and Badawi, R.D. (2002) Use of positron emission tomography in oncology and its potential role to assess response to imatinib mesylate therapy in gastrointestinal stromal tumors (GIST). *Eur. J. Cancer*, **38** (Suppl. 5), 60–65.
38. Weber, W.A. et al. (2003) Positron emission tomography in non-small-cell-lung cancer: prediction of response to chemotherapy by quantitative assessment of glucose use. *J. Clin. Oncol.*, **21**, 2651–2657.
39. Bombardieri, E. (2006) The added value of metabolic imaging with FDG-PET in oesophageal cancer: prognostic role and prediction of response to treatment. *Eur. J. Nucl. Med. Mol. Imaging*, **33**, 753–758.
40. Filmont, J.-E. et al. (2003) Conventional imaging and 2-deoxy-2-[^{18}F]fluoro-D-glucose positron emission tomography for predicting the clinical outcome of previously treated non-Hodgkin's lymphoma patients. *Mol. Imaging Biol.*, **5**, 232–239.
41. Hawkins, D.S. et al. (2005) [^{18}F]Fluorodeoxyglucose positron emission tomography predicts outcome for Ewing sarcoma family of tumors. *J. Clin. Oncol.*, **23**, 8828.
42. Hoekstra, C.J. (2005) Prognostic relevance of response evaluation using [^{18}F]-2-fluoro-2-deoxy-D-glucose positron emission tomography in patients with locally advanced non-small-cell lung cancer. *J. Clin. Oncol.*, **23**, 8362–8370.
43. Kostakoglu, L. et al. (2002) PET predicts prognosis after 1 cycle of chemotherapy in aggressive lymphoma and Hodgkin's disease. *J. Nucl. Med.*, **43**, 1018–1027.
44. Levine, E.A. et al. (2006) Predictive value of 18-fluoro-deoxy-glucose positron emission tomography (^{18}F-FDG-PET) in the identification of responders to chemoradiation therapy for the treatment of locally advanced esophageal cancer. *Ann. Surg.*, **243**, 472–478.
45. Kostakoglu, L. (2008) FDG-PET evaluation of response to treatment. *PET Clinics*, **3**, 37–75.
46. Dunphy, M.P.S. and Lewis, J.S. (2009) Radiopharmaceuticals in preclinical and clinical development for monitoring of therapy with PET. *J. Nucl. Med.*, **50** (Suppl. 1), 106S–121S.
47. Herrmann, K. et al. (2007) Early response assessment using 3′-deoxy-3′-[^{18}F]fluorothymidine-positron emission tomography in high-grade non-Hodgkin's lymphoma. *Clin. Cancer Res.*, **13**, 3552–3558.
48. Kenny, L. et al. (2007) Imaging early changes in proliferation at 1 week post chemotherapy: a pilot study in breast cancer patients with 3′-deoxy-3′[^{18}F]fluorothymidine positron emission tomography. *Eur. J. Nucl. Med. Mol. Imaging*, **34**, 1339–1347.
49. Fischman, E. and Jeffrey, R.B. (eds) (2003) *Multidetector Computed Tomography: Principles, Techniques, and Clinical Applications*, Lippincott Williams & Wilkins, Baltimore, MD.
50. Hashemi, R.H., Bradley, W.G., and Lisanti, C.J. (2004) *MRI: The Basics*, Lippincott Williams & Wilkins, Baltimore, MD.
51. Kalra, M.K., Saini, S., and Rubin, G.D. (2010) *MDCT: From Protocols to Practice*, Springer, Milan.
52. Mahmood, U. (2004) Near infrared optical applications in molecular imaging. Earlier, more accurate assessment of disease presence, disease course, and efficacy of disease treatment. *IEEE Eng. Med. Biol.*, **23**, 58–66.
53. Mettler, F.A. and Guiberteau, M.J. Jr. (2006) *Essentials of Nuclear Medicine*

54. Rumack, C., Wilson, S., Charboneau, J.W., and Johnson, J.A. (eds) (2004) *Diagnostic Ultrasound*, 3rd edn, Mosby, St. Louis, MO.
55. Alford, R. et al. (2009) Molecular probes for the *in vivo* imaging of cancer. *Mol. Biosyst.*, **5**, 1279–1291.
56. Haubner, R. et al. (2005) Noninvasive visualization of the activated alphav-beta3 integrin in cancer patients by positron emission tomography and [^{18}F]galacto-RGD. *Plos Med.*, **2**, e70.
57. Padhani, A.R. and Khan, A.A. (2010) Diffusion-weighted (DW) and dynamic contrast-enhanced (DCE) magnetic resonance imaging (MRI) for monitoring anticancer therapy. *Target. Oncol.*, **5**, 39–52.
58. Bradbury, M. and Hricak, H. (2005) Molecular MR imaging in oncology. *Magn. Reson Imaging Clin. N. Am.*, **13**, 225.
59. Cai, Q.-Y. et al. (2007) Colloidal gold nanoparticles as a blood-pool contrast agent for X-ray computed tomography in mice. *Invest. Radiol.*, **42**, 797–806.
60. Miyamoto, A. et al. (2006) Development of water-soluble metallofullerenes as X-ray contrast media. *Eur. Radiol.*, **16**, 1050–1053.
61. Popovtzer, R. et al. (2008) Targeted gold nanoparticles enable molecular CT imaging of cancer. *Nano Lett.*, **8**, 4593–4596.
62. Miles, K.A. and Griffiths, M.R. (2003) Perfusion CT: a worthwhile enhancement? *Br. J. Radiol.*, **76**, 220–231.
63. Weyman, A.E. (2009) Future directions in echocardiography. *Rev. Cardiovasc. Med.*, **10**, 4–13.
64. Deshpande, N., Pysz, M.A., and Willmann, J.K. (2010) Molecular ultrasound assessment of tumor angiogenesis. *Angiogenesis*, **13**, 175–188.
65. Pochon, S. et al. (2010) BR55: a lipopeptide-based VEGFR2-targeted ultrasound contrast agent for molecular imaging of angiogenesis. *Invest. Radiol.*, **45**, 89–95.
66. Pysz, M.A. et al. (2010) Antiangiogenic cancer therapy: monitoring with molecular US and a clinically translatable contrast agent (BR55). *Radiology*, **256**, 519–527.
67. Voigt, J.-U. (2009) Ultrasound molecular imaging. *Methods*, **48**, 92–97.
68. Alford, R. et al. (2009) Toxicity of organic fluorophores used in molecular imaging: literature review. *Mol. Imaging*, **8**, 341–354.
69. Xing, Y., Xia, Z., and Rao, J. (2009) Semiconductor quantum dots for biosensing and *in vivo* imaging. *IEEE Trans. Nanobiosci.*, **8**, 4–12.
70. Xing, Y. et al. (2008) Improved QD-BRET conjugates for detection and imaging. *Biochem. Biophys. Res. Commun.*, **372**, 388–394.
71. Hilderbrand, S.A. and Weissleder, R. (2010) Near-infrared fluorescence: application to *in vivo* molecular imaging. *Curr. Opin. Chem. Biol.*, **14**, 71–79.
72. Kobayashi, H. et al. (2010) New strategies for fluorescent probe design in medical diagnostic imaging. *Chem. Rev.*, **110**, 2620–2640.
73. Sheth, R.A. and Mahmood, U. (2010) Optical molecular imaging and its emerging role in colorectal cancer. *Am. J. Physiol. Gastrointest Liver Physiol.*, **299**, G807–G820.
74. Blankenberg, F.G. et al. (2006) *In vivo* tumor angiogenesis imaging with site-specific labeled ^{99m}Tc-HYNIC-VEGF. *Eur. J. Nucl. Med. Mol. Imaging*, **33**, 841–848.
75. Li, S. et al. (2004) Iodine-123-vascular endothelial growth factor-165 (^{123}I-VEGF165). Biodistribution, safety and radiation dosimetry in patients with pancreatic carcinoma. *Q. J. Nucl. Med. Mol. Imaging*, **48**, 198–206.
76. Perik, P.J., Lub-de Hooge, M.N., and Gietema, J.A. (2006) Indium-111-labeled trastuzumab scintigraphy in patients with human epidermal growth factor receptor 2-positive metastatic breast cancer. *J. Clin. Oncol.*, **24**, 2276–2282.
77. Blankenberg, F.G. et al. (1999) Imaging of apoptosis (programmed cell death) with ^{99m}Tc annexin V. *J. Nucl. Med.*, **40**, 184–191.

78. Saleem, A. et al. (2003) Metabolic activation of temozolomide measured *in vivo* using positron emission tomography. *Cancer Res.*, **63**, 2409–2415.
79. Saleem, A., Charnley, N., and Price, P. (2006) Clinical molecular imaging with positron emission tomography. *Eur. J. Cancer*, **42**, 1720–1727.
80. Saleem, A. et al. (2001) Pharmacokinetic evaluation of *N*-[2-(dimethylamino)ethyl]acridine-4-carboxamide in patients by positron emission tomography. *J. Clin. Oncol.*, **19**, 1421–1429.
81. Garner, R.C. (2005) Less is more: the human microdosing concept. *Drug Discov. Today*, **10**, 449–451.
82. Farley, J. and Rose, P.G. (2010) Trial design for evaluation of novel targeted therapies. *Gynecol. Oncol.*, **116**, 173–176.
83. Xue, F. et al. (2006) F-18 fluorodeoxyglucose uptake in primary cervical cancer as an indicator of prognosis after radiation therapy. *Gynecol. Oncol.*, **101**, 147–151.
84. Byrne, A.M. et al. (2004) Positron emission tomography in the staging and management of breast cancer. *Br. J. Surg.*, **91**, 1398–1409.
85. Shankar, L.K. et al. (2009) Considerations for the use of imaging tools for phase II treatment trials in oncology. *Clin. Cancer Res.*, **15**, 1891–1897.
86. Van den Abbeele, A.D. and Ertuk, M. (2008) FDG-PET to measure response to targeted therapy: the example of gastrointestinal stromal tumor and imatiib mesylate (Gleevec). *PET Clinics*, **3**, 77–87.
87. Galldiks, N. et al. (2006) Use of ^{11}C-methionine PET to monitor the effects of temozolomide chemotherapy in malignant gliomas. *Eur. J. Nucl. Med. Mol. Imaging*, **33**, 516–524.
88. Terakawa, Y. et al. (2008) Diagnostic accuracy of ^{11}C-methionine PET for differentiation of recurrent brain tumors from radiation necrosis after radiotherapy. *J. Nucl. Med.*, **49**, 694–699.
89. Pauleit, D. et al. (2006) ^{18}F-FET PET compared with ^{18}F-FDG PET and CT in patients with head and neck cancer. *J. Nucl. Med.*, **47**, 256–261.
90. Schuster, D.M. et al. (2007) Initial experience with the radiotracer anti-1-amino-3-^{18}F-fluorocyclobutane-1-carboxylic acid with PET/CT in prostate carcinoma. *J. Nucl. Med.*, **48**, 56–63.
91. Direcks, W.G. et al. (2008) [^{18}F]FDG and [^{18}F]FLT uptake in human breast cancer cells in relation to the effects of chemotherapy: an *in vitro* study. *Br. J. Cancer*, **99**, 481–487.
92. Dehdashti, F. et al. (2003) Assessing tumor hypoxia in cervical cancer by positron emission tomography with ^{60}Cu-ATSM: relationship to therapeutic response – a preliminary report. *Int. J. Radiat. Oncol. Biol. Phys.*, **55**, 1233–1238.
93. Dietz, D.W. et al. (2008) Tumor hypoxia detected by positron emission tomography with ^{60}Cu-ATSM as a predictor of response and survival in patients undergoing neoadjuvant chemoradiotherapy for rectal carcinoma: a pilot study. *Dis. Colon. Rectum.*, **51**, 1641–1648.
94. Takahashi, N. et al. (2000) Evaluation of ^{62}Cu labeled diacetyl-bis(N^4-methylthiosemicarbazone) as a hypoxic tissue tracer in patients with lung cancer. *Ann. Nucl. Med.*, **14**, 323–328.
95. Rasey, J.S. et al. (1996) Quantifying regional hypoxia in human tumors with positron emission tomography of [^{18}F]fluoromisonidazole: a pretherapy study of 37 patients. *Int. J. Radiat. Oncol. Biol. Phys.*, **36**, 417–428.
96. Rajendran, J.G. et al. (2004) Hypoxia and glucose metabolism in malignant tumors: evaluation by [^{18}F]fluoromisonidazole and [^{18}F]fluorodeoxyglucose positron emission tomography imaging. *Clin. Cancer Res.*, **10**, 2245–2252.
97. Rasey, J.S. et al. (1989) Radiolabeled fluoromisonidazole as an imaging agent for tumor hypoxia. *Int. J. Radiat. Oncol. Biol. Phys.*, **17**, 985–991.
98. Dehdashti, F. et al. (2009) PET-based estradiol challenge as a predictive biomarker of response to endocrine therapy in women with

estrogen-receptor-positive breast cancer. *Breast Cancer Res. Treat.*, **113**, 509–517.

99. Mortimer, J.E. et al. (2001) Metabolic flare: indicator of hormone responsiveness in advanced breast cancer. *J. Clin. Oncol.*, **19**, 2797–2803.

100. Lassau, N. et al. (2003) Gastrointestinal stromal tumors treated with imatinib: monitoring response with contrast-enhanced sonography. *Am. J. Roentgenol.*, **187**, 1267–1273.

101. Wang, H. et al. (2007) A new PET tracer specific for vascular endothelial growth factor receptor 2. *Eur. J. Nucl. Med. Mol. Imaging*, **34**, 2001–2010.

102. Reshef, A. et al. (2010) Small-molecule biomarkers for clinical PET imaging of apoptosis. *J. Nucl. Med.*, **51**, 837–840.

103. Schoenberger, J. et al. (2008) Innovative strategies in in vivo apoptosis imaging. *Curr. Med. Chem.*, **15**, 187–194.

104. Caruthers, S.D. et al. (2005) Targeted magnetic resonance imaging contrast agents. *Methods Mol. Med.*, **124**, 387–400.

105. DeVries, A.F. et al. (2003) Tumor microcirculation and diffusion predict therapy outcome for primary rectal carcinoma. *Int. J. Radiat. Oncol. Biol. Phys.*, **56**, 958–965.

106. Dzik-Jurasz, A. et al. (2002) Diffusion MRI for prediction of response of rectal cancer to chemoradiation. *Lancet*, **360**, 307–308.

107. Hein, P.A. et al. (2003) [Diffusion-weighted MRI – a new parameter for advanced rectal carcinoma]. *Rofo*, **175**, 381–386.

108. Thoeny, H.C. et al. (2005) Diffusion-weighted magnetic resonance imaging allows noninvasive in vivo monitoring of the effects of combretastatin a-4 phosphate after repeated administration. *Neoplasia*, **7**, 779–787.

109. Moffat, B.A. et al. (2005) Functional diffusion map: a noninvasive MRI biomarker for early stratification of clinical brain tumor response. *Proc. Natl. Acad. Sci. USA*, **102**, 5524–5529.

110. Tomura, N. et al. (2006) Diffusion changes in a tumor and peritumoral tissue after stereotactic irradiation for brain tumors: possible prediction of treatment response. *J. Comput. Assist. Tomogr.*, **30**, 496–500.

111. Kremser, C. et al. (2003) Preliminary results on the influence of chemoradiation on apparent diffusion coefficients of primary rectal carcinoma measured by magnetic resonance imaging. *Strahlenther. Onkol.*, **179**, 641–649.

112. Theilmann, J. et al. (2004) Changes in water mobility measured by diffusion MRI predict response of metastatic breast cancer to chemotherapy. *Neoplasia*, **6**, 831–837.

113. Uhl, M. et al. (2006) Evaluation of tumour necrosis during chemotherapy with diffusion-weighted MR imaging: preliminary results in osteosarcomas. *Pediatr. Radiol.*, **36**, 1306–1311.

114. Lee, K.C. et al. (2007) A feasibility study evaluating the functional diffusion map as a predictive imaging biomarker for detection of treatment response in a patient with metastatic prostate cancer to the bone. *Neoplasia*, **9**, 1003–1011.

115. Beloueche-Marbai, M. et al. (2010) Metabolic assessment of the action of targeting cancer therapeutics using magnetic resonance spectroscopy. *Br. J. Cancer*, **8**, 1–7.

116. Beloueche-Babari, M. et al. (2006) Identification of magnetic resonance detectable metabolic changes associated with inhibition of phosphoinositide 3-kinase signaling in human breast cancer cells. *Mol. Cancer Ther.*, **7**, 187–196.

117. Manton, D.J. et al. (2006) Neoadjuvant chemotherapy in breast cancer: early response prediction with quantitative MR imaging and spectroscopy. *Br. J. Cancer*, **94**, 427–435.

118. Meisamy, S. et al. (2004) Neoadjuvant chemotherapy of locally advanced breast cancer: predicting response with in vivo ^{1}H MR spectroscopy – a pilot study at 4 T. *Radiology*, **233**, 424–431.

119. Preul, M.C. et al. (2000) Using proton magnetic resonance spectroscopic imaging to predict in vivo response of recurrent malignant gliomas to tamoxifen chemotherapy. *Neurosurgery*, **46**, 306–318.

120. Schwarz, A.J. *et al.* (2002) Early *in vivo* detection of metabolic response: a pilot study of ^{1}H MR spectroscopy in extracranial lymphoma and germ cell tumours. *Br. J. Radiol.*, **75**, 959–966.
121. Wu, B. *et al.* (2006) In vivo ^{1}H magnetic resonance spectroscopy in evaluation of hepatocellular carcinoma and its early response of transcatheter arterial chemoembolization. *Chin. Med. Sci. J.*, **21**, 258–264.
122. Shukla-Dave, A. *et al.* (2002) Prediction of treatment response of head and neck cancers with P-31 MR spectroscopy from pretreatment relative phosphomonoester levels. *Acad. Radiol.*, **9**, 688–694.
123. George, M.L. *et al.* (2001) Non-invasive methods of assessing angiogenesis and their value in predicting response to treatment in colorectal cancer. *Br. J. Surg.*, **88**, 1628–1636.
124. Mayr, N.A. *et al.* (1996) Tumor perfusion studies using fast magnetic resonance imaging technique in advanced cervical cancer: a new non-invasive predictive assay. *Int. J. Radiat. Oncol. Biol. Phys.*, **36**, 623–633.
125. Boss, E.A. *et al.* (2001) Post-radiotherapy contrast enhancement changes in fast dynamic MRI of cervical carcinoma. *J. Magn. Res. Imaging*, **13**, 600–606.
126. Ohno, Y. *et al.* (2005) Prognostic value of dynamic MR imaging for non-small-cell lung cancer patients after chemoradiotherapy. *J. Magn. Res. Imaging*, **21**, 775–783.
127. Tomura, N. *et al.* (2005) Dynamic contrast-enhanced magnetic resonance imaging in radiotherapeutic efficacy in the head and neck tumors. *Am. J. Otolaryngol.*, **26**, 163–167.
128. Liu, G. *et al.* (2005) Dynamic contrast-enhanced magnetic resonance imaging as a pharmacodynamic measure of response after acute dosing of AG-013736, an oral angiogenesis inhibitor, in patients with advanced solid tumors: results from a phase I study. *J. Clin. Oncol.*, **23**, 5464–5473.
129. Wedam, S.B. *et al.* (2006) Antiangiogenic and antitumor effects of bevacizumab in patients with inflammatory and locally advanced breast cancer. *J. Clin. Oncol.*, **24**, 769–777.
130. Zhang, M. and Kono, M. (1997) Solitary pulmonary nodules: evaluation of blood flow patterns with dynamic CT. *Radiology*, **205**, 471–478.
131. Miles, K.A., Griffiths, M.R., and Fuentes, M.A. (2001) Standardized perfusion value: universal CT contrast enhancement scale that correlates with FDG PET in lung nodules. *Radiology*, **220**, 548–553.
132. Herman, R. *et al.* (1997) Non-invasive tumor perfusion measurement by dynamics CT: preliminary results. *Radiother. Oncol.*, **44**, 159–162.
133. Harvey, C. *et al.* (1999) Imaging of tumour therapy responses by dynamic CT. *Eur. J. Radiol.*, **30**, 221–226.
134. Harvey, C. *et al.* (2001) Functional CT imaging of the acute hyperemic response to radiation therapy of the prostate gland: early experience. *J. Comput. Assist. Tomogr.*, **25**, 43–49.
135. Goetti, R. *et al.* (2010) Quantitative computed tomography liver perfusion imaging using dynamic spiral scanning with variable pitch: feasibility and initial results in patients with cancer metastases. *Invest. Radiol.*, **45**, 419–426.
136. Herman, R. *et al.* (2003) Tumor perfusion rate determined non-invasively by dynamic computed tomography predicts outcome in head-and-neck cancer after radiotherapy. *Int. J. Radiat. Oncol. Biol. Phys.*, **57**, 1351–1356.
137. McCollough, C.H. *et al.* (2009) Strategies for reducing radiation dose in CT. *Radiol. Clin. N. Am.*, **47**, 27–40.
138. Bonvento, M. *et al.* (2003) CT angiography with gadolinium-based contrast media. *Acad. Radiol.*, **10**, 979–985.
139. Moriyasu, F. and Itoh, K. (2009) Efficacy of perflubutane microbubble-enhanced ultrasound in the characterization and detection of focal liver lesions. Phase 3 multicenter clinical trial. *Am. J. Roentgenol.*, **193**, 86.
140. Hwang, M. *et al.* (2009) Sonographic assessment of tumor response from *in vivo* models to clinical applications. *Ultrasound Q.*, **2009**, 175–183.

141. Suren, A. et al. (2010) Visualization of blood flow in small ovarian tumor vessels by transvaginal color doppler sonography after echo enhancement with injection of Lovovist. *Gynecol. Obstet. Invest.*, **38**, 210–212.
142. Lamuraglia, M. et al. (2006) To predict progression-free survival and overall survival in metastatic renal cancer treated with sorafenib: pilot study using dynamic contrast-enhanced Doppler ultrasound. *Eur. J. Cancer*, **42**, 2472–2479.
143. Batchelor, T.T. et al. (2007) AZD2171, a pan-VEGF receptor tyrosine kinase inhibitor, normalizes tumor vasculature and alleviates edema in glioblastoma patients. *Cancer Cell.*, **11**, 83–95.
144. Jain, R.K. (2005) Normalization of tumor vasculature: an emerging concept in antiangiogenic therapy. *Science*, **307**, 58–62.
145. Willmann, J.K. et al. (2008) US imaging of tumor angiogenesis with microbubbles targeted to vascular endothelial growth factor receptor type 2 in mice. *Radiology*, **246**, 508–518.
146. Willmann, J.K. et al. (2008) Dual-targeted contrast agent for US assessment of tumor angiogenesis *in vivo*. *Radiology*, **248**, 936–944.
147. Dufort, S. et al. (2010) Optical small animal imaging in the drug discovery process. *Biochim. Biophys. Acta*, **1798**, 2266–2273.
148. Torigian, D.A. et al. (2007) Functional imaging of cancer with emphasis on molecular techniques. *CA Cancer J. Clin.*, **57**, 206–224.
149. Manning, H.C. et al. (2008) Molecular imaging of therapeutic response to epidermal growth factor receptor blockade in colorectal cancer. *Clin. Cancer Res.*, **14**, 7413–7422.
150. Ogawa, M. et al. (2009) Fluorophore-quencher based activatable targeted optical probes for detecting *in vivo* cancer metastases. *Mol. Pharm.*, **6**, 386–395.
151. Edgington, L.E. et al. (2009) Noninvasive optical imaging of apoptosis by caspase-targeted activity-based probes. *Nat. Med.*, **15**, 973–980.
152. Choi, C.Y.H. et al. (2008) Molecular imaging of hypoxia-inducible factor 1a and von Hippel-Lindau interaction in mice. *Mol. Imaging*, **7**, 139–147.
153. Rosenthal, E.L. et al. (2007) Use of fluorescent label anti-epidermal growth factor receptor antibody to image head and neck squamous cell carcinoma xenografts. *Mol. Cancer Ther.*, **6**, 1230–1238.
154. Shan, L. et al. (2008) Visualizing head and neck tumors *in vivo* using near-infrared fluorescent transferring conjugate. *Mol. Imaging*, **7**, 42–59.
155. Li, W. et al. (2008) Noninvasive imaging and quantification of epidermal growth factor receptor kinase activation *in vivo*. *Cancer Res.*, **68**, 4990–4997.
156. Badr, C.E. et al. (2009) Real-time monitoring of nuclear factor κB activity in cultured cells and in animal models. *Mol. Imaging*, **8**, 278–291.
157. Moskaug, J.O., Carlsen, H., and Blomhoff, R. (2008) Noninvasive *in vivo* imaging of protein kinase A activity. *Mol. Imaging*, **8**, 35–42.
158. Ogawa, M. et al. (2009) *In vivo* molecular imaging of cancer with a quanching near-infrared fluorescent probe using conjugates of monoclonal antibodies and indocyanine green. *Cancer Res.*, **69**, 1268–1272.
159. Scherer, R.L. et al. (2008) Optical imaging of matrix metalloproteinase-7 activity *in vivo* using a proteolytic nanobeacon. *Mol. Imaging*, **7**, 118–132.
160. Pysz, M.A., Gambhir, S.S., and Willmann, J.K. (2010) Molecular imaging: current status and emerging strategies. *Clin. Radiol.*, **65**, 500–516.

8
Magnetic Nanoparticles in Magnetic Resonance Imaging and Drug Delivery

Patrick D. Sutphin, Efrén J. Flores, and Mukesh Harisinghani

8.1
Introduction

Prognosis and selection of treatment strategies in cancer patients is closely related to anatomical staging, which is a measure of disease burden and extent of spread. For example, rectal cancer, TNM (tumor–node–metastasis) stage I disease, which is characterized by disease confined to the rectal wall (T1–T2), has an estimated 5-year survival rate of more than 90%, whereas stage IV disease, defined as disease with distant metastases, has an estimated 5-year survival rate of 5–7% [1]. Additionally, anatomical staging of rectal cancer guides the therapeutic strategy. The treatment for disease confined to the rectal wall is surgical resection alone, whereas extension through the rectal wall or lymph node involvement is an indication for neoadjuvant chemo- and radiation therapy followed by excision of tumor. Prior to the integration of cross-sectional imaging into the clinical management of rectal cancer, in the absence of laparotomy, the physical exam, barium enema, and sigmoidoscopy were limited in the ability to stage rectal cancer beyond the rectal wall [2]. The addition of computed tomography (CT) to the clinical management protocol enabled evaluation of areas beyond the rectal wall that were anatomical blindspots to prior methodologies of noninvasive staging for more accurate pretherapeutic staging.

Despite the improvement in anatomical staging of cancer patients with CT, limitations remain in accurately characterizing disease for the application of the appropriate treatment. In the case of rectal cancer, nodal staging is critical in choosing the appropriate therapy. Evaluation of lymph node size is the most widely used criteria for determining whether a lymph node is positive for cancer based on imaging findings. However, no universally accepted size criteria exists for determining if a lymph node is positive for cancer. A retrospective radiologic–pathologic correlation in nodal staging of rectal cancer was performed and found an accuracy of 74% when a 7-mm (long-axis) size cutoff was used in patients prior to surgery alone as a therapy [3]. These results demonstrate that a substantial amount of disease is inaccurately classified as not all positive lymph nodes are enlarged and that lymph nodes may be enlarged for reasons other than metastatic disease. This problem is not unique to rectal cancer, as can be seen in Figure 8.1 where

Drug Delivery in Oncology: From Basic Research to Cancer Therapy, First Edition.
Edited by Felix Kratz, Peter Senter, and Henning Steinhagen.
© 2012 Wiley-VCH Verlag GmbH & Co. KGaA. Published 2012 by Wiley-VCH Verlag GmbH & Co. KGaA.

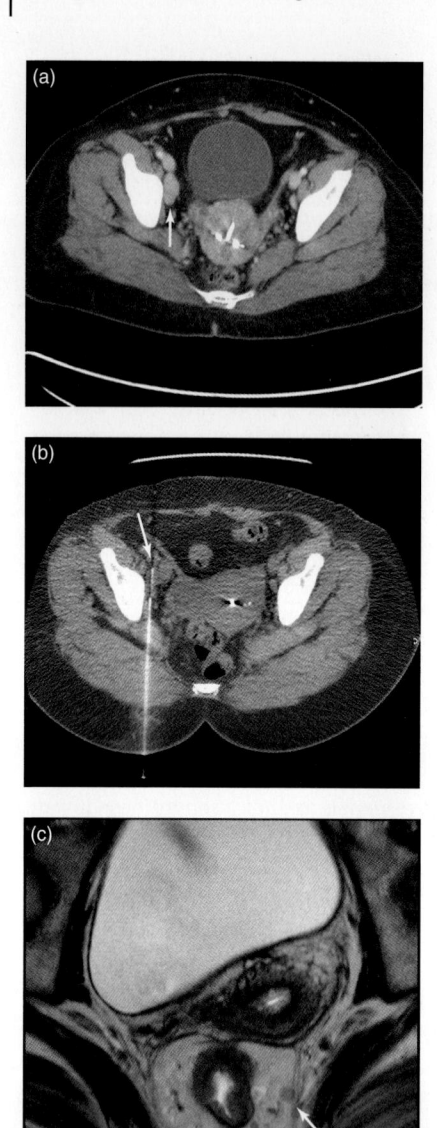

Figure 8.1 (a)–(c) Categorization of lymph nodes into benign or malignant by size criteria. (a) Axial contrast-enhanced CT image shows an enlarged right obturator node (white arrow) in a patient with cervical cancer. The node was interpreted as metastatic based on size criterion, but was proved to be benign on biopsy as shown in (b) (white arrow). (c) Axial T_2-weighted MR image shows two normal-sized perirectal lymph nodes (white arrows) in a patient with rectal cancer. The nodes were interpreted as benign on the basis of size criterion, but proved to be malignant at surgery.

lymph nodes were also misclassified in a patient with cervical cancer based on size criteria (Figure 8.1a and b). An example of misclassified lymph nodes in a patient with rectal cancer on magnetic resonance imaging (MRI) staging is also seen in Figure 8.1c. Therefore, techniques that rely solely on anatomic enlargement or distortion, including evaluation by ultrasound and MRI, are inherently limited in accurately detecting disease, highlighting the need for alternative imaging methods that evaluate functional characteristics.

Functional imaging techniques to improve detection of metastatic disease are an active area of investigation. The application of 2-^{18}F-fluoro-2-deoxyglucose (FDG)-positron emission tomography (PET)/CT to pretherapeutic staging has been used to provide functional information to the anatomical data provided by CT. PET, however, is limited by low resolution and metastatic disease cannot be definitively excluded in lymph nodes less than 1 cm. In addition, the sensitivity for the detection of metastases less than 5 mm in metastatic lymph nodes is poor. This was demonstrated in a study by Choi *et al.* using a rabbit model of lymph node metastasis, where zero of seven lymph nodes with metastatic disease less than 5 mm were detected by FDG-PET/CT [4]. An alternate strategy, which will be discussed in detail, is the use of magnetic nanoparticles in MRI of metastatic disease through both passive and active methodologies. In addition, the mechanisms employed to actively target metastatic disease for imaging purposes may also be used to target drugs to metastatic disease.

8.2
Passive Targeting of Nanoparticles

Lymphotropic superparamagnetic iron oxide (SPIO) nanoparticles serve as novel MRI contrast agents and allow for the characterization of structural and functional cellular changes. These are a relatively new class of MR contrast agents that were first described in 1990 [5, 6]. Originally developed for imaging, conventional SPIO particles (30–1000 nm) were used to image the mononuclear phagocytic system of the liver and spleen. It was hypothesized that the biodistribution of the particles could be altered by reducing the size of the particles through size fractionation. The initial report demonstrated that the ultra-small SPIO (USPIO) particles (70% less than 10 nm) were small enough in size to migrate across the capillary walls and localize within the mononuclear phagocytic system of the lymph nodes (Figure 8.2). Since the initial proof-of-concept study in rats, the use of SPIO nanoparticles has been applied to the imaging of lymph nodes in patients with a variety cancers, including colorectal, breast, prostate, and head and neck cancer among others [7]. A meta-analysis of the use of ferumoxtran-10-enhanced MRI found it to be both sensitive and specific for the detection of lymph node metastases with a higher diagnostic precision than unenhanced MRI for the variety of cancers examined in the meta-analysis [7].

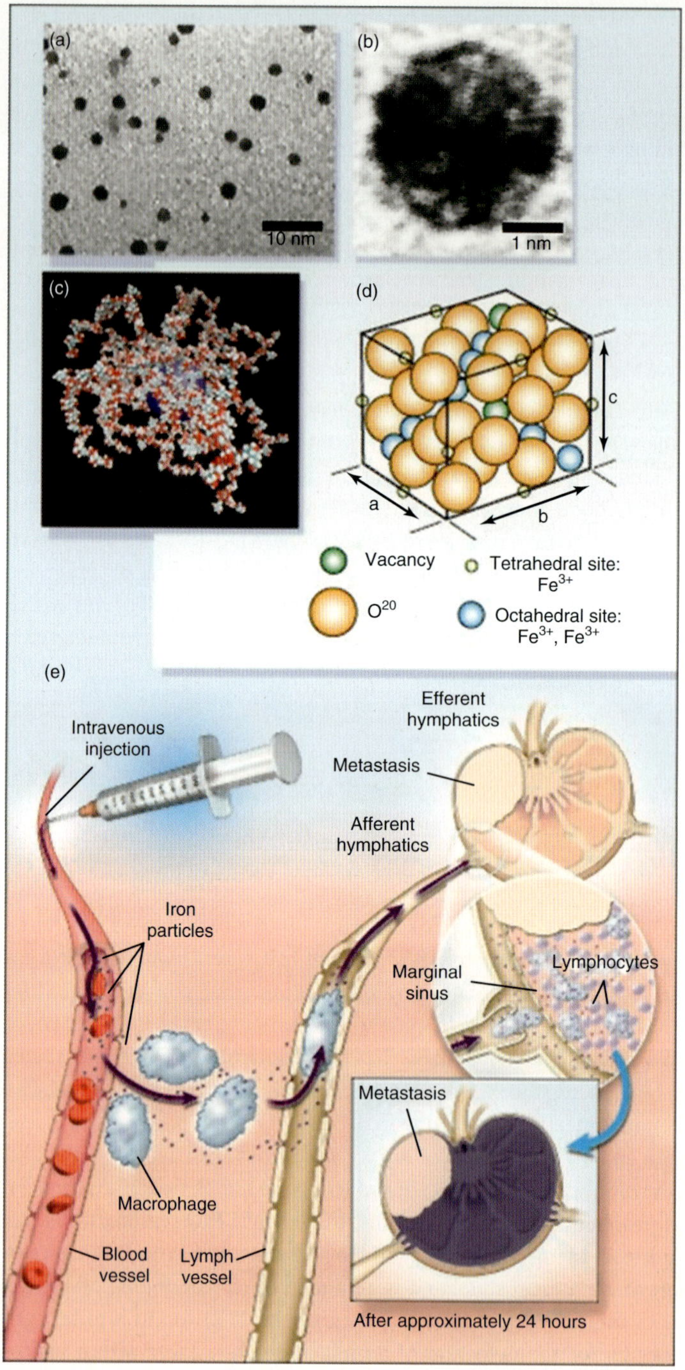
(a)
10 nm
(b)
1 nm
(c)
(d)
c
a
b
Vacancy
Tetrahedral site: Fe^{3+}
O^{20}
Octahedral site: Fe^{3+}, Fe^{3+}
(e)
Efferent hymphatics
Intravenous injection
Metastasis
Afferent hymphatics
Iron particles
Marginal sinus
Lymphocytes
Metastasis
Macrophage
Blood vessel
Lymph vessel
After approximately 24 hours

Figure 8.2 Electron micrographs of hexagonal lymphotropic superparamagnetic nanoparticles (a) and (b), molecular model of surface-bound 10-kDa dextrans and packing of iron oxide crystals (c) and (d), and mechanism of action of lymphotropic superparamagnetic nanoparticles. The model lymphotropic superparamagnetic nanoparticles shown here measure 2–3 nm on average (a) and (b). The mean overall particle size of 10-kDa dextran is 28 nm (c) and (d). In (e), the systemically injected long-circulating particles gain access to the interstitium and are drained through lymphatic vessels. Disturbances in lymph flow or in nodal architecture caused by metastases lead to abnormal patterns of accumulation of lymphotropic superparamagnetic nanoparticles, which are detectable by MRI. (Reprinted with permission from [8].)

8.2.1
Mechanism of Action

Ferumoxtran-10 is a SPIO particle with an iron oxide crystalline core, which measures 4.3–6.0 nm, coated with a low-molecular-weight dextran. Shortly after the intravenous administration of the USPIO nanoparticles, the particles are slowly extravasated from the blood vessels into the interstitial space (Figure 8.2). From the interstitial space the nanoparticles are transported to the lymph nodes. Transport to the lymph nodes occurs via two mechanisms. The first mechanism is through the direct transcapillary passage from venules into the medullary sinuses of lymph nodes. The second mechanism involves the nonselective endothelial transcytosis into the interstitial space; the particles then drain into the lymph nodes via the lymphatic system. The USPIO nanoparticles are absorbed by the macrophages and accumulate in normal lymph nodes. The accumulation of the superparamagnetic particles results in a decrease in signal intensity on T_2- and T_2^*-weighted MRI secondary to the magnetic moment and high dipolar relaxivity. Metastatic lymph nodes, in contradistinction, with either partially or complete infiltration by malignant cells demonstrate normal signal intensity because of the disruption of the mononuclear phagocytic system and the inability of the metastatic lymph nodes to accumulate the USPIO nanoparticles (see Figure 8.4) [8].

8.2.2
Lymphotropic Nanoparticle MRI

Lymphotropic nanoparticle enhanced MRI (LNMRI) is a developing technology for the identification of metastatic lymph nodes in cancer patients. Similar to conventional intravenous contrast agents, pre-nanoparticle images and post-nanoparticle contrast images are obtained. As the localization of the USPIO nanoparticles within in the lymph nodes is a slow process and the approximate half-life of the nanoparticles is approximately 25–30 h, images are obtained just prior to the intravenous administration of the nanoparticles and then again the following day. Identical imaging protocols are performed to acquire images to allow for the direct comparison of lymph nodes on the pre- and postcontrast studies. The nanoparticles distribute symmetrically throughout the body after intravenous administration, thus allowing for a comprehensive nodal evaluation independent of the injection site. As shown in Figure 8.3a, precontrast axial T_2^*-weighted images from a bladder cancer patient demonstrate an enlarged hyperintense left external iliac lymph node. Axial T_2^*-weighted images obtained 24 h after the administration of ferumoxtran-10 demonstrate homogeneous decrease in signal intensity in the benign left external iliac lymph (Figure 8.3b). In contrast, malignant lymph nodes do not demonstrate a decrease in signal intensity on postcontrast images. Precontrast axial T_2^*-weighted images were obtained from a patient with prostate cancer demonstrate an enlarged hyperintense left posterior obturator lymph node (Figure 8.1c). Axial T_2^*-weighted images obtained 24 h after the administration of ferumoxtran-10 show minimal peripheral signal loss with the bulk of the lymph node remaining hyperintense, consistent with a malignant lymph node (Figure 8.3d). Established guidelines for

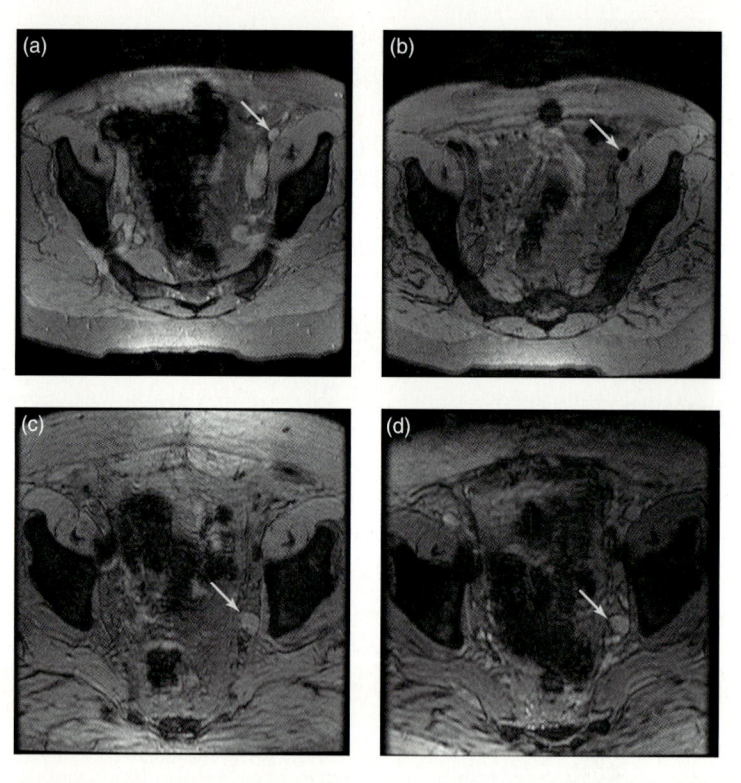

Figure 8.3 (a)–(d) Example of MR lymphangiography in patients. (a) T_2^*-weighted GRE MR image shows hyperintense left external iliac node (arrow) in a patient with bladder cancer that was characterized as metastatic on the basis of size criterion. (b) Axial MR image obtained 24 h after the administration of ferumoxtran-10 shows a homogeneous decrease in the signal intensity of the left external iliac node (arrow) indicating benignity. (c) T_2^*-weighted GRE MR image shows hyperintense left posterior obturator node (arrow) in a patient with prostate cancer. (d) Axial MR image obtained 24 h after the administration of ferumoxtran-10 demonstrates minimal peripheral signal drop, but the bulk of the node shows lack of darkening indicating malignant infiltration, which was pathologically proven.

characterization of lymph nodes based on the pattern of negative enhancement with ferumoxtran-10 are seen in Figure 8.4 [9–11].

Imaging sequences in LNMRI include gradient echo (GRE) T_1-weighted, fast spin-echo (FSE) T_2-weighted, and GRE T_2^*-weighted sequences. These have been described previously [12]. The T_2^* sequence is a heavily T_2-weighted GRE sequence that has been shown to be superior to FSE T_2 sequences for characterization of nodal involvement [10]. The T_1 shortening effect is predominantly seen in the vessels and this information can be used to generate anatomical vascular maps to superimpose on the nodal information acquired from the T_2 and T_2^* sequences. T_1-weighted images additionally provide information regarding the location of the nodal fatty hilum that can mimic a metastatic deposit on T_2-weighted images. Characterization of nodal involvement is performed primarily through analysis of the T_2^* images, as these have been shown to be superior to FSE T_2 sequences for the characterization of nodal involvement. Analysis of lymph nodes on GRE T_2^* and FSE T_2 sequences was performed by two reviewers, demonstrating improved accuracy of analysis of GRE T_2^* (TE 21 ms) over FSE T_2 sequences: 82.8 versus

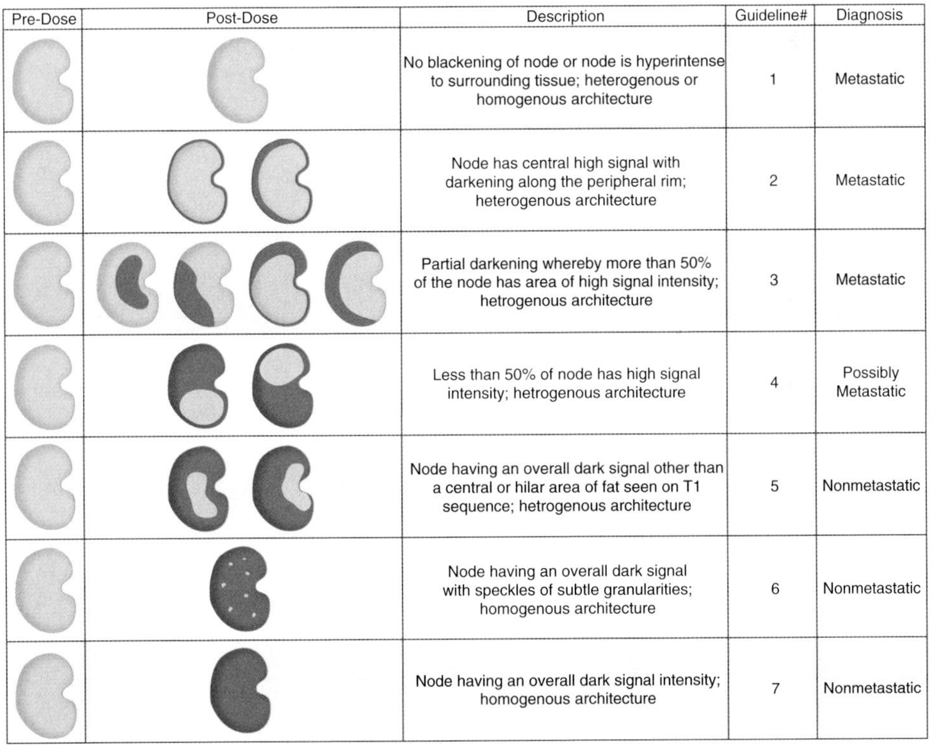

Pre-Dose	Post-Dose	Description	Guideline#	Diagnosis
		No blackening of node or node is hyperintense to surrounding tissue; heterogenous or homogenous architecture	1	Metastatic
		Node has central high signal with darkening along the peripheral rim; heterogenous architecture	2	Metastatic
		Partial darkening whereby more than 50% of the node has area of high signal intensity; hetrogenous architecture	3	Metastatic
		Less than 50% of node has high signal intensity; hetrogenous architecture	4	Possibly Metastatic
		Node having an overall dark signal other than a central or hilar area of fat seen on T1 sequence; hetrogenous architecture	5	Nonmetastatic
		Node having an overall dark signal with speckles of subtle granularities; homogenous architecture	6	Nonmetastatic
		Node having an overall dark signal intensity; homogenous architecture	7	Nonmetastatic

Figure 8.4 Example of guidelines used for nodal characterization on lymphotropic nanoparticle-enhanced MRI for characterization of benign versus malignant lymph nodes. (Adapted from [9].)

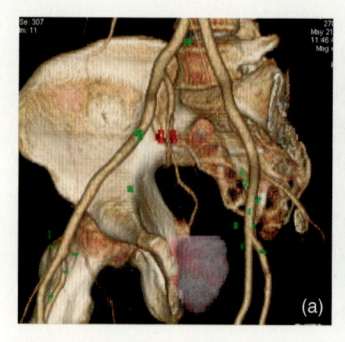

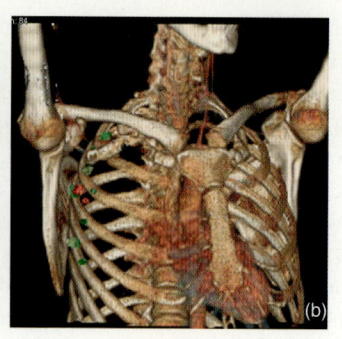

Figure 8.5 (a) and (b) Surface-rendered three-dimensional MRI of lymph nodes in a patient with prostate cancer. (a) Surface-rendered three-dimensional MR image from a patient with prostate cancer shows iliac vessels, which are enhanced due to the effect of ferumoxtran-10 on the T_1 sequence. Malignant nodes are coded in red and benign nodes are coded in green. (b) Surface-rendered three-dimensional MR image from a patient with breast cancer shows axillary vessels, which are enhanced due to the effect of ferumoxtran-10 on the T_1 sequence. Malignant nodes are coded in red and benign nodes are coded in green.

68.5% accuracy, respectively [10]. Three-dimensional sequences can be performed in addition to the above sequences which can be used to generate three-dimensional maps to aid in surgical planning as seen in Figure 8.5.

8.3
Active SPIO Nanoparticle Targeting

Size fractionation of standard SPIO particles for the creation of USPIO nanoparticles resulted in an alteration in the biodistribution of intravenously injected SPIO particles, from accumulating in the reticuloendothelial system of the liver and spleen to accumulating in the lymph nodes, thus enabling LNMRI. This demonstration that the biodistribution of these particles could be modified raised the possibility that the distribution of these particles could be more finely controlled. In addition, the relatively long blood half-life of USPIO nanoparticles as well as the ability of the nanoparticles to migrate across the capillary endothelium are characteristics that were encouraging for the concept that with the appropriate modification these nanoparticles could be selectively targeted [13]. The selective targeting of nanoparticles was first demonstrated by Weissleder *et al.* in which the USPIO nanoparticles were targeted to the asialoglycoprotein (ASG) receptor on hepatocytes. The nanoparticles in this study were modified through the conjugation of arabinogalactan, a galactose-terminated polysaccharide and ligand for the ASG receptor. The selective targeting of the nanoparticles was demonstrated through the *in vitro* binding of the nanoparticles to hepatocytes shown through electron microscopy as well as the *in vivo* targeting of the liver in rats with MRI [13]. Finally, the ASG–USPIO nanoparticles were used for the detection of liver tumors in rat model of liver cancer where the uptake of ASG–USPIO nanoparticles by normal hepatocytes resulted in decreased liver signal intensity relative to liver tumors that did not accumulate nanoparticles [14].

Selective targeting of the ASG–USPIO nanoparticles to the ASG receptor on hepatocytes was an important proof of concept that the USPIO nanoparticles could be modified to target a specific tissue type as well as identify disease entities such as cancer. This paved the way for conjugating additional tissue-specific and disease-specific targeting ligands to SPIO particles to promote the selective imaging of target tissues. Disease-specific imaging would thus then allow for the molecular profiling and early detection of disease. Information gleaned from such a study could be used to customize therapeutic regimens as well as monitor patients through their course of treatment.

8.3.1
Creating the Targeted Imaging Agents

Specific SPIO imaging agents can be developed by conjugating the respective targeting agents directly onto the surface of the SPIO surface or its hydrophilic coating. Additionally, the SPIO polymer coating may be modified to include reactive moieties such as amines, sulfhydryls, or carboxyls, which facilitate chemical coupling of biological ligands or antibodies [15].

A major consideration in the design of targeted nanoparticles is the selection of the target for imaging. In order for adequate contrast in MRI a sufficient focal concentration of nanoparticles must be achieved at the targeted site. This requires not only the selective overexpression of the biomarker relative to surrounding background tissues, but also requires that the targeted receptor undergo receptor-mediated endocytosis upon binding with the ligand–SPIO, resulting in the intracellular trapping of the ligand–SPIO particle. In fact, ASG was selected for the proof of concept as the ASG receptor system was not only well-characterized, but there is abundant expression of the receptor with as many as 500 000 surface ligand-binding sites per cell [16]. Strategies have been developed to circumvent low-level expression of the target receptor through the amplification of signal. One such strategy employs a two-step amplification technique whereby a biotinylated targeting antibody is administered that localizes to the disease-specific site. Subsequently, streptavidin-conjugated SPIO particles are administered that bind to the biotinylated antibody with high affinity. Since the initial biotinylated targeted antibody contains multiple high-affinity sites for streptavidin-conjugated SPIO particles, multiple particles bind to each cell ligand, thus amplifying the signal [17]. A schematic representation of this biotin–streptavidin-based two-step amplification technique can be seen in Figure 8.6. This strategy has been successful both *in vitro* and in human lymphoma xenografts in immune-deficient mice demonstrated by MRI, but has yet to be demonstrated in humans [18].

8.3.1.1 Transferrin–USPIO Nanoparticles
Early detection and the accurate anatomic staging of cancer is a fundamental goal of diagnostic imaging. To this end, numerous biomarkers have been the subject

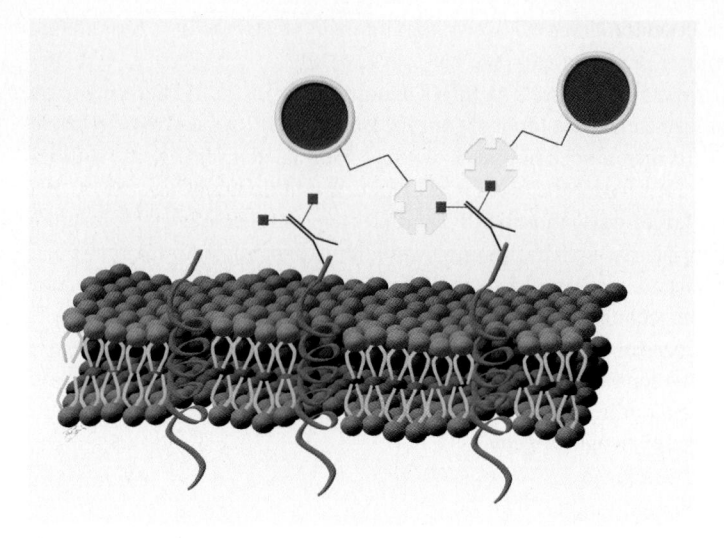

Figure 8.6 Schematic representation of the labeling of HER2/neu-expressing cells with targeted SPIO nanoparticles using the biotin–streptavidin linker. The native receptor seen on the left is labeled following the intravenous injection of biotinylated antibody (middle receptor). Following a second intravenous injection of a streptavidin–SPIO nanoparticle complex, the streptavidin–SPIO nanoparticle complex binds to the biotinylated antibody attached to the receptor on the right, labeling the HER2/neu-expressing cells for imaging.

of investigation for targeting by ligand-directed SPIO for the specific imaging of cancer [19]. One of the most widely studied targets is the transferrin receptor (TfR). The TfR is involved in the cellular uptake of iron. Iron, an essential element in cell proliferation, is insoluble at physiologic pH and is transported by the iron-chelating protein transferrin (Tf) to the cellular surface. Iron-bound Tf is recognized by the TfR at the cell surface and the Tf–iron complex is transported intracellularly via receptor-mediated endocytosis. The TfR is an attractive target for tumor-specific imaging as it is overexpressed in a variety of tumor types, including breast, glioma, prostate, transitional cell carcinoma of the bladder, and lung adenocarcinoma. For example, evaluation of TfR expression in 27 breast cancer patients demonstrated that the TfR mRNA was overexpressed in 74% of the patients, and of these patients, 41% expressed the TfR by 5-fold or greater relative to nontransformed cells [20]. Targeting of the human TfR has been successful with a Tf–USPIO nanoparticle in an *in vivo* rat model of breast cancer. The chemically induced, poorly differentiated rat mammary gland carcinoma SMT/2A cells were implanted near the mammary line of female Wistar-Furth rats. MRI following the injection of Tf–USPIO nanoparticles resulted in a 40% reduction in tumor signal intensity, compared to imaging with free USPIO and human serum albumin–USPIO, which demonstrated only a 10% reduction in signal intensity [21].

8.3.1.2 Folate Receptor

Another receptor system that has been well studied as a target for tumor-specific imaging is the folate receptor system. Folate is involved in nucleotide biosynthesis, and thus plays a critical role in DNA replication and cellular proliferation. Given the prominent role of folate in DNA biosynthesis and cell proliferation, the actions of folate have been the target of anticancer medications, the most notable of which is methotrexate. Methotrexate inhibits dihydrofolate reductase, thereby blocking the conversion of dihydrofolate to tetrahydrofolate, the active form of folate, reducing the ability of cells to synthesize DNA. Rapidly dividing cells, such as malignant cells, are more susceptible to the adverse effects of inhibition of DNA synthesis. As the rapidly dividing cells depend on folate for the production of the raw materials for DNA synthesis, the expression of the folate-binding protein has been found to be correspondingly increased in a variety of tumor types, including renal cell carcinoma, lung cancer, and breast cancer among others. In comparison, nonproliferating cells have a relative lack of folate receptors, with a few exceptions including cells of the choroid plexus, placenta, and low levels in the lung, thyroid, and kidney. Therefore, the expression of the folate receptor represents a means by which to selectively target tumor cells.

This strategy has most recently been applied to the targeted imaging of breast cancer. In the study by Meier *et al.* [22], USPIO particles were coated with folate moieties to create the folate receptor-targeted MR contrast agent P1133. P904 is the identical USPIO nanoparticle without the attached folate moiety. In the study, the authors demonstrated that folate receptor-targeted USPIO nanoparticles (P1133) resulted in negative enhancement of folate receptor-positive breast cancer xenografts in immune-deficient mice on MR images 24 h after administration. The control nanoparticle, P904, did not. These findings suggest that the P1133 nanoparticles were successfully targeted and retained in folate receptor-positive breast cancers *in vivo*. The targeted imaging of folate receptor-positive breast cancers has important clinical implications, as folate receptor overexpression may provide prognostic information as it has been correlated with histologic tumor grade and S-phase fraction. In addition, tumor-specific imaging of folate-receptor positive tumors may lead to earlier diagnosis, detection of tumor recurrence or metastatic disease, and differentiation between normal from cancerous tissue.

8.3.1.3 Integrins

Nanoparticles have been used to image integrins in endothelial cells, particularly the endothelial cells of angiogenic blood vessels [23–29]. In one study, cyclic RGD peptide magnetofluorescent cross-linked iron oxide nanoparticles were targeted at $\alpha_v\beta_3$ integrin-expressing tumor cells *in vivo* and were detectable by fluorescence reflectance imaging, fluorescence molecular tomography, and MRI [30]. This approach was successful on a BT-20 tumor model, a human breast carcinoma cell line, while another cell line (9L cells, a rat gliosarcoma cell line) did not express the integrin. It was argued that factors permitting the imaging of tumor integrins included the well-vascularized nature of the BT-20 tumor, the long nanoparticle blood half-life, and the ability of nanoparticles to slowly escape the vasculature.

Such integrin-targeted magnetofluorescent nanoparticles could not only provide precontrast MR images, but also intraoperative fluorescent images providing a more accurate margin delineation [31].

8.4
Nanoparticles in Targeted Therapy

The research for medical applications of magnetic nanoparticles has significantly increased because of their unique characteristics, such as small size (nanometer-sized to 1 µm), nontoxicity, biocompatibility, injectability, and high-level accumulation in the target tissue by applying an external magnetic field [32]. The use of nanoparticles for drug delivery was initially proposed in the 1970s by Widder, Senyel, and colleagues [33]. The basic principle is that therapeutic agents are attached to SPIO particles. SPIO particles contain a polymer coating that may be modified to include reactive moieties such as amines, sulfhydryls, or carboxyls that facilitate the attachment of cytotoxic drugs for targeted chemotherapy or therapeutic DNA to correct a genetic defect. In addition, this modification of the polymer allows chemical coupling of biological ligands or antibodies and facilitates targeting of neoplastic cell receptors that are overexpressed on neoplastic cells. In addition, the magnetic properties of SPIO serve as MRI contrast agents and as magnetic vectors that can be directed by field gradients in the case of targeted drug delivery. These properties serve as the basis for the role of SPIO in targeted drug delivery and therapy.

There are several mechanisms by which SPIO therapy can reach the target. The SPIO–therapeutic agent complex can be injected into the bloodstream and high magnetic fields are focused over the target site, which allows the particles to be extravasated and captured at the target (Figure 8.7) [34].Once at the targeted site the conjugated agent is released from the nanoparticle, creating a high focal concentration in the tumor tissue while minimizing exposure of normal tissues to drugs [35]. Although the use of magnetic nanoparticles for targeted drug delivery has been proposed for years, this has progressed slowly, and most of this work has been performed in animal studies and in a few clinical trials. While conceptually simple, the application of magnetic drug targeting has been limited by several factors, including magnetic field strength, depth of target tissue, complex tumor geometry, vascular supply, conjugation of drug to the nanoparticles as well as controlling the release of the drug from the nanoparticles [36]. Lubbe et al. were one of the first groups to conduct a phase I clinical trial [37–39]. Their work consisted of 4'-epidoxorubicin coupled to magnetic nanoparticles in the treatment of advanced solid tumors (i.e., breast cancer, chondrosarcoma, Ewing's sarcoma, squamous cell carcinoma, and malignant histiocytoma) in 14 patients. They were able to target therapy in six of these patients using high-energy magnetic fields over the tumor sites. Koda et al. in 2002 (30 patients) and Wilson et al. in 2004 (four patients) also performed clinical trials in patients with hepatocellular carcinomas, using magnetic nanoparticles coupled to doxorubicin [40, 41]. These complexes

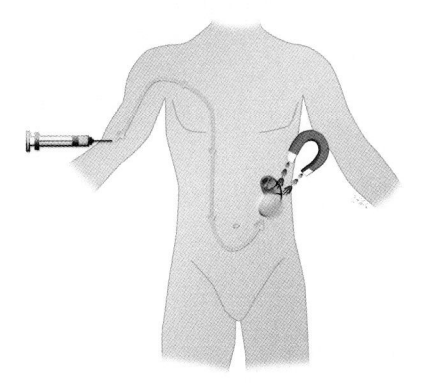

Figure 8.7 Magnetic drug targeting. The SPIO–therapeutic agent complex is injected intravascularly and a high magnetic field is applied to the tumor, resulting in the localization and accumulation of the therapeutic complex in the targeted area. Once at the targeted site the therapeutic agent is released, creating high focal concentrations of the therapeutic agent and thus minimizing exposure to normal tissues.

were delivered via hepatic artery catheterization and were focused at the tumor site using high-energy magnetic fields. In the study by Wilson *et al.*, the angiographic suite was coupled with a magnet that served to target therapy at the tumor site and allowed them to acquire images immediately after therapy, demonstrating the expected signal loss seen with SPIO confirming the presence of these complexes within the tumor. Although performed with a small group of patients, this study by Wilson *et al.* provides a glimpse of the virtues of SPIO – real-time visualization of targeted therapy.

8.4.1
Nanoparticles in Gene Therapy

Magnetofection is a method to enhance the introduction of gene vectors into cells by coupling magnetic nanoparticles with DNA and its vector [42]. Similar to targeted drug delivery with magnetic fields, SPIO–DNA complexes are then concentrated within the target site or cells using an external high-energy magnetic field. This allows delivery of the genetic material to the target cell surface receptors and DNA is then released into the cytoplasm [43]. Magnetofection has also been used successfully to deliver antisense oligonucleotides *in vitro* and *in vivo* [44]. This mechanism has many applications such as localized gene delivery for cancer therapy and development of tumor vaccines among others [45]. For example, Hirao *et al.* [46] developed a gene-delivery system combining magnetic cationic liposomes and magnetic induction that resulted in enhanced transfection efficiency in human osteosarcoma cells. Similarly, Rad *et al.* [47] developed a SPIO–AC133$^+$ progenitor cell (a subpopulation of CD34$^+$ stem cells) complex that enabled them to deliver the human sodium iodide symporter gene to the sites of implanted breast cancer cells. SPIO coupling allow them real-time *in vivo* tracking of these cells during gene delivery [47]. These are some of the many techniques where SPIO complexes play a key role in targeted gene therapy.

8.4.2
Nanoparticles in Molecularly Targeted Drug Delivery

A principle objective of both selective imaging and targeted drug delivery is to isolate disease *in vivo* on the background of functioning normal tissue without disrupting or altering normal physiologic processes for diagnostic and therapeutic purposes, respectively. Both of these processes depend on identifying a biomarker or disease characteristic that can be targeted to achieve this goal. The ideal target of selective imaging and targeted drug delivery has many overlapping features. As disease specificity is essential for both selective imaging and targeted therapy, the biomarker ideally would be unique to the pathology of interest. Similarly, high disease sensitivity is also critically important in the application of these methods. Therefore, the targeted biomarker ideally would have a high prevalence in the disease of interest, making it nearly universal to the disease entity. The targeting of a biomarker that is both unique and universal to the disease entity would thus accordingly translate into a high diagnostic and therapeutic yield at the bedside.

While many similarities exist in the features of the ideal biomarker, subtle differences remain. For diagnostic purposes the specificity of the imaging technique is less critical than for therapeutic purposes. In the imaging of disease, if normal tissues are concomitantly imaged, so long as the imaging of the normal tissues is recognized and does not obscure the detection of pathology, such as the physiologic uptake of FDG in brain or heart as in FDG-PET, lack of specificity can be tolerated. In the case of therapeutics, however, the nonspecific delivery of toxic agents to the brain or heart could result in effects ranging from minor adverse effects to catastrophic consequences in a patient undergoing the cancer treatments.

Another important difference in imaging versus therapy is the abundance of expression of the biomarker being targeted. For imaging purposes, the diagnostic quality of the images is directly proportional to the accumulation of the total number of SPIO nanoparticles. The magnitude of the accumulation of the nanoparticles is directly related to both the absolute number of receptors as well as the rate of receptor-mediated endocytosis for the accumulation or trapping of the nanoparticles within the cell. Therefore, the greater the number of receptors mediating the rapid internalization of nanoparticles, the higher the probability of generating adequate image contrast for successful imaging. Even with strategies used to amplify the signal, as described above, receptors with low-level expression or those that lack the ability to internalize and trap molecules will fail to accumulate SPIO particles in sufficient numbers to result in enough contrast for successful imaging. From the therapeutic perspective, however, there is no requisite for receptor internalization, as in the targeting of the CD20 antigen with antibodies such as rituximab, nor is the high-level of expression an important a factor as in imaging [48, 49].

8.4.3
Conversion of Therapeutic Agent to Imaging Agent

Monoclonal antibodies (mAbs) have recently been introduced into the clinical arena for the treatment of cancer. Rituximab, a genetically engineered chimeric (mouse/human) mAb designed to target the CD20 antigen found on malignant B-cells, was the first such therapy to receive US Food and Drug Administration (FDA) approval for the treatment of cancer in 1997 [50]. Since then multiple additional mAbs have been approved by the FDA for the treatment of cancer including trastuzumab (Herceptin®), approved 1998; bevacizumab (Avastin®), approved 2004; and cetuximab (Erbitux®), approved 2004. As these FDA-approved mAbs have been directed against molecules related to specific tumor types, have been rigorously tested for both toxicity and efficacy, and can be easily conjugated to USPIO nanoparticles, the conversion of these therapeutic mAbs into imaging agents is a logical application. The use of therapeutic mAb-conjugated USPIO nanoparticles may be used to selectively image disease as well as to monitor therapy in real-time. Additionally, it is conceivable that mAbs in clinical development can be conjugated to USPIO nanoparticles and evaluated by MRI imaging for the identification of unintended targets, such as the heart or brain, of the mAbs for the prediction of potential adverse effects.

The therapeutic mAb trastuzumab (Herceptin) has been adapted for imaging with the conjugation of Herceptin to SPIO nanoparticles [51]. The Herceptin–SPIO nanoparticles were designed for the imaging of breast cancer cell lines that express the HER2/*neu* receptor, thus allowing for the noninvasive characterization of breast cancer. Binding of the Herceptin–SPIO nanoparticles to HER2/*neu*-positive breast cancer cells was confirmed *in vitro* through immunohistochemistry. The Herceptin–SPIO nanoparticles were then examined for their ability to detect HER2/*neu*-positive breast cancer cells *in vivo* using a mouse xenograft model of breast cancer. The HER2/*neu*-positive human breast cancer cell line SKBR-3 was implanted into the left flank and the HER2/*neu*-negative human nasopharyngeal epidermal carcinoma was implanted into the right flank. MRI following the administration of the Herceptin–SPIO nanoparticles demonstrated a 45% decrease in signal intensity in the HER2/*neu*-positive SKBR-3 tumor compared to a 3% signal decrease in the KB tumor, consistent with the successful targeting of the HER2/*neu*-expressing tumor with the Herceptin–SPIO nanoparticles. As the study was designed for the detection of HER2/*neu*-positive cells through imaging with SPIO nanoparticles the authors did not evaluate the antitumor efficacy of the agent *in vivo*. A low level of toxicity was, however, detected in their *in vitro* studies, suggesting that Herceptin–SPIO nanoparticles may serve as both a therapeutic and diagnostic agent allowing for the real-time monitoring of therapy.

8.4.4
Toxic Payload

Traditional chemotherapeutic cytotoxins are notoriously nonspecific and the associated dose-limiting adverse effects, such as bone marrow suppression, of these agents often arise from the unintended consequences of toxicity to normal tissues. With the more precise delivery of these agents to neoplastic tissue, the expectation is that there will be a reduction in the dose-limiting side effects allowing increased delivery of drug to diseased tissues and increased antitumor efficacy. In addition to the magnetic field localization of therapeutic agents, as detailed above, an additional possibility is the use of a receptor–ligand system to target the toxic payload to tumor tissue. This would require the conjugation of a targeting ligand such as Tf or folate to the iron oxide nanoparticle conjugated to the chemotherapeutic agent. An example of such a particle was created by Dilnawaz *et al.* in which a glycerol monooleate-coated magnetic nanoparticle (GMO-MNP) was conjugated to the HER2 antibody for targeted delivery to HER2/*neu*-positive MCF-7 cells [52]. The HER2-GMO-MNP used in the study was loaded with paclitaxel and/or rapamycin, and showed enhanced uptake and antiproliferative effect in MCF-7 cells. Furthermore, the magnetization properties of the magnetic nanoparticles were not affected by the modifications and should retain the imaging features, although this was not specifically demonstrated in the study [52].

8.5
Conclusions

SPIO nanoparticles offer a multitude of potential applications in both the diagnosis and treatment of cancer. Table 8.1 presents a brief overview of applications in both clinical and preclinical development. The most-studied application is the use of SPIO nanoparticles as a contrast agent in LNMRI. LNMRI offers the opportunity to increase the accuracy of diagnostic imaging beyond that achievable with anatomic imaging alone. While numerous small studies have demonstrated increased diagnostic accuracy in the identification of malignant lymph nodes, the technology has yet to be adapted to routine clinical use. One obstacle to the adaptation of this technology is that neither of the contrast agents, ferumoxtran-10 or ferumoxytol, have FDA approval for the specific application to LNMRI.

Selective targeting of SPIO nanoparticles offers the potential of detecting malignancy beyond the lymph node. Through the use of ligand–target interactions, SPIO nanoparticles can be targeted to specific tissue types or disease entities allowing for the detection of primary tumor lesions as well as metastatic foci beyond the lymph nodes. While this concept has not been evaluated in humans, results from preclinical studies have been promising. The same techniques used to target tumor tissue for imaging purposes have been applied to the therapeutic delivery of anticancer agents to cancer cells in preclinical studies. In the therapeutic context, the SPIO nanoparticle serves as a scaffold to which therapeutic agents

Table 8.1 Application of SPIO nanoparticles in clinical and preclinical development.

Application	Description	Stage of development	Associated figure
Imaging			
LNMRI – ferumoxtran-10, ferumoxytol	imaging of malignant lymph nodes by the passive uptake of iron oxide nanoparticles	clinical	Figures 8.2–8.5
Active targeting	selective targeting of nanoparticles to specific tissues or disease entities such as cancer through ligand–target interactions	research/ preclinical	–
Therapeutic			
Magnetic guided	use of magnetic field to guide and localize nanoparticles to a specific anatomic location such as a tumor	clinical	Figure 8.7
Drug conjugated	conjugation of chemotherapeutic agents such as doxorubicin to nanoparticles and the targeted release of these agents in tumor tissue	clinical	–
Antibody conjugated	conjugation of therapeutic antibodies to nanoparticles for the selective targeting of the nanoparticle to the receptor of the antibody	research/ preclinical	Figure 8.6
Gene therapy	magnetofection is the method of introduction of genes into cells by the conjugation of nanoparticles to DNA and its vector	research/ preclinical	–
Two-step amplification	method of amplifying the number of nanoparticles targeted to the tissue using the biotin–streptavidin system	research/ preclinical	Figure 8.6

"Clinical" denotes in clinical development, including pilot studies and/or phase I/II clinical trials in humans; none are in routine clinical use. "Research/preclinical" refers to agents tested in animals, but not yet in humans.

such chemotherapeutic drugs, therapeutic antibodies, or DNA for gene therapy are conjugated to the nanoparticle. The therapeutic nanoparticles are then directed to the diseased cells where the therapeutic payloads are released. Ideally, such an approach would result in maximal local concentrations of therapeutic agent in the diseased tissue while minimizing the exposure of normal tissue, in effect maximizing antitumor effect while reducing the dose-limiting adverse effects.

In conclusion, the clinical applications of SPIO nanoparticles for both the diagnosis and treatment of cancer hold great promise. Recent advances in nanotechnology, molecular cell biology, and small-animal imaging have resulted in the rapid development and proliferation of potential applications of this technology. Unfortunately, translating this technology from the bench to the bedside has been sluggish with human studies limited to small pilot studies or early clinical trials. The lack of an FDA-approved agent for imaging purposes may be partially to blame for this slow development. In June 2009, ferumoxytol was approved as an intravenous treatment for iron deficiency anemia in adult patients with chronic kidney disease [53]. While this does not apply directly to imaging, FDA approval of ferumoxytol does offer a stable agent in the marketplace for the development of this exciting technology and translation to routine clinical use. Once SPIO nanoparticles are in routine clinical use, the transition of additional SPIO applications to the clinic will be greatly facilitated, ideally benefiting patients with earlier cancer detection and a more individualized targeted therapy.

References

1. Meyerhardt, J.A. and Mayer, R.J. (2005) Systemic therapy for colorectal cancer. N. Engl. J. Med., 352, 476–487.
2. Thoeni, R.F., Moss, A.A., Schnyder, P., and Margulis, A.R. (1981) Detection and staging of primary rectal and rectosigmoid cancer by computed tomography. Radiology, 141, 135–138.
3. Pomerri, F., Maretto, I., Pucciarelli, S., Rugge, M., Burzi, S., Zandonà, M., Ambrosi, A., Urso, E., Muzzio, P.C., and Nitti, D. (2009) Prediction of rectal lymph node metastasis by pelvic computed tomography measurement. Eur. J. Surg. Oncol., 35, 168–173.
4. Choi, S.H., Moon, W.K., Hong, J.H., Son, K.R., Cho, N., Kwon, B.J., Lee, J.J., Chung, J., Min, H.S., and Park, S.H. (2007) Lymph node metastasis: ultrasmall superparamagnetic iron oxide-enhanced MR imaging versus PET/CT in a rabbit model. Radiology, 242, 137–143.
5. Weissleder, R., Elizondo, G., Wittenberg, J., Lee, A.S., Josephson, L., and Brady, T.J. (1990) Ultrasmall superparamagnetic iron oxide: an intravenous contrast agent for assessing lymph nodes with MR imaging. Radiology, 175, 494–498.
6. Weissleder, R., Elizondo, G., Wittenberg, J., Rabito, C.A., Bengele, H.H., and Josephson, L. (1990) Ultrasmall superparamagnetic iron oxide: characterization of a new class of contrast agents for MR imaging. Radiology, 175, 489–493.
7. Will, O., Purkayastha, S., Chan, C., Athanasiou, T., Darzi, A.W., Gedroyc, W., and Tekkis, P.P. (2006) Diagnostic precision of nanoparticle-enhanced MRI for lymph-node metastases: a meta-analysis. Lancet Oncol., 7, 52–60.
8. Harisinghani, M.G., Barentsz, J., Hahn, P.F., Deserno, W.M., Tabatabaei, S., van de Kaa, C.H., de la Rosette, J., and Weissleder, R. (2003) Noninvasive detection of clinically occult lymph-node metastases in prostate cancer. N. Engl. J. Med., 348, 2491–2499.
9. Harisinghani, M.G., Saksena, M.A., Hahn, P.F., King, B., Kim, J., Torabi, M.T., and Weissleder, R. (2006) Ferumoxtran-10-enhanced MR lymphangiography: does contrast-enhanced imaging alone suffice for accurate lymph node characterization? Am. J. Roentgenol., 186, 144–148.
10. Saksena, M., Harisinghani, M., Hahn, P., Kim, J., Saokar, A., King, B., and Weissleder, R. (2006) Comparison of lymphotropic nanoparticle-enhanced MRI sequences in patients with various primary cancers. Am. J. Roentgenol., 187, W582–W588.
11. Anzai, Y., Piccoli, C.W., Outwater, E.K., Stanford, W., Bluemke, D.A., Nurenberg, P., Saini, S., Maravilla, K.R., Feldman, D.E., Schmiedl, U.P., Brunberg, J.A., Francis, I.R., Harms, S.E., Som, P.M., and Tempany, C.M. (2003) Evaluation of neck and body metastases to nodes with ferumoxtran 10-enhanced MR imaging: phase III safety and efficacy study. Radiology, 228, 777–788.

12. Harisinghani, M.G., Dixon, W.T., Saksena, M.A., Brachtel, E., Blezek, D.J., Dhawale, P.J., Torabi, M., and Hahn, P.F. (2004) MR lymphangiography: imaging strategies to optimize the imaging of lymph nodes with ferumoxtran-10. *Radiographics*, **24**, 867–878.

13. Weissleder, R., Reimer, P., Lee, A.S., Wittenberg, J., and Brady, T.J. (1990) MR receptor imaging: ultrasmall iron oxide particles targeted to asialoglycoprotein receptors. *Am. J. Roentgenol.*, **155**, 1161–1167.

14. Reimer, P., Weissleder, R., Lee, A.S., Wittenberg, J., and Brady, T.J. (1990) Receptor imaging: application to MR imaging of liver cancer. *Radiology*, **177**, 729–734.

15. Thorek, D.L.J., Chen, A.K., Czupryna, J., and Tsourkas, A. (2006) Superparamagnetic iron oxide nanoparticle probes for molecular imaging. *Ann. Biomed. Eng.*, **34**, 23–38.

16. Weissleder, R., Reimer, P., Lee, A.S., Wittenberg, J., and Brady, T.J. (1990) MR receptor imaging: ultrasmall iron oxide particles targeted to asialoglycoprotein receptors. *AJR Am. J. Roentgenol.*, **155**, 1161–1167.

17. Artemov, D., Mori, N., Okollie, B., and Bhujwalla, Z.M. (2003) MR molecular imaging of the Her-2/neu receptor in breast cancer cells using targeted iron oxide nanoparticles. *Magn. Reson. Med.*, **49**, 403–408.

18. Baio, G., Fabbi, M., Salvi, S., de Totero, D., Truini, M., Ferrini, S., and Neumaier, C.E. (2010) Two-step in vivo tumor targeting by biotin-conjugated antibodies and superparamagnetic nanoparticles assessed by magnetic resonance imaging at 1.5 T. *Mol. Imaging Biol.*, **12**, 305–315.

19. Islam, T. and Josephson, L. (2009) Current state and future applications of active targeting in malignancies using superparamagnetic iron oxide nanoparticles. *Cancer Biomark.*, **5**, 99–107.

20. Högemann-Savellano, D., Bos, E., Blondet, C., Sato, F., Abe, T., Josephson, L., Weissleder, R., Gaudet, J., Sgroi, D., Peters, P.J., and Basilion, J.P. (2003) The transferrin receptor: a potential molecular imaging marker for human cancer. *Neoplasia*, **5**, 495–506.

21. Kresse, M., Wagner, S., Pfefferer, D., Lawaczeck, R., Elste, V., and Semmler, W. (1998) Targeting of ultrasmall superparamagnetic iron oxide (USPIO) particles to tumor cells in vivo by using transferrin receptor pathways. *Magn. Reson. Med.*, **40**, 236–242.

22. Meier, R. et al. (2010) Breast cancers: MR imaging of folate-receptor expression with the folate-specific nanoparticle P1113. *Radiology*, **255**, 527–535.

23. Winter, P.M., Morawski, A.M., Caruthers, S.D., Fuhrhop, R.W., Zhang, H., Williams, T.A., Allen, J.S., Lacy, E.K., Robertson, J.D., Lanza, G.M., and Wickline, S.A. (2003) Molecular imaging of angiogenesis in early-stage atherosclerosis with alpha$_v$beta$_3$-integrin-targeted nanoparticles. *Circulation*, **108**, 2270–2274.

24. Hood, J.D., Bednarski, M., Frausto, R., Guccione, S., Reisfeld, R.A., Xiang, R., and Cheresh, D.A. (2002) Tumor regression by targeted gene delivery to the neovasculature. *Science*, **296**, 2404–2407.

25. Hallahan, D., Geng, L., Qu, S., Scarfone, C., Giorgio, T., Donnelly, E., Gao, X., and Clanton, J. (2003) Integrin-mediated targeting of drug delivery to irradiated tumor blood vessels. *Cancer Cell*, **3**, 63–74.

26. Anderson, S.A., Rader, R.K., Westlin, W.F., Null, C., Jackson, D., Lanza, G.M., Wickline, S.A., and Kotyk, J.J. (2000) Magnetic resonance contrast enhancement of neovasculature with alpha$_v$beta$_3$-targeted nanoparticles. *Magn. Reson. Med.*, **44**, 433–439.

27. Arap, W., Pasqualini, R., and Ruoslahti, E. (1998) Cancer treatment by targeted drug delivery to tumor vasculature in a mouse model. *Science*, **279**, 377–380.

28. Yu, X., Song, S.K., Chen, J., Scott, M.J., Fuhrhop, R.J., Hall, C.S., Gaffney, P.J., Wickline, S.A., and Lanza, G.M. (2000) High-resolution MRI characterization of human thrombus using a novel fibrin-targeted paramagnetic nanoparticle contrast agent. *Magn. Reson. Med.*, **44**, 867–872.

29. Schmieder, A.H., Winter, P.M., Caruthers, S.D., Harris, T.D., Williams, T.A., Allen, J.S., Lacy, E.K., Zhang, H., Scott, M.J., Hu, G., Robertson, J.D., Wickline, S.A., and Lanza, G.M. (2005) Molecular MR imaging of melanoma angiogenesis with alphanubeta3-targeted paramagnetic nanoparticles. *Magn. Reson. Med.*, **53**, 621–627.

30. Montet, X., Montet-Abou, K., Reynolds, F., Weissleder, R., and Josephson, L. (2006) Nanoparticle imaging of integrins on tumor cells. *Neoplasia*, **8**, 214–222.

31. Kircher, M.F., Mahmood, U., King, R.S., Weissleder, R., and Josephson, L. (2003) A multimodal nanoparticle for preoperative magnetic resonance imaging and intraoperative optical brain tumor delineation. *Cancer Res.*, **63**, 8122–8125.

32. Barakat, N.S. (2009) Magnetically modulated nanosystems: a unique drug-delivery platform. *Nanomedicine*, **4**, 799–812.

33. Widder, K.J., Senyel, A.E., and Scarpelli, G.D. (1978) Magnetic microspheres: a model system of site specific drug delivery in vivo. *Proc. Soc. Exp. Biol. Med.*, **158**, 141–146.

34. Kubo, T., Sugita, T., Shimose, S., Nitta, Y., Ikuta, Y., and Murakami, T. (2000) Targeted delivery of anticancer drugs with intravenously administered magnetic liposomes in osteosarcoma-bearing hamsters. *Int. J. Oncol.*, **17**, 309–315.

35. Douziech-Eyrolles, L., Marchais, H., Hervé, K., Munnier, E., Soucé, M., Linassier, C., Dubois, P., and Chourpa, I. (2007) Nanovectors for anticancer agents based on superparamagnetic iron oxide nanoparticles. *Int. J. Nanomed.*, **2**, 541–550.

36. Sun, C., Lee, J.S.H., and Zhang, M. (2008) Magnetic nanoparticles in MR imaging and drug delivery. *Adv. Drug Deliv. Rev.*, **60**, 1252–1265.

37. Lübbe, A.S., Bergemann, C., Riess, H., Schriever, F., Reichardt, P., Possinger, K., Matthias, M., Dörken, B., Herrmann, F., Gürtler, R., Hohenberger, P., Haas, N., Sohr, R., Sander, B., Lemke, A.J., Ohlendorf, D., Huhnt, W., and Huhn, D. (1996) Clinical experiences with magnetic drug targeting: a phase I study with 4¢-epidoxorubicin in 14 patients with advanced solid tumors. *Cancer Res.*, **56**, 4686–4693.

38. Lübbe, A.S., Bergemann, C., Huhnt, W., Fricke, T., Riess, H., Brock, J.W., and Huhn, D. (1996) Preclinical experiences with magnetic drug targeting: tolerance and efficacy. *Cancer Res.*, **56**, 4694–4701.

39. Lübbe, A.S., Alexiou, C., and Bergemann, C. (2001) Clinical applications of magnetic drug targeting. *J. Surg. Res.*, **95**, 200–206.

40. Koda, J., Venoo, A., Walser, E., and Goodwin, S. (1990) A multicenter, phase I/II trial of hepatic intra-arterial delivery of doxorubicin hydrochloride adsorbed to magnetic targeted carriers in patients with hepatocellular carcinoma. *Eur. J. Cancer*, **38**, S18.

41. Wilson, M.W., Kerlan, R.K., Fidelman, N.A., Venook, A.P., LaBerge, J.M., Koda, J., and Gordon, R.L. (2004) Hepatocellular carcinoma: regional therapy with a magnetic targeted carrier bound to doxorubicin in a dual MR imaging/conventional angiography suite – initial experience with four patients. *Radiology*, **230**, 287–293.

42. Scherer, F., Anton, M., Schillinger, U., Henke, J., Bergemann, C., Krüger, A., Gänsbacher, B., and Plank, C. (2002) Magnetofection: enhancing and targeting gene delivery by magnetic force in vitro and in vivo. *Gene Ther.*, **9**, 102–109.

43. Goodwin, S.C., Bittner, C.A., Peterson, C.L., and Wong, G. (2001) Single-dose toxicity study of hepatic intra-arterial infusion of doxorubicin coupled to a novel magnetically targeted drug carrier. *Toxicol. Sci.*, **60**, 177–183.

44. Krötz, F., de Wit, C., Sohn, H.Y., Zahler, S., Gloe, T., Pohl, U., and Plank, C. (2003) Magnetofection – a highly efficient tool for antisense oligonucleotide delivery in vitro and in vivo. *Mol. Ther.*, **7**, 700–710.

45. Plank, C., Schillinger, U., Scherer, F., Bergemann, C., Rémy, J., Krötz, F., Anton, M., Lausier, J., and Rosenecker, J. (2003) The magnetofection method: using magnetic force to enhance gene delivery. *Biol. Chem.*, **384**, 737–747.

46. Hirao, K., Sugita, T., Kubo, T., Igarashi, K., Tanimoto, K., Murakami, T., Yasunaga, Y., and Ochi, M. (2003) Targeted gene delivery to human osteosarcoma cells with magnetic cationic liposomes under a magnetic field. *Int. J. Oncol.*, **22**, 1065–1071.
47. Rad, A.M., Iskander, A.S.M., Janic, B., Knight, R.A., Arbab, A.S., and Soltanian-Zadeh, H. (2009) AC133$^+$ progenitor cells as gene delivery vehicle and cellular probe in subcutaneous tumor models: a preliminary study. *BMC Biotechnol.*, **9**, 28.
48. Pedersen, I.M., Buhl, A.M., Klausen, P., Geisler, C.H., and Jurlander, J. (2002) The chimeric anti-CD20 antibody rituximab induces apoptosis in B-cell chronic lymphocytic leukemia cells through a p38 mitogen activated protein-kinase-dependent mechanism. *Blood*, **99**, 1314–1319.
49. Cartron, G., Watier, H., Golay, J., and Solal-Celigny, P. (2004) From the bench to the bedside: ways to improve rituximab efficacy. *Blood*, **104**, 2635–2642.
50. Leget, G.A. and Czuczman, M.S. (1998) Use of rituximab, the new FDA-approved antibody. *Curr. Opin. Oncol.*, **10**, 548–551.
51. Chen, T., Cheng, T., Chen, C., Hsu, S.C.N., Cheng, T., Liu, G., and Wang, Y. (2009) Targeted Herceptin-dextran iron oxide nanoparticles for noninvasive imaging of HER2/*neu* receptors using MRI. *J. Biol. Inorg. Chem.*, **14**, 253–260.
52. Dilnawaz, F., Singh, A., Mohanty, C., and Sahoo, S.K. (2010) Dual drug loaded superparamagnetic iron oxide nanoparticles for targeted cancer therapy. *Biomaterials*, **31**, 3694–3706.
53. Lu, M., Cohen, M.H., Rieves, D., and Pazdur, R. (2010) FDA report: ferumoxytol for intravenous iron therapy in adult patients with chronic kidney disease. *Am. J. Hematol.*, **85**, 315–319.

9
Preclinical and Clinical Tumor Imaging with SPECT/CT and PET/CT

Andreas K. Buck, Florian Gärtner, Ambros Beer, Ken Herrmann, Sibylle Ziegler, and Markus Schwaiger

9.1
Introduction

The introduction of nuclear imaging technologies to clinical medicine has influenced the management of patients with cancer. In most industrialized countries, single photon emission computed tomography (SPECT) and, more recently, positron emission tomography (PET) are accepted as both useful and economic diagnostic imaging modalities for the characterization of indeterminate lesions, initial staging, restaging, and assessment of response to therapy in a variety of cancers. Combination of a SPECT or PET scanner with spiral computed X-ray tomography in a single examination (SPECT/CT,PET/CT) allows integrated functional (SPECT, PET) and morphologic (CT) imaging (Figure 9.1). Additionally to the results returned by individual modalities, coregistration of CT allows precise localization of PET or SPECT lesions. The addition of functional imaging data to CT leads to an increase of sensitivity as well as specificity. Moreover, CT data can be used for attenuation correction, which leads to a significant reduction of scanning time as compared to traditional attenuation correction methods, making nuclear imaging more comfortable for the patient. A standard examination with PET/CT including the head, thorax, abdomen, and pelvis can be performed within 20 min.

Since its introduction to clinical medicine in 2001, PET/CT has been one of the fastest growing imaging modalities. The Centers of Medicare and Medicaid Services (CMS) approved a variety of clinical indications, including staging and restaging of non-small-cell lung cancer (NSCLC), esophageal, colorectal, breast, and head and neck cancers, malignant lymphoma, and melanoma. Monitoring response to treatment in breast cancer is also covered. Recently, the CMS announced to provide widespread coverage of PET when examinations are part of prospective clinical trials. Recently, due to the clinical success of hybrid PET/CT devices, integrated SPECT/CT scanners have been made available. SPECT/CT has an additional value in sentinel lymph node (SLN) mapping, especially in head and neck tumors, and tumors draining into pelvic lymph nodes. Regarding the growing number of studies demonstrating an added value of hybrid SPECT/CT over single imaging

(a) SPECT/CT

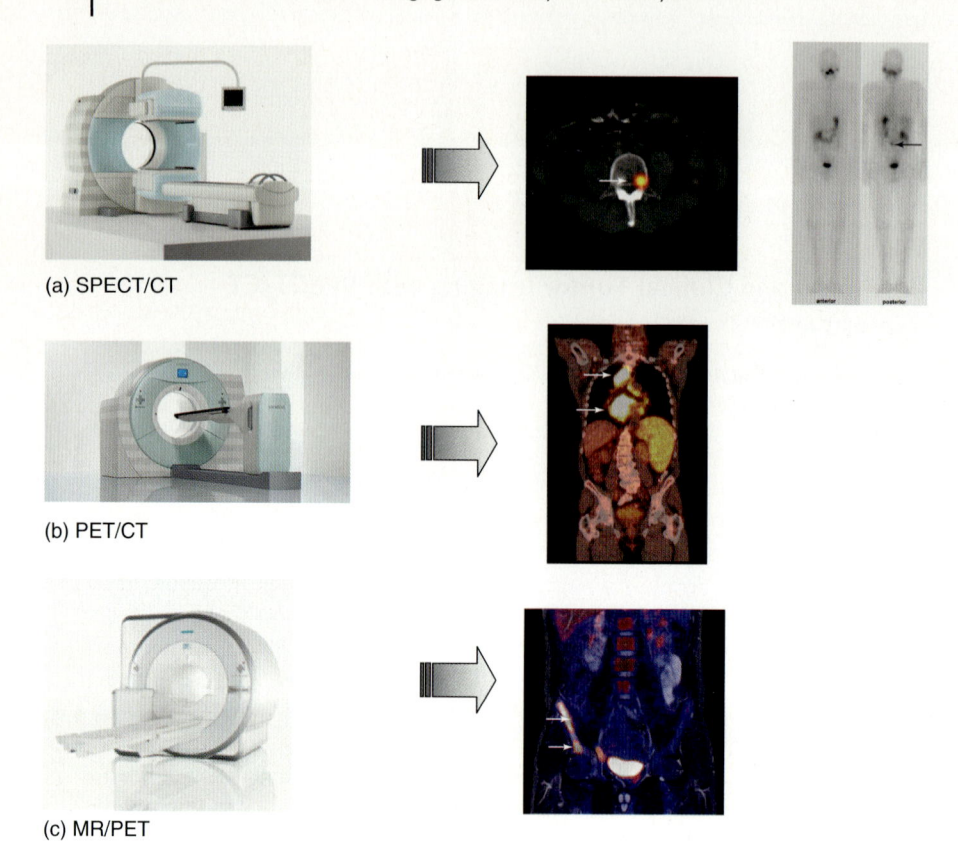

(b) PET/CT

(c) MR/PET

Figure 9.1 Overview of hybrid imaging modalities designed for clinical use. Clinical examples are shown on the right. (a) Clinical SPECT/CT device is shown on the left. The clinical example on the right shows a small bone metastasis in a patient with thyroid cancer (lumbar vertebra, arrow), as detected by fused tomographic SPECT/CT using ^{131}I as radionuclide. The planar whole-body scintigraphy has a similar sensitivity (arrow), but markedly reduced anatomic resolution, potentially leading to misinterpretation. (b) Clinical PET/CT scanner. The clinical example shows mediastinal manifestation of lymphoma (arrows). (c) Hybrid MRI/PET scanner. The clinical example shows malignant involvement of bone marrow (arrows). (Scanner images courtesy of Siemens Medical Solutions, Erlangen, Germany.)

modalities, it appears likely that this promising technique will play an increasingly important role in clinical routine practice. The broad spectrum of existing SPECT tracers and their widespread availability suggest that SPECT/CT will be able to play a complementary role to PET/CT imaging procedures.

SPECT/CT and PET/CT technology has been downscaled to allow molecular imaging also of small animals (Figure 9.2). Modern devices enable noninvasive whole-body imaging with a resolution of several hundreds of micrometers (SPECT) up to 1.5 mm (PET, SPECT), thus transferring nuclear imaging also to translational cancer research.

9.2 Technical Aspects of Functional and Molecular Imaging with SPECT and PET

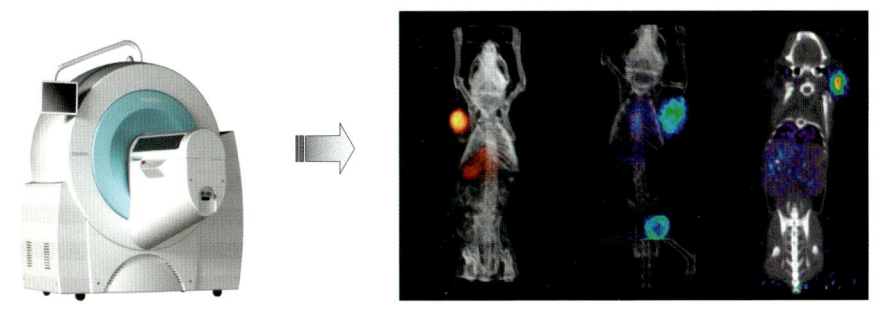

(a) Small-animal SPECT/CT

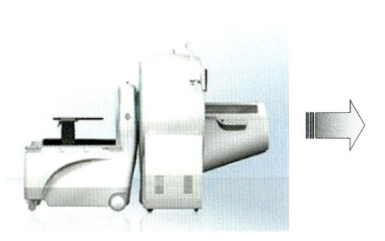

(b) Small-animal PET/CT

Figure 9.2 Examples of small-animal hybrid scanners designed for preclinical studies. (a) Hybrid SPECT/CT device. Several hybrid scans of mice with tumor xenotransplants in the shoulder region are demonstrated on the right. (b) Small-animal PET/CT device with corresponding CT, ^{18}F-FDG-PET, and ^{18}F-FDG-PET/CT scans of a mouse. (Scanner images courtesy of Siemens Medical Solutions, Erlangen, Germany.)

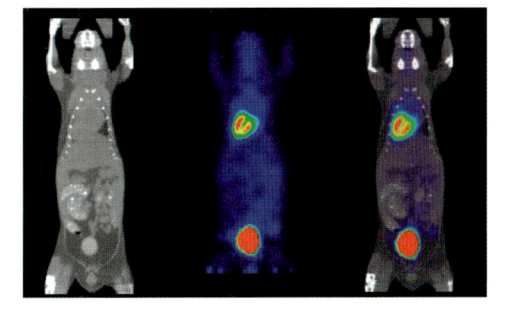

9.2
Technical Aspects of Functional and Molecular Imaging with SPECT and PET

9.2.1
Principles of Clinical PET and Hybrid PET/CT Imaging

PET allows noninvasive assessment of the three-dimensional distribution of a positron-labeled compound within the living body. Positrons are antiparticles of electrons and originate from β^+ decay of radioactive isotopes such as ^{11}C, ^{13}N, ^{15}O, ^{18}F, ^{68}Ga, ^{86}Y, or ^{124}I. During β^+ decay a positron and a neutrino are emitted, both sharing a certain amount of kinetic energy. Once the positron is slowed down, a positronium consisting of a positron and an electron is created. The positronium has a very short half-life of 10^{-10} s, and the masses of the positron and the electron are finally transferred into energy. This annihilation results in two γ quanta with an energy of 511 keV each. Decay events are detected by coincidence registration, enabling the measurement of activity distribution in a specific transaxial section of the body. Activity distribution can be calculated from respective projections after correction for scatter, attenuation, dead time, and random coincidences. Attenuation correction can be performed using a radioactive transmission source rotating around the patient, but this has been replaced in most centers by using coregistered CT data. Emission and transmission scanning from the skull to mid thigh usually takes 30–45 min, whole-body scans 60–90 min. The radiation dose of a standard PET examination is low at approximately 7.4 mSv and similar to a spiral CT of the thorax. Using integrated PET/CT systems, the scanning time can be markedly reduced. Nowadays, a PET/CT scan from the head to the mid thigh can be performed within 20 min.

9.2.2
Biomarkers for PET and PET/CT Imaging

Depending on the clinical situation, various radiolabeled pharmaceuticals can be utilized for tumor imaging (Table 9.1 and Figure 9.3). The most important biomarker for functional diagnosis of tumors is the glucose analog $2'$-^{18}F-fluoro-$2'$-deoxy-D-glucose (FDG). Since conventional imaging modalities such as CT, magnetic resonance imaging (MRI), or ultrasound detect malignant lesions because of characteristic morphological alterations, ^{18}F-FDG-PET enables the diagnosis of malignant tumors due to an increased glucose metabolism in malignant cells. After intravenous administration, ^{18}F-FDG is predominantly taken up by tumor cells. After enzymatic conversion of ^{18}F-FDG to ^{18}F-FDG-6-monophosphate by hexokinase, the metabolite cannot be further metabolized, resulting in an intracellular "trapping" of ^{18}F-FDG.

There are many other radiopharmaceuticals capable of assessing distinct pathophysiologic processes (Table 9.1 and Figures 9.4–9.8). As an example, radiolabeled nucleoside analogs such as $3'$-deoxy-$3'$-^{18}F-fluorothymidine (FLT) can be used to noninvasively assess the proliferative activity of tumors (Figures 9.8–9.10). With the positron emitter ^{15}O, H_2^{15}O can be synthesized and used for assessment of tumor blood flow. A variety of radiolabeled amino acids such as ^{11}C-methionine (^{11}C-MET), ^{11}C-leucine (^{11}C-LEU), or ^{18}F-fluoroethyltyrosine (^{18}F-FET) can be used to evaluate transport rates of amino acids and/or protein biosynthesis (Figure 9.11). Imidazole derivatives such as ^{18}F-fluoromisonidazole (^{18}F-FMISO) can be used to delineate hypoxic tissue areas of the tumor, which is particularly useful for radiation treatment planning (Figure 9.12). Synthesis of phospholipids is increased in many neoplasms, leading to increased uptake of ^{18}F- and ^{11}C-choline (^{18}F- and ^{11}C-CHO) (Figure 9.13). ^{68}Ga-DOTA-TOC (DOTA–D-Phe^1–Tyr^3–octreotide (OC); DOTA = 1,4,7,10-tetraazacyclododecane-1,4,7,10-tetraacetic acid) specifically binds to somatostatin receptors (SSTRs) and is therefore highly sensitive for detection of neuroendocrine tumors. ^{18}F-galacto-RGD has a high affinity to the vitronectin receptor $\alpha_v\beta_3$ and can be used as potential surrogate marker of neoangiogenesis (Figures 9.5 and 9.6). These and many other radiopharmaceuticals specifically address metabolic pathways or bind to specific target structures, and therefore

Table 9.1 Radiopharmaceuticals (tracers) used for PET imaging.

Tracer	Native molecule	Uptake mechanism in cancer	Clinical applications
^{18}F-fluorodeoxyglucose (FDG)	glucose	glucose transport, phosphorylation by hexokinase	diagnosis, (re-)staging (cancer of the lung, breast, colon, pancreas, rectum; lymphoma, melanoma); monitoring of response to treatment (lymphoma, breast, gastrointestinal tract, lung cancer)
^{18}F-fluoroethyltyrosine (FET)	tyrosine	amino acid transport, protein biosynthesis	diagnosis, (re-)staging of brain tumors; differentiation of scar/local recurrence, monitoring response in various tumors
^{11}C-methionine (MET)	methionine	amino acid transport, protein biosynthesis	diagnosis, (re-)staging of brain tumors; differentiation of scar/local recurrence, monitoring response in various tumors
^{11}C-choline (CHO), ^{18}F-fluorocholine	choline	uptake by active transport and phosphorylation by choline kinase; incorporation into phospholipids (cellular membrane)	(re-)staging (e.g., prostate cancer, bladder cancer); monitoring of response to treatment (prostate cancer, bladder cancer)
^{18}F-fluoroethylcholine (FEC)	choline	uptake by active transport and phosphorylation by choline kinase; incorporation into phospholipids (cellular membrane)	(re-)staging (e.g., prostate cancer, bladder cancer); monitoring of response to treatment (prostate cancer, bladder cancer)
^{11}C-acetate	acetate	lipid biosynthesis, key enzyme fatty acid synthase	(re-)staging monitoring response to treatment in several tumor entities
^{68}Ga-DOTA-TOC, ^{68}Ga-DOTA-TATE	octreotide (somatostatin analog)	binding to somatostatin receptors (predominantly SSTR2)	diagnosis, (re-)staging of neuroendocrine tumors

(continued overleaf)

Table 9.1 (continued).

Tracer	Native molecule	Uptake mechanism in cancer	Clinical applications
^{18}F-DOPA	dihydroxyphenyl-alanine	uptake in tumors facilitating DOPA decarboxylation	diagnosis, (re-)staging of neuroendocrine and brain tumors
^{18}F-fluorothymidine (FLT), ^{11}C-thymidine (THY)	thymidine	DNA synthesis, tumor cell proliferation	assessment of tumor proliferation (monitoring response to cytotoxic treatment in lymphoma, sarcoma, breast cancer)
^{18}F-galacto-RGD	peptide containing the sequence RGD	binding to integrin $\alpha_v\beta_3$ (vitronectin receptor), expressed on activated endothelial cells	assessment of tumor angiogenesis (melanoma, sarcoma, head and neck cancer, breast cancer), monitoring response to antiangiogenic treatment
^{18}F-fluoroazamycine arabinoside (FAZA), ^{18}F-fluoromisonidazole (FMISO)	hypoxia markers (no biologic analog)	passive diffusion into hypoxic cells; reactive intermediates are formed by intracellular nitroreductase and trapped within the cell	assessment of tumor hypoxia (for use in tumors of the head and neck), radiation treatment planning
^{18}F-fluoro-17-β-estradiol (FES)	estradiol	binding to estrogen receptors	monitoring of response to antihormone treatment (breast cancer)
^{18}F-fluoride	fluoride	bone mineralization	screening for bone metastases

enable molecular imaging of cancer. Specific radiotracers are especially helpful for evaluation of new drugs and early response assessment in cancer.

9.2.3
Principles of Clinical SPECT and Hybrid SPECT/CT Imaging

Before the introduction of dedicated SPECT/CT cameras, various software algorithms had been established to allow image fusion of anatomical (CT, MRI) and functional (SPECT) imaging [1]. In the early 1980s, many efforts had been made to allow image fusion in brain studies. Current software algorithms permit highly accurate coregistration of anatomical and functional datasets. This kind of nonrigid

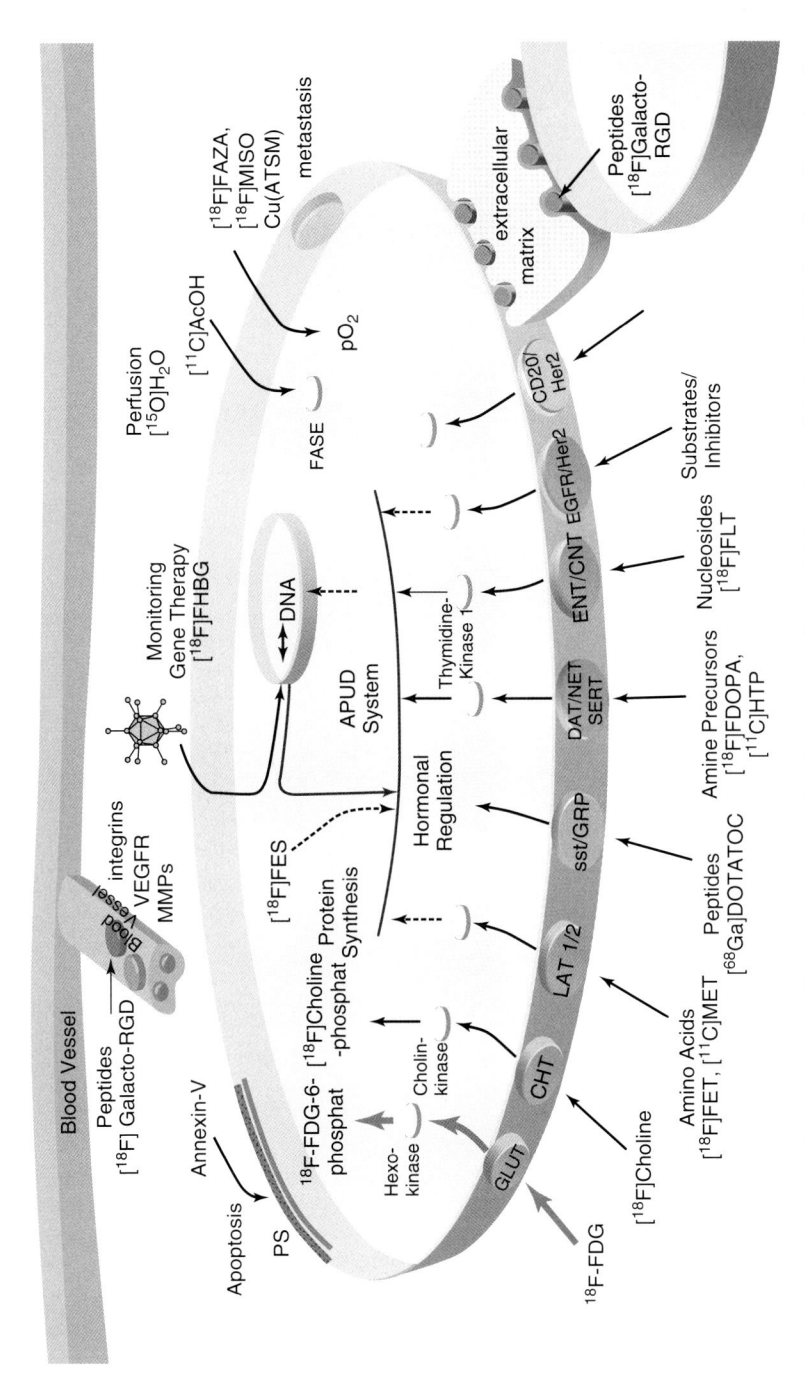

Figure 9.3 Overview of PET tracers enabling noninvasive molecular imaging of tumor biology in preclinical and clinical studies. (Reproduced with permission of the AACR [2]).

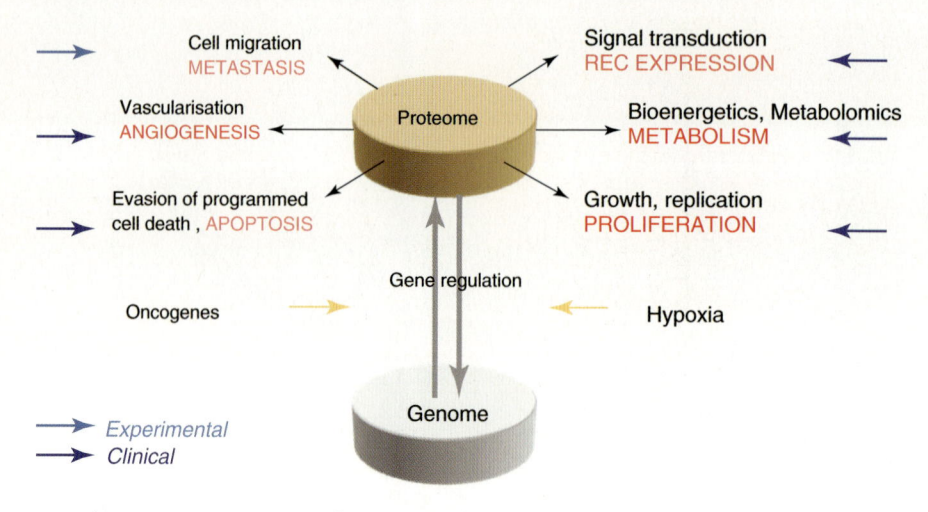

Figure 9.4 Imaging targets for imaging hallmarks of cancer and monitoring of cancer therapies that can be addressed by specific PET tracers.

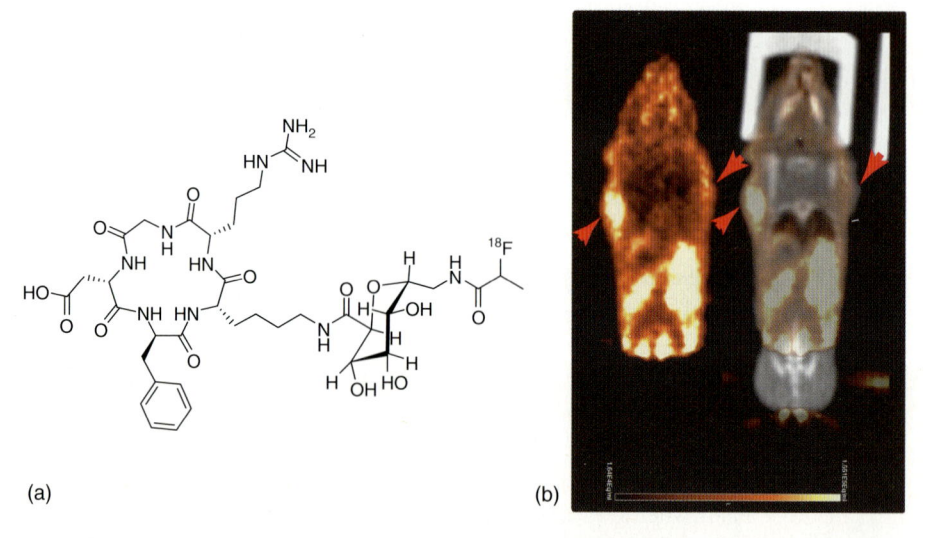

Figure 9.5 Small-animal microPET/CT with ^{18}F-galacto-RGD of a nude mouse. (a) Molecular structure of ^{18}F-galacto-RGD. (b) Nude mouse with tumor xenograft consisting of highly $\alpha_v\beta_3$-overexpressing M21 cells (arrow closed tip) and α_v-defective M21L cells (arrow open tip). Note that while the M21 tumor shows intense tracer accumulation, the M21L tumor shows only faint tracer uptake, corresponding to the different levels of $\alpha_v\beta_3$ expression.

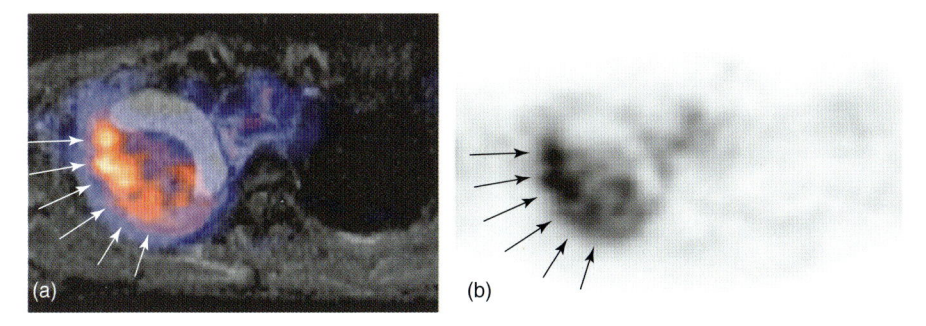

Figure 9.6 Example of ^{18}F-galacto-RGD PET examination in a patient with NSCLC of the right lung (arrows): image fusion with MRI (a) and PET (b). Note intense tracer accumulation predominantly in the periphery of the tumor, suggesting intense peripheral $\alpha_v\beta_3$ expression within the lesion.

Figure 9.7 Molecular structure of ^{18}F-fluciclatide – an RGD peptide used as a PET tracer for molecular imaging of neoangiogenesis.

image coregistration is therefore a regular component in daily clinical practice (e.g., for image-guided surgery or imaging-guided planning of radiotherapy). However, motion artifacts heavily affect image fusion in the thorax, abdomen, pelvis, or head and neck region when CT and SPECT acquisition are performed separately [3, 4]. Functional images of the thorax or the abdomen contain little or no anatomical landmarks that can be correlated to anatomic reference points. Moreover, the chest and abdomen do not represent rigid structures. Differences in patient positioning and respiratory motion make the correct alignment of anatomical and functional images even more complicated. More recently, three-dimensional elastic transformations or nonlinear warping have been established to further improve the accuracy of image fusion. With these modern approaches, the accuracy of software-based

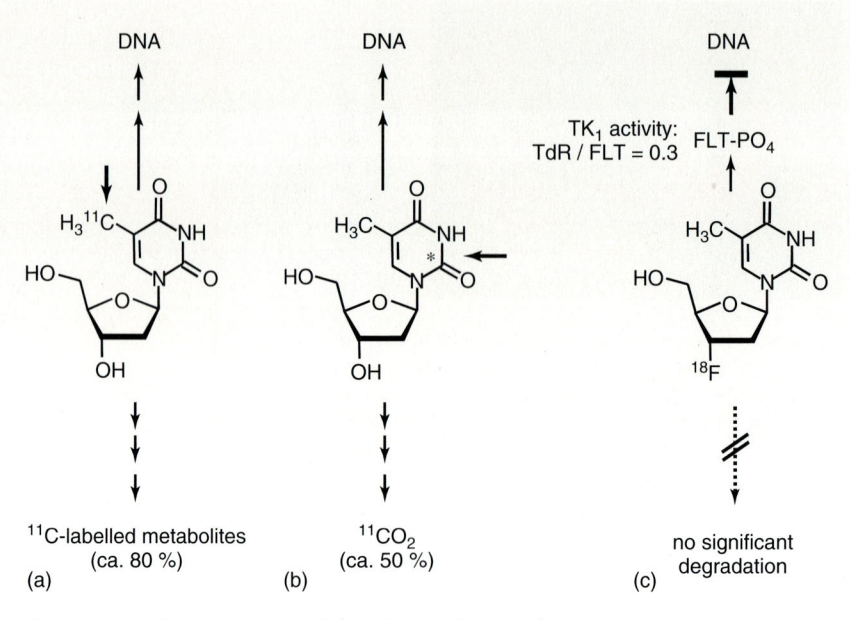

Figure 9.8 Molecular structure of thymidine analogs used for imaging proliferation. (a) ^{11}C-labeled thymidine molecule undergoing rapid serum degradation. (b) native thymidine molecule, and (c) metabolically stable thymidine analog ^{18}F-FLT.

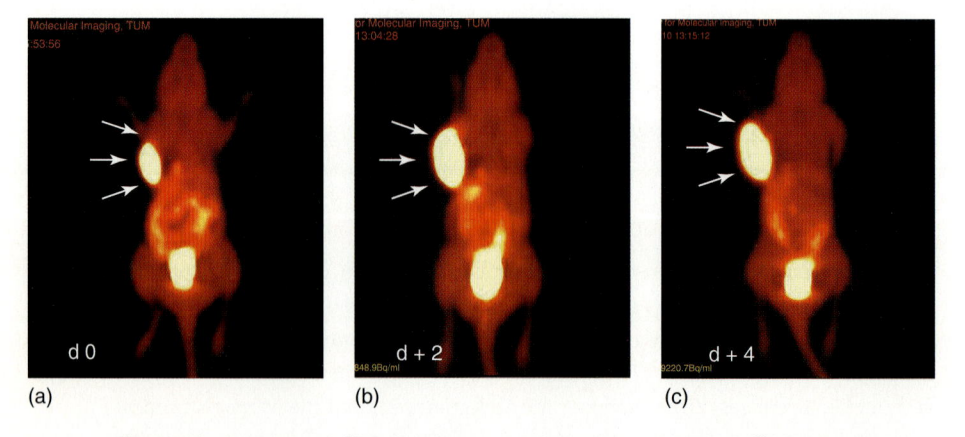

Figure 9.9 Assessment of response to treatment with ^{18}F-FLT-PET in an animal model of lymphoma (arrows). (a) PET prior to treatment indicating intense uptake of the radiotracer (arrows) and, hence, a high proliferation fraction. (b) and (c) PET demonstrates increasing ^{18}F-FLT-uptake in the transplanted tumor (at day +2 and day +4) which indicates resistance to treatment with the mammalian target of rapamycin (mTOR) inhibitor RAD001.

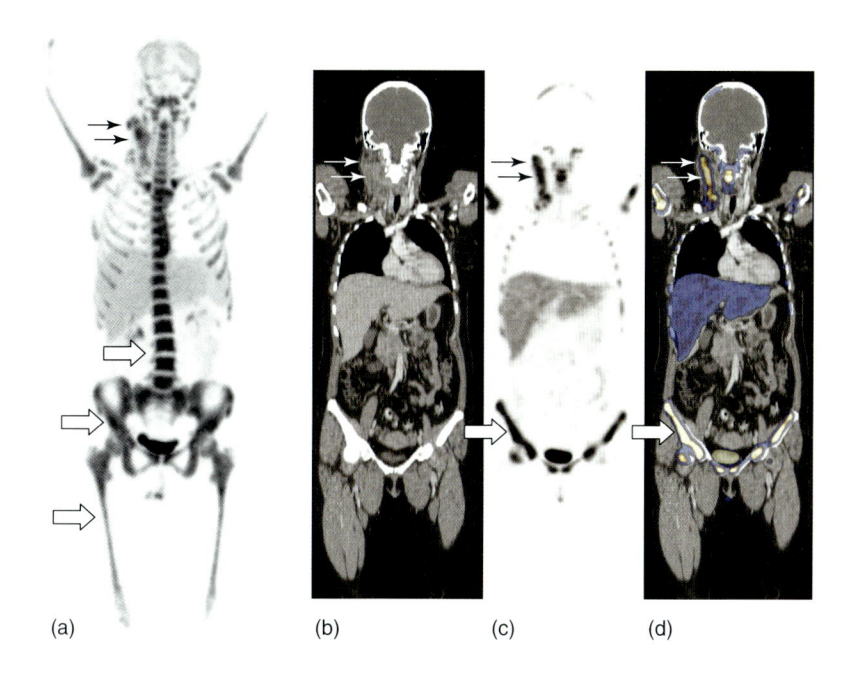

Figure 9.10 ^{18}F-FLT-PET scan in a patient with malignant lymphoma. (a) Intense focal tracer uptake in the right cervical region indicates malignant lymphoma (maximum intensity projection of ^{18}F-FLT-PET), (b) coronal CT, (c) coronal PET, and (d) fused PET/CT sections. High physiologic ^{18}F-FLT uptake can be seen in the proliferating bone marrow (lumbar, thoracic vertebra, ribs, femora, and humeri.)

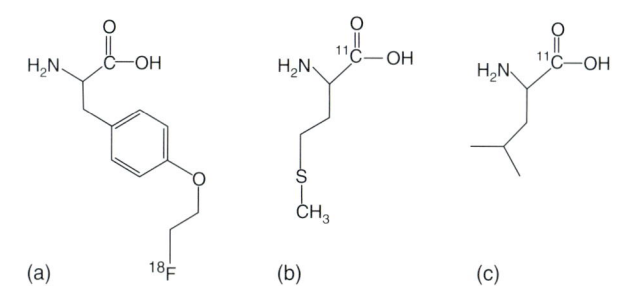

Figure 9.11 PET tracers for imaging amino acid transport and/or protein biosynthesis. (a) ^{18}F-FET, (b) ^{11}C-MET, and (c) ^{11}C-LEU.

image coregistration is in the range of 5 mm. Whereas software algorithms did not reach widespread clinical use for image coregistration of the abdomen or thorax, this technology will still play an important role to allow correction of misregistrations due to patient motion or breathing artifacts that may also arise from integrated SPECT/CT scanners.

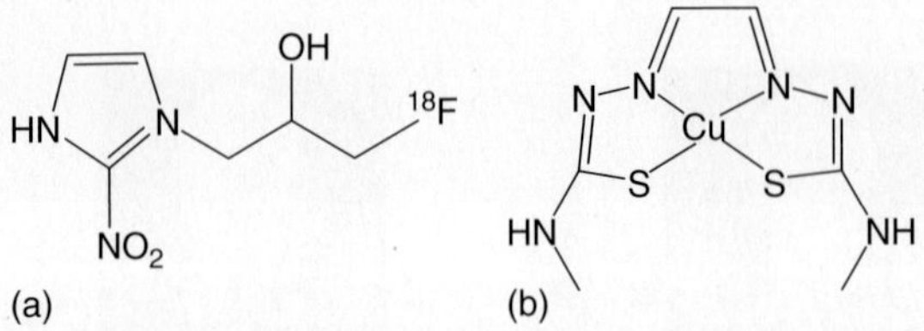

Figure 9.12 PET tracers used for molecular imaging of hypoxia. (a) ^{18}F-FMISO. (b) ^{64}Cu-ATSM.

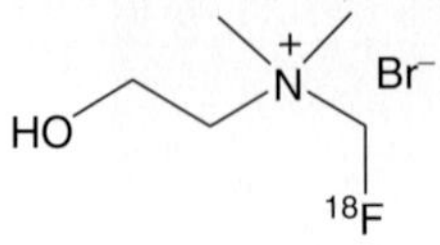

Figure 9.13 PET tracer ^{18}C-CHO for imaging biosynthesis of phospholipids.

9.2.4
Biomarkers for SPECT and SPECT/CT Imaging

A variety of radioisotopes and radiopharmaceuticals are available for SPECT imaging. A list of biomarkers relevant for preclinical cancer research and established clinical applications is given in Table 9.2. In the clinical setting, ^{123}I or ^{131}I represent important biomarkers for staging and detection of local recurrence or distant metastases from differentiated thyroid cancers. Planar scintigraphy and SPECT using ^{99m}Tc-labeled phosphate are still regarded as standard imaging modalities for whole-body screening for bone metastases. For the management of rare cancer types such as neuroendocrine tumors and pheochromocytoma, imaging biomarkers enable specific detection of SSTR expression (^{111}In-OC) or tumoral uptake of noradrenaline analogs (^{123}I-*meta*-iodobenzylguanidine (^{123}I-MIBG). Recently, less-specific radiopharmaceuticals such as ^{201}Th or ^{67}Gallium-citrate have become less relevant. In most centers, these techniques have been replaced by PET and PET/CT imaging. Radiolabeled antibodies specifically binding to carcinoembryonic antigen (anti-CEA) or prostate-specific membrane antigen (anti-PSMA) offer very high specificity, but superiority to PET and PET/CT imaging has not been demonstrated so far. Therefore, these compounds are exclusively used in clinical or preclinical studies.

9.2.5
Principles of Preclinical Imaging with SPECT and PET

Similar to the clinical devices, small-animal SPECT cameras consist of a collimator, a scintillator crystal, a light guide, and a number of photomultiplier tubes (PMTs). Segmented scintillator crystals and position-sensitive PMTs are also used in current systems in order to improve spatial resolution in preclinical applications. A typical SPECT device contains one, two, or more γ-cameras that rotate around the animal. Furthermore, systems are available using a stationary system rotating the animal within the field of view. Block detectors are used in clinical PET, consisting of a

Table 9.2 Radiopharmaceuticals (tracers) used for SPECT imaging.

Tracer	Native molecule/isotope	Uptake mechanism in cancer	Clinical applications
^{123}I, ^{131}I	iodine	natrium iodide symporter, peroxidase (thyroid peroxidase)	(re-)staging of differentiated thyroid cancer (papillary, follicular)
^{99m}Tc-phosphate HDP	phosphate	bone mineralization	detection of bone metastases (cancer of prostate, breast, lung, colorectal; sarcoma; melanoma); monitoring response to therapy
^{99m}Tc-nanocoll	albumin	transport in lymphatic vessels	detection of SLNs (breast and prostate cancer, melanoma)
^{111}In-octreotide	octreotide (somatostatin analog)	binding to somatostatin receptors	diagnosis, (re-)staging of neuroendocrine tumors
^{123}I-meta-iodobenzylguanidine (MIBG), ^{131}I-MIBG	borepinephrine (guanethidine)	human noradrenaline transporter	detection, (re-)staging of pheochromocytoma, neuroblastoma, paraganglioma
^{201}Th	thallium	active transport (Na/K-ATPase)	detection, (re-)staging of lymphoma and various solid cancers
^{67}Ga-citrate	gallium	transferrin adsorption, binding to transferrin receptors (located at tumor cell surface)	detection, (re-)staging of lymphoma, seminoma
^{111}In-satumomab	–	binding to glycoprotein 72 (TAG-72)	detection, (re-)staging of colon cancer
^{111}In-architumomab	–	binding to CEA	detection, (re-)staging of colon cancer
^{111}In-labeled PSMA-specific antibodies	–	binding to PSMA	detection, (re-)staging of prostate cancer

number of individual crystal elements read out by a small number of PMTs. The sum of four PMT signals is used to determine the energy information. Another option is the read-out of a large number of crystals with a continuous light guide in an array of PMTs. An alternative to the block detector concept is the individual crystal read-out that can be achieved using more compact photon detectors such as avalanche photodiodes. The thickness of the crystal is critical for both PET and SPECT imaging. A thick crystal increases the γ detection efficiency and, hence, the sensitivity of the imaging device. However, in SPECT, large thickness enhances the spread of the scintillation light before reaching the PMT. In PET, especially in small-animal systems, making use of the depth of interaction (DOI) information plays an important role in the improvement of spatial resolution. DOI measurement is not yet a standard feature of commercial systems, but is likely to become more available in the future.

Tomographic image reconstruction is based on measured integrals of a radiotracer distribution, as seen under different angles (projections). The algorithms used for SPECT and PET for reconstructing the underlying activity distribution are entirely the same. Filtered back-projection has long been the most widely used analytical reconstruction algorithm. Quantification of activity concentration in reconstructed images is most important, especially if changes in the accumulation are used for monitoring a therapeutic effect. While PET is widely accepted as a quantitative imaging method, this is not the case for SPECT. The major effects determining the quantification of radioactivity are attenuation and scatter in the object of interest as well as the spatial resolution of the imaging device. Both in PET and SPECT, attenuation and scatter correction algorithms rely on the availability of structural information such as CT. The highest spatial resolution in preclinical SPECT is in the range of a few hundreds of micrometers that can be achieved using pinhole collimators, although these have a low sensitivity. In order to increase sensitivity, several detectors are used. The spatial resolution of a commercial PET device for small-animal imaging is in the range of 1–1.5 mm (Figures 9.2, 9.5, and 9.9).

9.3
Preclinical and Clinical Developments

9.3.1
Imaging Neoangiogenesis

Angiogenesis is a process involving the growth of new blood vessels from pre-existing vessels. Numerous disorders are characterized by an imbalance or upregulation of the angiogenic process, including tumor growth. Great efforts are being made to develop antiangiogenic drugs as novel cancer therapeutics. However, currently available imaging techniques are limited in monitoring treatment using this class of drugs. Therefore, new methods are needed for planning and monitoring of treatments targeting the angiogenic process. There are different approaches currently studied, including MRI, Doppler ultrasound, and scintigraphic techniques.

9.3.1.1 VEGF/VEGFR Imaging

The probes currently used for imaging vascular endothelial growth factor (VEGF)/VEGF receptor (VEGFR) pathways fall into two categories. The first category includes antibodies against VEGF. VEGF121 is freely soluble, VEGF165 is secreted, whereas a significant fraction remains localized to the extracellular matrix, such as for VEGF189 and VEGF206 [5]. This will most likely lead to locally high VEGF levels. Noninvasive measurement of VEGF in the tumor might give insight to the available target for VEGF-dependent antiangiogenic therapy and thus assist in tumor response prediction. The humanized monoclonal antibody bevacizumab blocks VEGF-induced endothelial cell proliferation, permeability, and survival, and it inhibits human tumor cell line growth in preclinical models. Small-animal PET imaging with ^{89}Zr-bevacizumab showed higher tumor uptake compared with human ^{89}Zr-IgG in a human SKOV-3 ovarian tumor xenograft. Similar results were observed with ^{124}I-labeled monoclonal antibody VG67e [6] that binds to human VEGF. huMV833, the humanized version of a mouse monoclonal anti-VEGF antibody MV833, was also labeled with ^{124}I, and the distribution and biological effects of huMV833 in patients in a phase I clinical trial were investigated [7]. These results demonstrated that the radiolabeled antibody is a new class of tracer for noninvasive *in vivo* imaging of VEGF in the tumor microenvironment. However, antibody distribution and clearance were quite heterogeneous not only between and within patients, but also between and within individual tumors [7]. In addition, radiolabeled antibody tumor accumulation is not always correlated with the level of VEGF expression in the tissue as determined by *in situ* hybridization and enzyme-linked immunosorbent assay. Furthermore, due to the large size of antibody, it is hard to penetrate into the center of the tumor and it usually takes several hours or even days before high-contrast images can be obtained for antibody-based tracers. Using engineered antibody fragments with compromised binding affinity can partially overcome this problem. The second category includes radiolabeled VEGF-A and its derivatives for imaging VEGFRs. Several PET studies have been reported on the use of appropriately labeled VEGF proteins for PET [8]. However, most of the reported wild-type VEGF-based imaging agents are unsuitable for clinical translation because of the unacceptably high major organ (e.g., liver and kidney) uptake [9] or uncertain binding activity of the protein, owing to damage caused by random radiolabeling or bioconjugation [10–13]. Therefore, optimization of VEGF protein-based probes without changing the conformation of the protein and compromising its functional activity is required.

The VEGF family is composed of seven members with a common VEGF homology domain [14]. VEGF-A is a dimeric, disulfide-bound glycoprotein existing in at least seven homodimeric isoforms. Apart from the difference in molecular weight, these isoforms also differ in their biological properties, such as the ability to bind to cell surface heparin sulfate proteoglycans [14]. Both VEGF165 and VEGF121 have been used for VEGFR imaging [12, 15]. The advantages of this class of tracers are that they are natural ligands for VEGFRs and have high binding affinity to the receptors. However, VEGF165 and VEGF121 bind to both VEGFR1 and VEGFR2; their binding affinity to VEGFR1 was even higher than that to VEGFR2, which resulted in high kidney retention – an organ that expresses a high level of VEGFR1. Compared with VEGF121, VEGF165 is less soluble and contains an extra domain for heparin binding, resulting in increased nonspecific binding and low tumor/background ratio. Therefore, optimization of VEGF protein probes is mainly based on VEGF121 protein instead of VEGF165 protein. Recombinant VEGF121 has been labeled with ^{64}Cu for PET imaging of tumor angiogenesis and VEGFR expression [16]. PEGylated VEGF121 site-specifically labeled with ^{64}Cu showed considerably prolonged blood clearance, higher tumor uptake, and lower kidney uptake. Overall, PET imaging using VEGF protein-based radiotracers is a feasible option to noninvasively detect VEGFR expression *in vivo*.

9.3.1.2 Radiolabeled Integrin Antagonists (RGD Peptides)

Integrins are cell adhesion receptors that are not only involved in mediating migration of endothelial cells, but are also important regulators of endothelial cell growth, survival, and differentiation [17, 18]. Integrin $\alpha_v\beta_3$ plays an essential role in the regulation of tumor growth, local invasiveness, and metastatic potential, but is also highly expressed on activated endothelial cells during angiogenesis. Integrin $\alpha_v\beta_3$ is a heterodimeric transmembrane glycoprotein consisting of two subunits. It is found that several extracellular matrix proteins like vitronectin, laminin, and fibronectin interact via the amino acid sequence Arg–Gly–Asp (RGD) with this integrin [19]. Based on these findings Kessler *et al.* developed the $\alpha_v\beta_3$-targeting pentapeptide cyclo(-Arg-Gly-Asp-dPhe-Val-) [20], which is the most prominent lead structure for the development of radiotracers for the noninvasive determination of this receptor [21]. Another lead structure is based on the sequence H-Lys-Cys-Arg-Gly-Asp-Cys-Phe-Cys-OH (NC-100717) including to bridging systems (N^α of Lys1 is bridged with Cys8 via a chloroacetyl moiety and Cys2–Cys6 via disulfide formation). The side-chain amino function of the lysine is used for derivatization allowing radiolabeling with ^{18}F, ^{99m}Tc, or other radiometals. C-terminal modifications include the introduction of a poly(ethylene glycol) (PEG) linker as biomodifier.

9.3.1.3 Monomeric Tracer Labeling Strategies

Due to its favorable β energy and half-life, ^{18}F is the most frequently used radionuclide in PET. The main approach to label peptides with ^{18}F involves prosthetic groups. The most prominent ^{18}F-labeled tracer for imaging $\alpha_v\beta_3$ expression is ^{18}F-galacto-RGD, which is labeled via conjugation of 4-nitrophenyl-2-^{18}F-fluoropropionate [22]. This compound resulted from an optimization strategy introducing sugar moieties to improve pharmacokinetics (see below). In murine tumor models as well as in patients (for details see also below) this tracer showed receptor-specific tumor accumulation and good elimination kinetics, resulting in high-contrast images demonstrating that noninvasive determination of $\alpha_v\beta_3$ expression and quantification with ^{18}F-labeled RGD peptides is feasible (Figures 9.5 and 9.6). However, synthesis of ^{18}F-labeled peptides using activated esters is complex and time-consuming, sometimes requiring complicated protection strategies, therefore chemoselective ^{18}F-labeling strategies based on oxime formation using 4-^{18}F-fluorobenzaldehyde [23, 24] and more recently also with ^{18}F-fluorosilyl benzaldehyde [25] have been introduced. The 4-^{18}F-fluorobenzaldehyde has also been used in combination with HYNIC (6-hydrazinonicotinic acid)-modified RGD peptides [26] resulting in 4'-^{18}F-fluorobenzylidenehydrazone-6-nicotinamide-c(RGDyK). ^{18}F-AH111585 is an aminooxy-funtionalized double-bridged RGD peptide that has already entered clinical trials (see below). Other strategies use thiol-reactive groups. For example 3,4,6-tri-O-acetyl-2-deoxy-2-^{18}F-fluoroglucopyranosylphenyl-thiosulfonate (Ac3-^{18}F-FGlc-PTS) [27] was used as a thiol-reactive glycosyl donor for ^{18}F-glycosylation of peptides. This approach would allow both introduction of the radiolabel and a pharmacokinetic modifier in one synthesis step (see below). Another group introduced N-2-(4-^{18}F-fluorobenzamido)ethyl-maleimide [28] as a thiol-reactive synthon. With this technique ^{18}F-labeling of a monomeric and dimeric thiolated RGD peptide at high specific activities and high radiochemical yields could be carried out. Recently, the Husigen [3 + 2] azide−alkyne cycloaddition (more prominent as "click chemistry") has found its way into radiopharmaceutical chemistry. The main advantages of this reaction, which can be carried out under mild copper-promoted reaction conditions, are selectivity, reliability, and short reaction time. A comparison of different strategies of chemoselective labeling of functionalized double-bridged RGD peptides confirmed that "click labeling" of peptides may be an attractive alternative to the aminooxyaldehyde condensation [29]. ^{18}F-RGD-K5, another "click chemistry"-derived RGD-based peptidomimetic PET tracer with high $\alpha_v\beta_3$ binding affinity, has already entered initial clinical trials [30] (see also below).

Some recent preclinical studies indicate the potential value of PET imaging of $\alpha_v\beta_3$ expression for response assessment. One study suggested that ^{64}Cu-RGD has the potential to monitor physiologic changes in the bone metastatic microenvironment after osteoclast-inhibiting bisphosphonate therapy. Another study in an animal model of Lewis lung cell cancer showed that PET imaging with ^{18}F-AH111585 (now called ^{18}F-fluciclatide, Figure 9.7) was able to visualize reduction of microvessel density during low-dose paclitaxel therapy, while uptake of ^{14}C-FDG did not decrease [31]. Thus, ^{18}F-AH111585 might be of potential value for assessment of response to antiangiogenic therapy. Clinical trials with this tracer are currently ongoing. Most clinical data, however, are currently still found for ^{18}F-galacto-RGD. ^{18}F-galacto-RGD was the first PET tracer applied in patients and could successfully image $\alpha_v\beta_3$ with good tumor/background ratios [32]. Further biodistribution studies have confirmed rapid clearance of ^{18}F-galacto-RGD from the blood pool and primarily renal excretion. Background activity in lung and muscle tissue was low, and the calculated effective dose was found to be similar to a ^{18}F-FDG scan [33]. Standardized uptake values and tumor/blood ratios correlated significantly with the intensity of immunohistochemical staining as well as with the microvessel density in 19 patients with solid tumors. Moreover, immunohistochemistry confirmed lack of $\alpha_v\beta_3$ expression in normal tissue and in the two tumors without tracer uptake. In squamous cell carcinoma of the head and neck (SCCHN), immunohistochemistry demonstrated predominantly vascular $\alpha_v\beta_3$ expression, suggesting that ^{18}F-galacto-RGD-PET might be used as a surrogate parameter of angiogenesis [34]. In patients with glioblastoma, normal brain tissue did not show significant tracer accumulation. In areas of highly proliferating glial tumor cells, tracer uptake in the PET images correlated with immunohistochemical $\alpha_v\beta_3$ expression of corresponding tumor samples [35]. Recently, the SPECT tracer ^{99m}Tc-NC100692 was introduced by GE Healthcare for imaging $\alpha_v\beta_3$ expression in humans and was first evaluated in breast cancer by Bach-Gansmo et al. [36]. Nineteen of 22 tumors could be detected with this agent, which was safe and well tolerated by the patients. Moreover, a PET imaging agent was also introduced. First studies with ^{18}F-AH111585 in humans have demonstrated favorable biodistribution of this tracer with predominantly renal excretion [37]. In seven patients with metastasized breast cancer all 18 tumors detected by CT were visible on the ^{18}F-AH111585-PET images [38]. Currently, a proof-of-concept study in up to 30 patients is being performed in patients with brain tumors, lung cancers, SCCHN, differentiated thyroid carcinoma, sarcoma, and melanoma to correlate dynamic and static ^{18}F-AH111585-PET imaging with histologic parameters of angiogenesis (including $\alpha_v\beta_3$ expression) and dynamic contrast-enhanced CT (*http://clinicaltrials.gov/ct2/show/NCT00565721*).

9.3.2
Imaging the Proliferative Activity of Tumors

According to Hanahan and Weinberg, proliferation is one of the key processes in oncology [39]. Therefore, a significant proportion of therapeutic drugs have been designed to inhibit cell proliferation and/or to induce apoptosis. Metabolic imaging with PET and the glucose analog ^{18}F-FDG has been demonstrated to sensitively detect malignant tumors, to identify responding tumors early in the course of anticancer treatment and to predict tumor response to therapy and patient survival. However, tumoral uptake of ^{18}F-FDG reflects proliferation only in part and is associated with false-positive findings due to unspecific tracer retention in inflammatory processes [40, 41]. One potential tracer to complement the information of ^{18}F-FDG is the thymidine analog ^{18}F-FLT, which was suggested for noninvasive assessment of proliferation and more specific tumor imaging, allowing a measurement of tumor growth and proliferative activity in malignant tumors [25]. The azidovudine-derived ^{18}F-FLT has been reported to be stable *in vitro*, and to accumulate in proliferating tissues and malignant tumors. Thymidine kinase 1 was identified as a key enzyme for the intracellular metabolism and trapping of ^{18}F-FLT (Figures 9.8–9.10) [42]. In a number of different tumor entities comprising breast cancer, colorectal cancer, lung cancer, gliomas, sarcomas, and lymphomas, a correlation of tumoral proliferation and ^{18}F-FLT uptake was shown (for review, see [43]). A clear advantage for use in the clinical routine is the well-established synthesis of ^{18}F-FLT – a procedure similar to that of the standard radiotracer ^{18}F-FDG [44].

As staging and detection of tumors still remains the domain of conventional imaging modalities and ^{18}F-FDG-PET (Figures 9.14–9.16) due to higher sensitivities compared to ^{18}F- FLT-PET, and therapy approaches comprising radio- and chemotherapy rapidly decrease proliferation rates in responding tumors, *in vivo* imaging of proliferation under therapy appears a promising indication [45]. A decrease of proliferation usually precedes changes of tumor size and therefore potentially allows an early assessment of response to therapy. This indication gains importance as many newly introduced targeted drugs have predominantly cytostatic effects and do not lead to rapid tumor shrinkage.

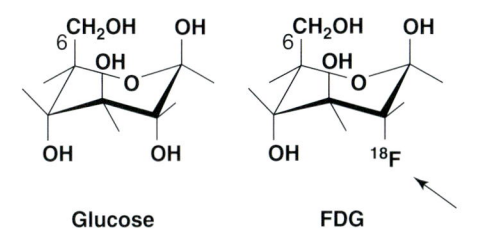

Figure 9.14 Standard PET tracer ^{18}F-FDG is used for cancer detection: structural similarity of ^{18}F-FDG and native glucose molecule.

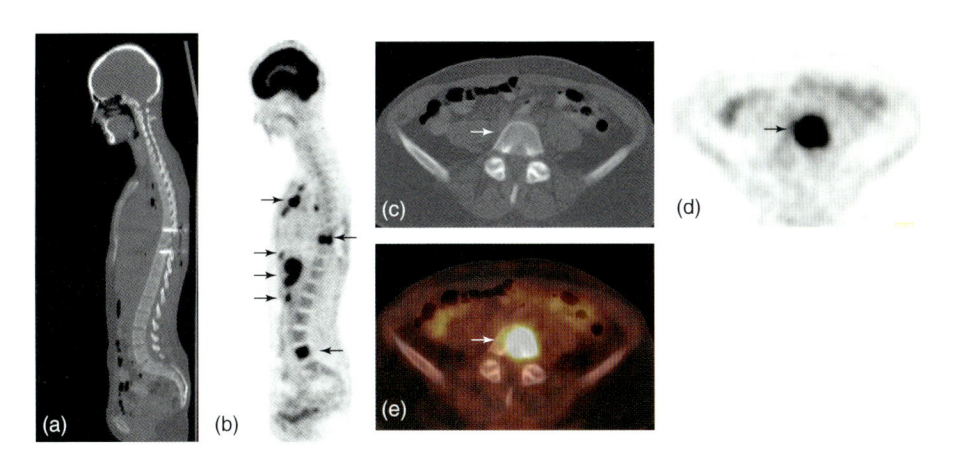

Figure 9.15 ^{18}F-FDG-PET/CT for staging malignant lymphoma. (a) Anatomically based imaging (spiral CT) indicates a single lesion in a thoracic vertebra that has been stabilized by a metal implant. (b) ^{18}F-FDG-PET indicates multiple lymphoma lesions in a lumbar vertebra (no. 5), sternum, and extraosseous lesions in the upper abdomen (arrows). (c) Normal anatomy of lumbar vertebra 5 (spiral CT, arrow). (d) Lymphoma manifestation of lumbar vertebra, as indicated by intense uptake of the glucose analog ^{18}F-FDG (arrow). (e) Further evidence of malignant bone involvement and precise anatomic delineation of the lesion using PET/CT hybrid imaging.

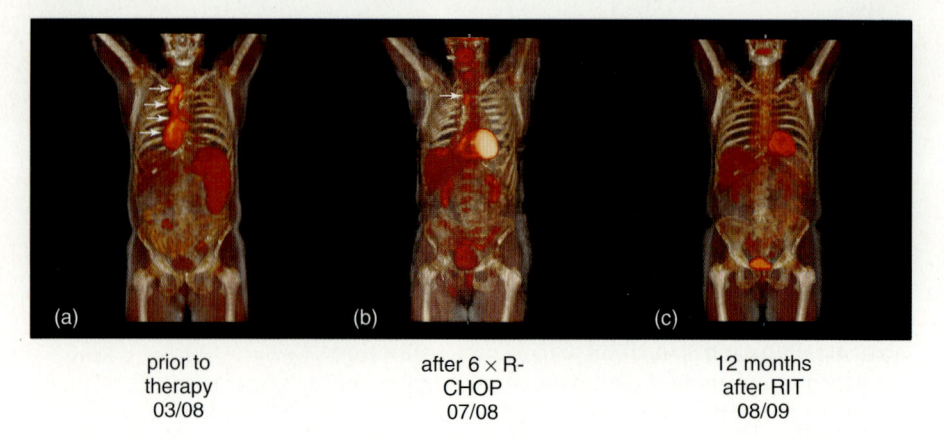

(a)	(b)	(c)
prior to therapy 03/08	after 6 × R-CHOP 07/08	12 months after RIT 08/09

Figure 9.16 ^{18}F-FDG-PET/CT for response monitoring in a patient with lymphoma. (a) Fused whole-body image with intense glucose uptake in the mediastinal lymphoma manifestation (arrows). (b) After standard chemotherapy (R-CHOP), residual ^{18}F-FDG uptake in the mediastinum indicates persisting vital tumor (arrow). (c) Due to the PET result, additional radioimmunotherapy (RIT) was performed and another follow-up PET/CT proved complete response 12 months after treatment.

In the preclinical setting it was shown in a number of studies that ^{18}F-FLT uptake decreases significantly in response to radiotherapy, cytotoxic chemotherapy, radiochemotherapy, and treatment with protein kinase inhibitors in a wide variety of different preclinical tumor models comprising esophageal cancer, lymphoma, fibrosarcoma, breast cancer, and glioblastoma (for review, see [45]). ^{18}F-FLT-PET for treatment monitoring in patients has also been studied in a number of different tumor entities. A necessary condition for repetitive imaging and assessment of therapy-induced changes is the reproducibility of the ^{18}F-FLT signal. Test–retest reproducibility for ^{18}F-FLT uptake was investigated in patients with NSCLC and head and neck cancers, and revealed to be less than 10% for standardized uptake values [46, 47]. So far it has been shown for breast cancer, lung cancer, and glioblastoma that changes of ^{18}F-FLT uptake predicted response to therapy and survival correctly [48–51]. In patients with diffuse large B-cell lymphoma ^{18}F-FLT uptake decreased significantly after CHOP administration; however, rituximab alone led to significant alteration of the ^{18}F-FLT uptake. Due to the low number of included patients and the efficient treatment it was impossible to draw any conclusions regarding prediction of response and survival [52]. In contrast, monitoring of response to treatment by ^{18}F-FLT-PET in patients with colorectal cancer undergoing neoadjuvant radiochemotherapy did not differentiate between responding and nonresponding patients. A more recently performed trial in patients with metastatic germ cell tumors undergoing chemotherapy response assessment by ^{18}F-FLT-PET did not separate responders from nonresponders [53]. It is important to mention that ^{18}F-FDG-PET was also investigated in this study population, showing comparably disappointing results as for ^{18}F-FLT-PET. In a further study in patients with non-small-lung cancer undergoing radiochemotherapy even a temporary increase of the ^{18}F-FLT signal after 2 Gy of radiation was observed and interpreted as a "flare" signal [54].

To date, the reported findings regarding therapy monitoring in patients with ^{18}F-FLT-PET are too preliminary to draw final conclusions. Reported results in varying tumor entities with different therapies indicate the need to consider disease- and drug-specific effects on the ^{18}F-FLT uptake. Interestingly, ^{18}F-FLT-PET has been reported to be more successful in monitoring palliative therapy than in neoadjuvant and highly effective, potentially curative treatments [45]. One possible interpretation is that high-dose radio-, chemoradio- or chemotherapies result in a significant decrease of the ^{18}F-FLT signal in most tumors, but that a enduring effect or complete response is only achieved in a subset of patients. Due to the low patient numbers in the majority of published studies it would be premature to draw final hypotheses, underlining the need for larger multicenter studies in a variety of tumor entities with clearly defined study protocols, valid endpoints, and in comparison to standard imaging modalities comprising CT, magnetic resonance tomography, and especially ^{18}F-FDG-PET.

9.3.3
Imaging the Hypoxic Cell Fraction of Tumors

Hypoxia is the result of an imbalance of oxygen supply and consumption in solid tumors. Factors leading to an inadequate oxygen supply are increased diffusion distances between the tumor blood vessels and tumor cells, impaired structure and function of the tumor microvasculature, and decreased oxygen transport capacity of the blood due to disease- or treatment-related anemia. Tumor hypoxia is of clinical interest as hypoxic tumors are associated with an increased local aggressiveness, a higher potential of developing distant metastasis, and an increased resistance to chemo- and radiotherapy, which has been shown for different tumor entities (e.g., SCCHN, cervical cancer, and soft-tissue sarcomas).

Hypoxic areas are typically distributed inhomogenously in solid tumors. Hypoxia-selective radiotracers labeled either with γ-emitting radioisotopes for SPECT imaging or positron-emitting isotopes (e.g., ^{18}F and ^{62}Cu) for PET imaging deliver three-dimensional maps of the hypoxia distribution in tumors. Most preclinical and clinical studies have been performed using hypoxia tracers for PET imaging, as this method delivers quantitative images and, compared to SPECT, a higher spatial resolution can be achieved in the clinical setting.

One group of hypoxia-selective radiotracers is based on 2-nitroimidazoles, comprised of an imidazole ring containing a nitro group at the 2′ position and different side-chains at the 1′ position determining their pharmacokinetic properties. In vital tissues, the nitro group is reduced enzymatically by nitroreductases and in normoxic tissues it is quickly reoxidized to its initial state in the presence of O_2. However, in hypoxic tissues, reoxidation is impaired and further reduction steps take place leading to a reactive alkylating amine metabolite covalently binding to intracellular macromolecules, irreversibly trapping the compound in these tissues. Due to the dependence of this mechanism on the availability of functional nitroreductases, this process only occurs in vital hypoxic tissues, not in areas of necrosis.

^{18}F-FMISO is the most extensively studied 2-nitroimidazole compound for PET imaging of hypoxia in the preclinical and clinical setting. ^{18}F-FMISO showed a 26-fold increased accumulation in hypoxic tumor cells compared to normoxic controls *in vitro* [55], and *in vivo* its hypoxia-dependent tissue accumulation has been demonstrated in a hepatic artery occlusion model in pigs. In xenograft tumor models, a good correlation between direct measurement of the partial pressure of oxygen (pO$_2$) with a polarographic needle electrode and ^{18}F-FMISO accumulation was reported [56], and ^{18}F-FMISO accumulation in xenograft tumors was increased in mice breathing room air compared to a group of mice breathing carbogen gas (95% O$_2$/5% CO$_2$). In cancer patients, positive correlations were also reported between direct pO$_2$ electrode measurements and ^{18}F-FMISO-PET uptake in SCCHN.

Other hypoxia-selective PET tracers based on the 2-nitroimidazole structure have been developed with the aim of enhancing their pharmacokinetic properties for *in vivo* PET imaging (e.g., by increasing their hydrophilicity). An ideal radiotracer for imaging of tissue hypoxia should possess balanced lipophilic/hydrophilic properties. On the one hand, it should be lipophilic enough to show a homogeneous tissue penetration, as hypoxia typically occurs in areas of impaired perfusion. On the other hand, it should be washed out of normoxic tissues at a suitable rate and should be excreted from the organism quickly preferably via the kidneys, which is the case for more hydrophilic compounds. Examples for more hydrophilic 2-nitroimidazoles than ^{18}F-FMISO are ^{18}F-fluoroazomycin-arabinofuranoside (^{18}F-FAZA), ^{18}F-fluoroerythronitroimidazole (^{18}F-FETNIM), or ^{18}F-fluoroetanidazole (^{18}F-FETA) [57], and superior biokinetics over ^{18}F-FMISO have been reported for ^{18}F-FAZA and ^{18}F-FETA *in vivo* [58, 59].

Cu-ATSM is a hypoxia-selective radiotracer that is not based on a nitroimidazole structure. Instead, it is comprised of a chelate of a Cu(II) ion complexed by diacetyl-bis(N^4-methylthiosemicarbazone) (ATSM). Complexion with a copper isotope that decays under positron emission (e.g., ^{60}Cu, ^{61}Cu, ^{62}Cu, or ^{64}Cu) enables its application as a PET tracer for hypoxia imaging. The mechanism of hypoxia-dependent accumulation of Cu-ATSM is based on the reduction of Cu(II) to Cu(I) in the mitochondria of hypoxic cells, leading to dissociation of the complex and subsequent trapping of the copper ion in the intracellular copper pool. PET images acquired by Cu-ATSM typically show a higher signal/noise ratio than ^{18}F-FMISO, which facilitates delineation of hypoxic tumor subvolumes. However, the uptake of Cu-ATSM in tumors might be dependent on other tissue-specific factors additional to the oxygenation status of the tumor, as in some cell lines no significant hypoxia-dependent tumor uptake of Cu-ATSM could be observed [60–62].

In clinical studies, the pretherapeutic tumor oxygenation status assessed by hypoxia PET was predictive of patient outcome in several tumor entities (e.g., SCCHN, lung, cervical and rectal cancer, and brain tumors). Tumor reoxygenation assessed by hypoxia PET during the course of chemo- or radiotherapy was also predictive of an increased survival [57, 63]. In the future, hypoxia PET might also prove to be of value in radiation therapy planning, especially with the aim of selective dose escalation to the potentially more radioresistant hypoxic tumor subvolumes. However, due to limitations of the method, such as the typically low signal/noise ratio in PET images delivered by many hypoxia-selective radiotracers, further clinical studies are needed to validate this approach.

9.3.4
Imaging Receptor Expression

Receptors specifically overexpressed on the surface of tumor cells pose a target for molecular imaging, which in oncology can be useful for tumor detection (staging), patient selection for receptor-targeted forms of therapy, or therapy monitoring. For *in vivo* receptor imaging, sensitive methods of tracer detection are required, as typically the receptor concentration and thus the amount of specifically bound ligand in the tissue is very low. The radiotracer approach with SPECT and especially PET techniques allows sensitive tracer detection in the femtomolar range, and can be employed for molecular imaging of receptor expression *in vivo* by radiolabeling physiologic receptor ligands or analog compounds. Some examples of receptors that have been successfully used for tumor imaging are SSTRs, epidermal growth factor receptors (EGFRs), bombesin receptors, estrogen and androgen receptors, steroid receptors, and integrins [64]. Since in the last decades imaging of SSTR expression has found its way into routine clinical management of patients with neuroendocrine tumors, this chapter will focus on imaging of this receptor type.

Neuroendocrine tumors are a heterogeneous group of tumors originating from cells of the disseminated endocrine system, including gastroenteropancreatic neuroendocrine tumors, carcinoids, paragangliomas, medullar thyroid carcinoma, and pituitary adenomas. Most frequently these tumors are localized in the gastrointestinal tract and in the lung. Overall, neuroendocrine tumors are of low incidence – only about 2% of all gastrointestinal malignancies are of neuroendocrine origin. One common feature of neuroendocrine tumors is the overexpression of SSTRs, a family of receptors comprised of five subtypes (SSTR1–5). SSTR2 is of special clinical interest as this subtype is most frequently overexpressed in neuroendocrine tumors, next to SSTR5 [65]. Somatostatin, the physiologic ligand of SSTRs, is a polypeptide existing in different splicing variants – one comprised of 14, the other of 28 amino acids. However, due to its susceptibility to degradation resulting in a short half-life *in vivo* of approximately 2 min [66], it is not feasible as a radiotracer for *in vivo* tumor imaging. The development of cyclic oligopeptides analogous to somatostatin by increasing their plasma half-life by protection against degradation *in vivo* while maintaining high affinity to the SSTR, especially SSTR2, led to compounds that are suitable for radionuclide imaging of SSTR expression *in vivo*.

About 15 years ago, pentetreotide was introduced into the clinic as a radiotracer approved by the US Food and Drug Administration for scintigraphic imaging of patients with neuroendocrine tumors. It can be labeled with the γ-emitting isotope ^{111}In (half-life 2.8 days) via the chelating substance diethylenetriaminepentaacetic acid (DTPA) for planar scintigraphy or SPECT imaging (^{111}In-DTPA-OC; Octreoscan®). Typically, scintigraphy is performed 4–6 h after tracer injection. Late images are acquired 24 h after tracer administration, characterized by better tumor/background contrast than the early images, although impaired by higher unspecific intestinal activity due to hepatobiliary excretion. The detection rate of neuroendocrine tumors by SSTR scintigraphy is to a large part influenced by the SSTR density on the cell surface and thus dependent on the grade of differentiation of the tumor. Accordingly, in a clinical study, the tumor detection sensitivity for ^{111}In-DTPA-OC scintigraphy was reported as 95% for highly differentiated neuroendocrine tumors, 86% for highly differentiated neuroendocrine carcinomas, and only 60% for low differentiated neuroendocrine carcinomas [67]. Radiotracers labeled with the γ emitter ^{99m}Tc (half-life 6.0 h) for *in vivo* SSTR imaging have also been developed (^{99m}Tc-EDDA/HYNIC-TOC/-TATE/-NOC), resulting in lower radiation exposure for the patient and potentially better image quality due to higher spatial resolution, especially with SPECT imaging [68]; however, none of these tracers have yet been officially approved for clinical routine use.

For PET and PET/CT imaging of neuroendocrine tumors (Figures 9.17 and 9.18), somatostatin analogs coupled to the chelator DOTA have been developed, which

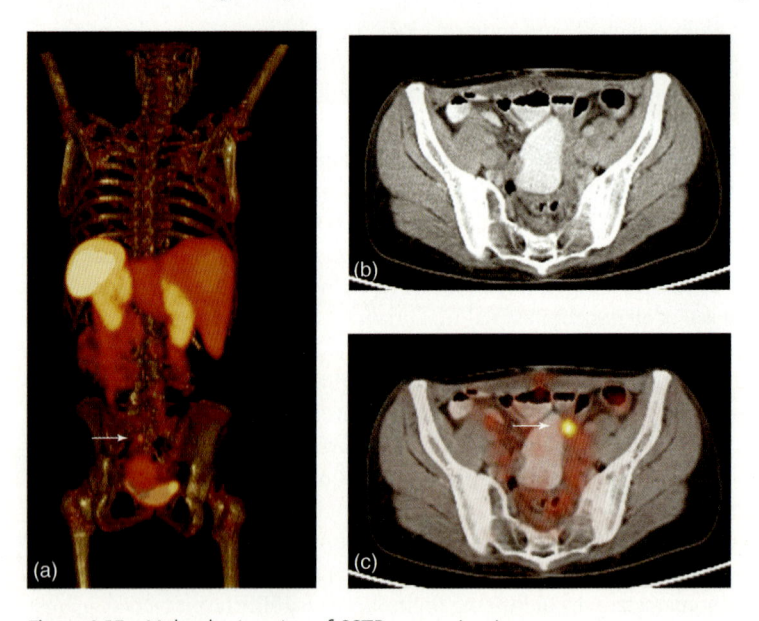

Figure 9.17 Molecular imaging of SSTR expression in a patient with neuroendocrine cancer. (a) Intense focal uptake of the somatostatin analog ^{68}Ga-DOTA-TOC indicates a small recurrent tumor lesion (less than 5 mm). (b) CT scan alone shows normal anatomic structures. (c) The tumor can be precisely delineated in fused images using ^{68}Ga-DOTA-TOC.

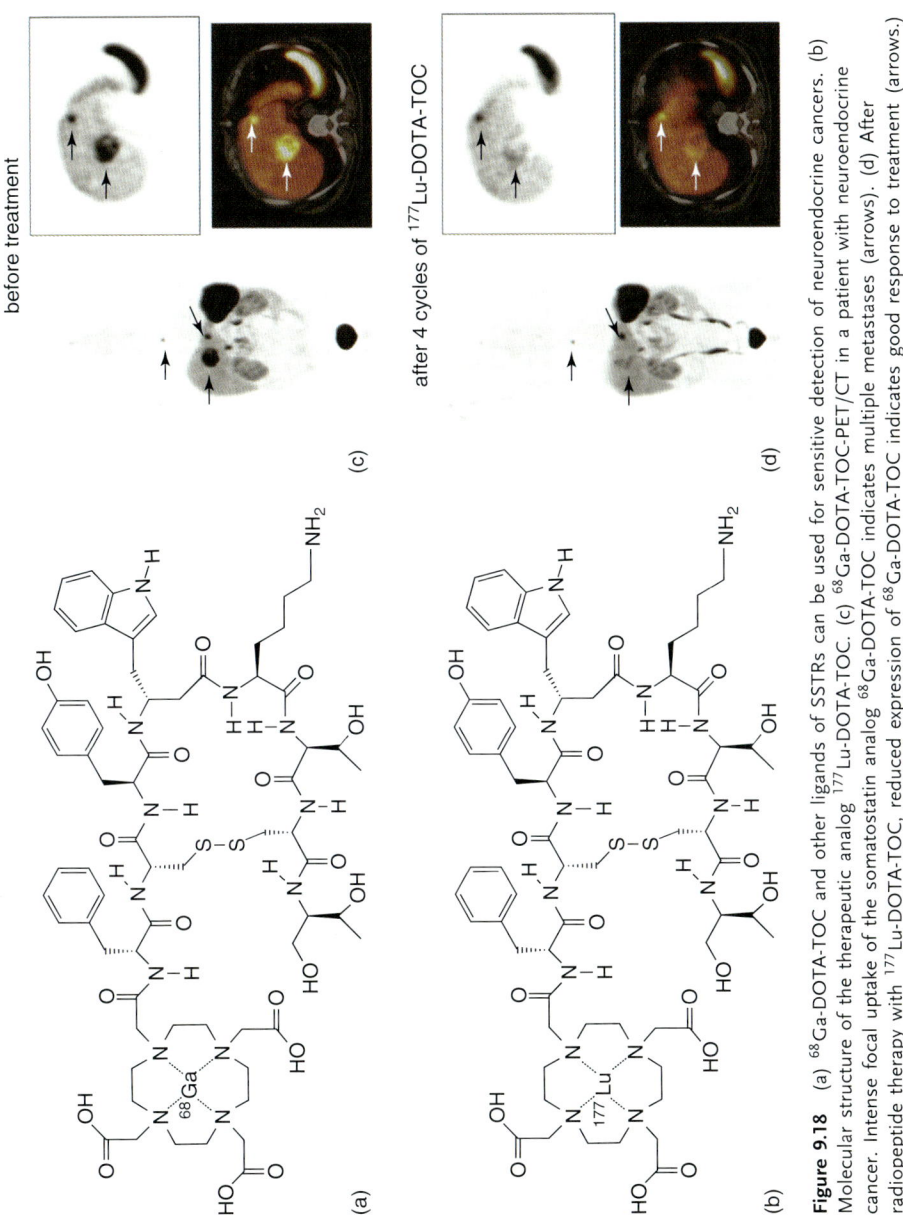

Figure 9.18 (a) ^{68}Ga-DOTA-TOC and other ligands of SSTRs can be used for sensitive detection of neuroendocrine cancers. (b) Molecular structure of the therapeutic analog ^{177}Lu-DOTA-TOC. (c) ^{68}Ga-DOTA-TOC-PET/CT in a patient with neuroendocrine cancer. Intense focal uptake of the somatostatin analog ^{68}Ga-DOTA-TOC indicates multiple metastases (arrows). (d) After radiopeptide therapy with ^{177}Lu-DOTA-TOC, reduced expression of ^{68}Ga-DOTA-TOC indicates good response to treatment (arrows.)

allows stable labeling with ^{68}Ga – a positron-emitting generator-produced metal isotope (half-life 68 min). Compared to SPECT imaging, PET delivers higher spatial resolution images and a higher tumor/background contrast in the clinical setting, thus resulting in a better image quality and higher sensitivity for detection of SSTR-overexpressing tumor tissue. Due to faster pharmacokinetics compared to ^{111}In-DTPA-OC used for planar scintigraphy and SPECT, PET images may be acquired already as early as 20 min after tracer injection, minimizing unspecific intestinal activity. Examples of PET tracers are DOTA-TOC, -TATE, or -NOC, which differ slightly in their amino acid sequence and their affinities to the SSTR subtypes; however, all of them show a high affinity to the SSTR subtype 2, which is of highest relevance for tumor imaging [69]. Patient studies have shown a good correlation between SSTR expression assessed by immunohistochemistry and ^{68}Ga-DOTA-TOC-PET uptake of neuroendocrine tumors [70]. As PET imaging allows quantitative assessment of tracer uptake, it could also be useful for monitoring of patients with neuroendocrine tumors undergoing therapy (Figure 9.18).

In the recent years, peptide receptor radionuclide therapy (PRRT) of neuroendocrine tumors has found its way into the clinic. By labeling somatostatin analogs with therapeutically active β-emitting radionuclides, like ^{90}Y or ^{177}Lu, encouraging results have already been reported in patients with inoperable metastasized neuroendocrine carcinoma treated with PRRT [71]. As ^{177}Lu also emits γ radiation suitable for radionuclide imaging, planar scintigraphy or SPECT imaging could potentially be used for dosimetric estimation of the radiation exposure of patients undergoing PRRT.

9.4
Clinical Applications of SPECT/CT and PET

9.4.1
Differentiation of Benign from Malignant Tumors and Cancer Detection

Due to the different glucose consumption of benign and malignant lesions, ^{18}F-FDG-PET allows assessment of undefined tumors detected by conventional imaging modalities such as CT or MRI. Furthermore, PET sometimes allows detection of malignant lesions even when no or only minimal morphologic alterations are present. Regarding evaluation of indeterminate pulmonary nodules, prospective studies reported sensitivity values for ^{18}F-FDG-PET between 89 and 100%, a specificity of 69–100%, and an overall accuracy of 89–96%. ^{18}F-FDG is not tumor-specific, leading also to nonspecific tracer accumulation in benign, predominantly inflammatory lesions [72]. However, surgery may be circumvented in patients with increased perioperative risk if the PET scan is negative. Dynamic data acquisition can further enhance the accuracy of PET imaging. In malignant lesions, a continuous increase of glucose uptake has been described, whereas benign lesions showed an increase of ^{18}F-FDG uptake followed by rapid efflux of ^{18}F-FDG. Dual-timepoint imaging or delayed PET imaging after 1 and 2 h contributes to better differentiate between benign and malignant tumors.

PET can also be used for detection of the malignant primary ("cancer of unknown primary"). PET is especially useful in detecting primary tumors in the head and neck region [73]. In the case of increased tumor markers or paraneoplastic syndromes, PET can aid in localizing the primary tumor manifestation site.

9.4.2
Staging of Cancer: Prognostic Potential of Imaging Biomarkers

For optimal treatment of patients with cancer, precise knowledge of the extent of the disease is crucial (Figure 9.15). If cancer is detected at a stage in which uncontrolled growth of tumor cells takes place, but no tumor manifestations are present in distant organs, surgery is usually performed to obtain ultimate cure. However, if the tumor has already spread to distant organs, cure can usually not be achieved by surgery alone. In this situation, surgery has to be replaced or supported by systemic chemo- and/or radiotherapy to entirely destroy the primary tumor and metastatic sites or to induce growth arrest in the tumor. In this context, PET has several advantages compared to conventional imaging modalities [74]. Small tumor manifestation sites, such as metastases in the bone, liver, lung, and adrenal gland, or in rare locations, such as soft tissues, thyroid, or (sub-)cutaneous lesions, can be detected. However, micrometastases or single tumor cells can also not be detected with PET. Also, small lung metastases may appear negative at ^{18}F-FDG-PET. In principal, staging of all tumors is possible. With the standard radiotracer ^{18}F-FDG, PET is highly accurate for staging of NSCLC, thyroid cancer, tumors of the head and neck region, colorectal and esophageal cancer, malignant lymphomas, sarcoma, and melanoma. PET has been demonstrated to cause a change in patient management in 15–40% depending on the type of cancer. Some tumors present without increased glucose consumption, such as prostate or neuroendocrine cancer. ^{11}C-CHO-PET and ^{11}C-CHO-PET/CT have been demonstrated to be highly accurate for staging and especially restaging of prostate cancer. ^{68}Ga-DOTA-TOC is a new PET tracer for imaging neuroendocrine tumors. A variety of molecular probes have been evaluated to address biologic targets or metabolic pathways *in vivo* (Table 9.1). In the majority of these compounds, clinical utility remains to be determined.

The most important prognostic factor is the tumor stage at initial presentation. However, risk stratification according to the tumor/node/metastasis (TNM) system is also subject to error, because patients with limited disease undergoing definite therapy may also develop recurrent disease. Other factors such as tumor aggressiveness or metabolic activity of tumors may aid in individual risk assessment. Several studies have correlated the intensity of ^{18}F-FDG uptake in the primary tumor to progression-free and overall survival in various cancers. In lung cancer, intensity of ^{18}F-FDG uptake turned out to be an independent prognostic marker.

The prognostic potential of PET has also been described for colorectal cancer, breast cancer, and malignant lymphoma.

9.4.3
Assessment of Response to Therapy

Therapeutic efficiency of chemo- and radiotherapeutic strategies varies significantly between individual patients. Therefore, noninvasive assessment of the performance of a therapeutic protocol in an individual patient is highly desirable. With conventional imaging modalities such as CT or MRI, response to therapy can be detected as early as a reduction in tumor size occurs. On the contrary, PET allows assessment of response to treatment at an earlier timepoint before tumor shrinkage can be detected by conventional imaging [75]. In responding tumors, metabolism of tumor cells is markedly decreased due to the cytotoxic effect of the respective therapeutic regimen. Concomitantly, accumulation of ^{18}F-FDG is reduced. This is a sign of an efficient treatment and has a high prognostic value regarding the success of further treatment. In the case of a nonresponding tumor, the therapeutic regimen can be altered by changing the combination of cytotoxic drugs or the radiation dose. In breast cancer, rapid decline of ^{18}F-FDG uptake already after one cycle of chemotherapy was demonstrated, whereas in nonresponding tumors increasing or unchanged ^{18}F-FDG uptake was described. A variety of other neoplasms including malignant lymphoma, gastric and esophageal cancer, head and neck, or NSCLC showed rapid reduction of ^{18}F-FDG uptake in responding tumors. Significantly better disease-free and overall survival was described in responders compared to tumors without significant reduction of tumoral ^{18}F-FDG uptake. Clinical studies are needed reporting on the clinical benefit of a PET-guided change of patient management.

9.4.4
Restaging of Cancer and Detection of Recurrence

After definite surgery or chemo/radiotherapy, examinations and imaging at follow-up is important to early detect disease recurrence originating from residual tumor cells. In daily clinical practice, differentiation between scar tissue and vital tumor tissue is a frequent problem. At anatomically based imaging modalities, both are present as indeterminate tissue formation and, frequently, biopsy is needed for further clarification. Differentiation of scar tissue from vital tumor tissue is a prerequisite of PET imaging. While new onset of cancer tissue is associated with increased metabolism causing increased uptake of, for example, ^{18}F-FDG, scar tissue is frequently associated with reduced metabolism compared to the surrounding normal tissue. PET is especially useful in the follow-up of tumor entities such as colorectal and esophageal cancer, NSCLC, breast cancer, tumors of the head and neck, brain tumors, melanoma, and malignant lymphoma. Restaging with PET is also approved for differentiated thyroid cancer with a negative ^{131}I whole-body scan and elevated tumor marker thyroglobulin.

9.4.5
PET for Radiation Treatment Planning

The use of metabolic information leads to biological target volumes that can have a substantial impact on radiation treatment planning by increasing or reducing the target volume [76]. The additional identification of tumor manifestation sites that are not visible at conventional staging causes an enlargement of respective target volume. On the other hand, the radiation field can be reduced when nonmalignant lesions such as atelectatic tissue can be reliably characterized as benign. Consecutively, radiation dose to surrounding normal tissue can be reduced. The use of PET for radiation treatment planning leads to a change of the target volume in up to 60% of patients. This is in part related to pretherapeutic detection of distant metastases, previously unknown metastases in locoregional lymph nodes, or characterization of suspicious lesions as benign. However, PET-based radiotherapy planning is not trivial. In particular, the delineation of the primary tumor is subject to a relevant interobserver variability. There is a need for standardized evaluation criteria of PET allowing also the quantification of metabolic changes. The recent introduction of PET/CT hybrid scanners has led to a reduction of errors concerning image coregistration. In several prospective studies it was shown that overall survival of patients receiving PET-guided radiation therapy was significantly longer compared to patients receiving standard treatment. Prospective randomized studies have to be performed demonstrating that the use of PET positively affects patient outcome and overall survival.

9.4.6
PET for Cancer Drug Development

PET imaging has unique properties for use in drug development. Therapeutic efficiency of a novel drug can be evaluated noninvasively by assessment of specific biologic endpoints [77], such as changes in cellular proliferation (e.g., by the use of ^{18}F-FLT), glucose utilization (^{18}F-FDG), tissue perfusion (^{15}O-H$_2$O), metabolism of amino acids (^{18}F-FET, ^{11}C-MET), or inhibition of angiogenesis (^{18}F-galacto-RGD). (Over)expression of the therapeutic target such as thymidylate synthase, VEGFR, ErbB2, or estrogen receptor status can be quantified with ^{11}C-THY, radiolabeled antibodies specifically binding to VEGF or ErbB2, or ^{18}F-fluoro-17-β-estradiol, respectively. Assessing biologic endpoints further provides proof of principle of the proposed mechanism of action. PET can also be utilized for *in vivo* evaluation of gene expression, for example, by the use of the substrate ^{124}I-fluoro-5-iodo-1-β-D-arabinofuranosyluracil (^{124}I-FIAU) for the detection of herpes simplex virus thymidine kinase type 1 or Na^{124}I for the detection of sodium iodide symporter expression.

Generic endpoints can also be studied by PET. Drugs or biochemical probes can be labeled with positron emitters such as small molecules, proteins, or antibodies. Drugs that have been evaluated so far include ^{18}F-fluorouracil, ^{18}F-tamoxifen, and ^{13}N-cisplatin. Pharmacokinetics of a drug can be investigated in tumors and normal tissues, in animal models, or as part of clinical phase I (or phase II) studies. In the future, PET will be increasingly used to assess the efficiency of novel anticancer drugs.

9.4.7
SPECT/CT for Mapping of SLNs

In cancer patients, accurate lymph node staging is mandatory for appropriate treatment planning. A combination of preoperative lymphoscintigraphy and intraoperative mapping with blue dye has been demonstrated as a practical approach to accurately localize the SLNs. However, planar scintigrams lack anatomic information, making a correct localization of SLNs problematic. Whereas most SLNs can be identified intraoperatively using a hand-held probe, SLN identification may be impossible in certain cases. Preoperative localization using CT coregistration may facilitate operative access and thus improves overall detection rates.

The added value of CT coregistration for SLN mapping has been demonstrated by many groups. Whereas inguinal and lower axillary nodes can be reliably detected on planar scintigrams, anatomic coregistration represents a valuable tool for SLN detection in the pelvis, the mediastinum, or the head and neck region. In patients with melanoma of the head and neck or the trunk, a pilot study indicated that SPECT/CT enables detection of SLNs in up to 43% of patients negative at planar scintigrams [78]. In patients with early-stage cervical cancer and invasive bladder cancer, superior detection of SLNs compared to planar scintigrams has been described. The CT portion of the examination was especially helpful for the intraoperative identification of SLNs. The clinical utility of SPECT/CT in head and neck cancers has been investigated by several groups. In 20 patients with oral squamous cell carcinoma, Khafif *et al.* showed a sensitivity of SPECT/CT of 87.5% [79]. SPECT/CT further improved SLN identification and localization compared to planar images in six patients (30%). In another series comprising 34 patients, SPECT/CT identified the SLN in 94% (32/34) and identified additional nodes in 47% (15/32). More accurate localization of SLN was also described by Keski-Santti in oral cavity squamous cell carcinoma [80]. Enhancement of topographic SLN assignment with SPECT/CT was described in a two further studies in head and neck cancer or melanoma [78, 81].

Husarik *et al.* examined the added value of SPECT/CT over planar scintigraphy in breast cancer [82]. In 41 consecutive patients, findings at planar scintigrams and SPECT/CT were identical in only seven patients (17%), whereas SPECT/CT indicated the correct anatomical localization in 29 patients (70%) according to the American Joint Committee on Cancer staging system. In six patients, additional SLNs were detected which were located in close proximity to the injection site and were not visible at planar scintigrams due to scatter radiation. Misinterpretation of planar scintigrams occurred in seven patients (17%) due to confusion of injection site or cutaneous contaminations and SLNs. In 26 patients (63%), exact anatomic localization could be derived exclusively by SPECT/CT and three SLNs close to the injection site not detected with SPECT could be clearly visualized with

SPECT/CT. Similar findings have been described recently by Lerman *et al.* [83]. In 157 consecutive patients, 13% of SLNs were visualized with SPECT/CT, but not with planar scintigrams. Unexpected sites of drainage and hotspots that were not node related were found at SPECT/CT in 33 patients. In another prospective series comprising 51 patients, SLNs could be assigned to axillary levels I–III using SPECT/CT data, but not planar images [84]. In a pilot study by van der Ploeg *et al.* [85], SPECT/CT was superior to SPECT regarding SLN detection. In four out of 31 patients, six additional SLN could be detected with SPECT/CT, leading to a change of management in 5% of patients. Furthermore, SPECT/CT was able to detect SLNs in three patients in whom planar images failed to demonstrate lymphatic drainage.

SPECT/CT has been shown to be especially useful in overweight patients. In a prospective study comprising 220 patients with breast cancer, 122 patients with a body mass index greater than 25 were identified [86]. In 49 patients (22%), planar images failed to identify a SLN. However, in 29 of these (59%), the SLNs could be identified with SPECT/CT. Overall, sensitivity of SPECT/CT in overweight patients was 89%. SPECT/CT was also superior to intraoperative blue dye labeling and identified the SLNs in 75% of patients in whom the blue dye technique failed to detect the SLNs.

9.4.8
SPECT/CT for Detection of Bone Metastases

For more than 30 years, planar bone scintigraphy and, more recently, SPECT have represented valuable methods to sensitively detect or characterize focal bone pathology [87]. Whereas functional bone imaging is a highly sensitive method, it lacks specificity [88]. Therefore, X-ray, CT, or MRI is frequently performed after bone scintigraphy to further characterize lesions evident at bone scans. Integrated SPECT/CT offers direct correlation of focal bone pathology to anatomic structures and therefore minimizes the number of equivocal findings.

Screening for bone metastases and evaluation of treatment response represents the most frequent indication for bone scanning. Whereas the majority of bone metastases appear as hotspots, several appear as cold lesions. Benign lesions such as hemangioma may also appear as "cold," making the differential diagnosis problematic. Differentiation of benign and malignant lesions can usually be achieved with coregistration of CT and is a major advantage of SPECT/CT. Furthermore, fused images can be used to further guide biopsy of bone lesions.

A normal tracer distribution at planar bone scans usually makes the use of SPECT/CT unnecessary. Whereas in many cases the correct diagnosis can already be derived from planar bone scans, SPECT/CT is necessary to make the correct diagnosis in the case of undefined lesions. In particular, scintigraphic lesions in the spine or pelvis can frequently not be exactly defined, requiring the additional use of CT or MRI. Recently, image coregistration was demonstrated to be superior to planar radiographic techniques or SPECT and proved useful in further characterizing benign skeletal abnormalities. The presence of accompanying complications such as fractures or compression of the spinal cord can also be diagnosed in a single examination [89].

The first report demonstrating the superiority of SPECT/CT over planar or SPECT imaging was published by Römer et al. [90]. In this retrospective study, SPECT-guided CT was reported to clarify more than 90% of bone lesions indeterminate at SPECT. Sixty-three percent of indeterminate findings could be definitely assigned as benign lesions, involving mostly osteochondrosis, spondylosis, or spondylarthrosis of the spine. Twenty-nine percent of all lesions could be clearly assigned to osteolytic or osteosclerotic bone metastases. Four lesions (8%) remained indeterminate also at SPECT/CT due to a missing anatomic correlate. The majority of these lesions were located in the ribs or scapula. Since performance of MRI in the thorax is also affected by motion artifacts, the authors concluded that even MRI may not be able to confirm or exclude bone metastases in such lesions. The study also indicates that exact matching of functional and anatomic data may be necessary, especially in small anatomic structures. Small osteolytic bone metastases were observed in close proximity to facet joints, potentially causing misinterpretation of SPECT lesions. The concept of Römer et al. included the use of SPECT data for determination of the field of view for CT scanning, resulting in reduced additional radiation exposure. On a patient basis, mean radiation exposure of additional CT scanning was as low as 2.3 mSv. "SPECT-guided CT" therefore results in acceptable overall radiation exposure. The use of CT data for attenuation correction may also increase the performance of SPECT, but this issue has not been studied in detail [91, 92].

Using a combination of a dual-head SPECT camera and a low-dose nondiagnostic CT scanner, Horger et al. were also able to correctly classify 85% of unclear foci compared to 36% using SPECT alone [93]. Integrated SPECT/CT seems also to be superior to side-by-side reading of SPECT and CT images. Using juxtaposed CT and SPECT scanners, Utsunomiya et al. demonstrated that fused images were superior for differentiation of malignant from benign lesions compared to side-by-side reading [94].

Bone metastases may be apparent at functional imaging only, which cannot be further confirmed by CT or planar radiographs. Lytic bone lesions do not become evident at CT or radiographs until more than 50–70% of the trabecular structure has been destroyed by the tumor. Nevertheless, SPECT/CT can usually provide the correct diagnosis also in indeterminate lesions, illustrating the benefit of combined SPECT/CT imaging in a one-step procedure.

9.4.9
SPECT/CT in Thyroid Cancer

In patients with differentiated thyroid carcinoma, whole-body imaging after oral administration of ^{131}I or ^{123}I is commonly performed to identify residual or metastatic disease. ^{131}I scintigraphy has a higher sensitivity compared to morphologically based imaging modalities. However, interpretation of ^{131}I images may be difficult due to the absence of anatomic landmarks. Therefore, precise localization of hotspots is frequently not possible. In addition, physiologic uptake of ^{131}I may cause false-positive findings (Figure 9.1). Integrated SPECT/CT imaging potentially allows differentiation of physiological, artificial, and pathological uptake of ^{131}I. In a retrospective study by Tharp et al., SPECT/CT had an incremental diagnostic value in 41 of 71 patients (57%) [95]. Especially in the neck region, SPECT/CT allowed the precise characterization of equivocal lesions in 14 of 17 patients and changed lesion location in five patients. SPECT/CT also improved the characterization of indeterminate findings as definitely benign in 13% (9/71), precise designation of metastases to the skeleton in 17% (12/71), and to the lungs versus mediastinum in 6% (5/71). SPECT/CT further optimized the designation of ^{131}I uptake to lymph node metastases versus remnant thyroid tissue and to lung versus mediastinal metastases. Overall, additional findings at SPECT/CT had an impact on patient management in 41%.

A study by Yamamoto in 17 patients with differentiated thyroid carcinoma demonstrated that SPECT/CT image fusion using external markers improved the diagnosis in 15 of 17 patients (88%) mainly due to better anatomic localization of scintigraphic findings and differentiation of physiologic from specific uptake [96]. Fused images caused a change in management in four of 17 patients (24%). A pilot study in 25 patients undergoing thyroablative radioiodine treatment also indicated an added value of SPECT/CT image fusion. Using an integrated SPECT/CT camera, Ruf et al. reported superior anatomic localization in 44% of suspicious lesions (17/39). The findings returned by fused imaging influenced the therapeutic management in 25% of patients (6/24) [97].

9.4.10
SPECT/CT for Imaging of Adrenocortical Tumors

Morphologic imaging modalities such as CT or MRI offer high sensitivity for detection of tumors of the sympathetic nervous system. Major advantages of radionuclide imaging such as ^{123}I-MIBG-SPECT are a high specificity that can be used for better characterization of lesions, and superior differentiation of scar tissue and residual tumor in a postoperative situation [98, 99]. Radionuclide imaging is also helpful for detection of extra-adrenal tumor sites. In a prospective study, Franzius et al. evaluated the clinical utility of ^{123}I-MIBG-SPECT/CT in 19 patients with a variety of tumors of the sympathetic nervous system including neuroblastoma and pheochromocytoma [100]. ^{123}I-MIBG-SPECT/CT showed a similar sensitivity of 93% compared to 99% achieved with PET/CT using ^{11}C-*meta*-hydroxyephedrine (^{11}C-HED) as tracer. ^{11}C-HED-PET/CT has been demonstrated to show a higher spatial resolution and to return the final diagnosis within 30 min. SPECT/CT was compromised by a longer examination time and the necessity to perform delayed imaging 24 h after tracer administration. However, no superiority of PET/CT over SPECT/CT was observed. Due to the high cost and reduced availability of ^{11}C, ^{123}I-MIBG-SPECT/CT seems therefore appropriate for imaging of tumors derived

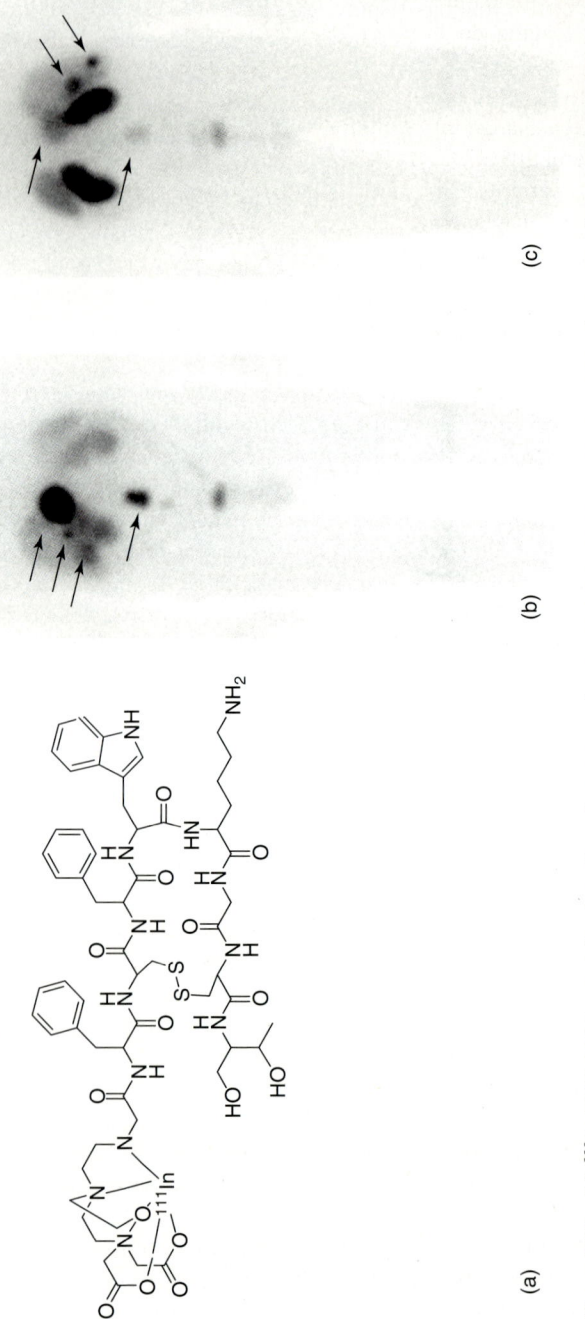

Figure 9.19 (a) ^{111}In-DTPA-OC is used for detection of somatostatin receptor expression using conventional scintigraphic or tomographic (SPECT) imaging. (b) Patient with neuroendocrine cancer in the pancreas as well as metastases in the liver and retroperitoneal lymph nodes (ventral view, arrows). (c) Dorsal view of the same patient. Imaging was performed 24 h after injection of ^{111}In-DTPA-OC.

from the sympathetic nervous system, such as neuroblastoma, pheochromocytoma, ganglioneuroblastoma, or paraganglioma.

Scintigraphic techniques also complement anatomically based imaging modalities for evaluation of adrenocortical disease. The impact of hybrid SPECT/CT imaging on the performance of functional imaging tests such as ^{75}Se-selenomethylnorcholesterol or ^{131}I-iodocholesterol remains to be determined since only few data can be derived from the literature. In a pilot study, Even-Sapir *et al.* reported a change in the clinical management in a few patients undergoing ^{75}Se-cholesterol-SPECT/CT [101]. Despite an obvious lack of clinical studies demonstrating the superiority of integrated SPECT/CT over separately performed imaging modalities, one may speculate that hybrid imaging will increase the diagnostic accuracy and may evoke a more frequent use of functional imaging techniques.

9.4.11
SPECT/CT in Neuroendocrine Tumors

Neuroendocrine tumors usually exhibit increased expression of SSTRs, enabling their detection due to specific binding of radiolabeled ligands, such as ^{111}In-DTPA^0-D-Phe^1-OC (Figure 9.19) or ^{111}In-pentetreotide. SSTR scintigraphy is predominantly used for detection of primary tumors, and hepatic or mesenteric metastases, but can also be used for assessment of response to treatment with somatostatin analogs. The number of publications illustrating the added value of CT coregistration to planar SSTR images or SSTR-SPECT is limited. The largest study so far performed SSTR-SPECT/CT in 72 patients with various neuroendocrine tumors, including 45 carcinoid tumors, medullary thyroid carcinoma, or islet cell tumors [102]. No additional information compared to planar images or SPECT was achieved in 48 patients, whereas SPECT/CT improved localization of scintigraphic findings in 23 patients (32%) and changed the clinical management in 14%. In another series comprising 27 patients with various neuroendocrine tumors, Even-Sapir *et al.* have demonstrated increased accuracy of SPECT-detected lesions undergoing ^{131}I-, ^{123}I-MIBG-, ^{75}Se-cholesterol-, or ^{111}In-penetreotide-SPECT/CT. In one-third of the patients, a change in clinical management was observed [101]. A significant impact of SPECT/CT on therapeutic management was also demonstrated by Hillel *et al.* in 29 patients with carcinoid and other neuroendocrine tumors [103]. Addition of clinically relevant information by SPECT/CT in 40% of patients compared to SPECT was described by Gabriel *et al.* [104].

9.5
Conclusions and Perspectives

PET and, more recently, PET/CT hybrid imaging have changed the diagnostic algorithm in a variety of cancers. Based on characteristic metabolic or molecular alterations, malignant tumors and distant metastases can be sensitively detected in the entire patient, thereby reducing futile curative interventions. The clinical benefit has been demonstrated in a number of indications. PET and PET/CT are also regarded as cost-effective modalities for cancer management. Coregistration of anatomic information such as CT increases specificity as well as sensitivity of PET imaging and is now regarded as standard for clinical care of cancer patients. Due to the unique option to define a biological target volume, PET/CT will play an increasing role for radiation treatment planning. The modality is also useful for estimation of response to chemo- and/or radiotherapy. However, prospective randomized trials are necessary to demonstrate a positive effect of PET- or PET/CT-based changes of the therapeutic management on the outcome of cancer patients. The role of SPECT and integrated SPECT/CT is also growing. The superiority of SPECT/CT over planar scintigrams and SPECT has also been clearly demonstrated.

Nowadays, there is a keen interest in techniques allowing noninvasive imaging of cancer biology, including receptor expression, proliferation, hypoxia, metastatic potential, or angiogenesis. Thus, a variety of approaches are currently studied, which include MRI, optical imaging, ultrasound imaging as well as tracer techniques such as SPECT and PET. However, further data including studies in patients are needed to demonstrate the potential usefulness of this class of tracers in clinical settings. Overall, it is likely that nuclear imaging will eventually be assessed not using a single parameter, target structure, or imaging technique, but rather a combination of parameters that allow for a multimodal/multiparametric imaging evaluation of the intricacies of the angiogenic cascade. Combined MRI/PET scanners might help in this respect, as they could provide functional imaging by dynamic contrast enhanced MRI and molecular imaging with PET in a one-stop-shop examination [105]. With PET MRI inserts for brain imaging already being in use and whole-body hybrid MRI/PET scanners being developed, assessing the different aspects of tumor biology at the structural, functional, and molecular levels before, during, and after targeted cancer therapy within one examination will likely become a reality and help further steps toward personalized medicine.

References

1. O'Connor, M.K. and Kemp, B.J. (2006) Single-photon emission computed tomography/computed tomography: basic instrumentation and innovations. Semin. Nucl. Med., **36**, 258–266.
2. Wester, HJ. (2007) Nuclear imaging probes: from bench to bedside. Clin Cancer Res., **13**(12), 3470–3481. in review.
3. Perault, C., Schvartz, C., Wampach, H., Liehn, J.C., and Delisle, M.J. (1997) Thoracic and abdominal SPECT-CT image fusion without external markers in endocrine carcinomas. J. Nucl. Med., **38**, 1234–1242.
4. Scott, A.M., Macapinlac, H., Zhang, J., Daghighian, F., Montemayor, N., Kalaigian, H. et al. (1995) Image registration of SPECT and CT images using an external fiduciary band and three-dimensional surface fitting in metastatic thyroid cancer. J. Nucl. Med., **36**, 100–103.
5. Park, J.E., Keller, G.A., and Ferrara, N. (1993) The vascular endothelial growth factor (VEGF) isoforms: differential deposition into the subepithelial extracellular matrix and bioactivity of extracellular matrix-bound VEGF. Mol. Biol. Cell., **4**, 1317–1326.
6. Collingridge, D.R., Carroll, V.A., Glaser, M., Aboagye, E.O., Osman, S., Hutchinson, O.C. et al. (2002) The development of [^{124}I]iodinated-VG76e: a novel tracer for imaging vascular endothelial growth factor in vivo using positron emission tomography. Cancer Res., **62**, 5912–5919.

7. Jayson, G.C., Zweit, J., Jackson, A., Mulatero, C., Julyan, P., Ranson, M. et al. (2002) Molecular imaging and biological evaluation of HuMV833 anti-VEGF antibody: implications for trial design of antiangiogenic antibodies. *J. Natl. Cancer Inst.*, **94**, 1484–1493.
8. Niu, G. and Chen, X. (2009) PET imaging of angiogenesis. *PET Clin.*, **4**, 17–38.
9. Lu, E., Wagner, W.R., Schellenberger, U., Abraham, J.A., Klibanov, A.L., Woulfe, S.R. et al. (2003) Targeted *in vivo* labeling of receptors for vascular endothelial growth factor: approach to identification of ischemic tissue. *Circulation*, **108**, 97–103.
10. Blankenberg, F.G., Mandl, S., Cao, Y.A., O'Connell-Rodwell, C., Contag, C., Mari, C. et al. (2004) Tumor imaging using a standardized radiolabeled adapter protein docked to vascular endothelial growth factor. *J. Nucl. Med.*, **45**, 1373–1380.
11. Li, S., Peck-Radosavljevic, M., Kienast, O., Preitfellner, J., Hamilton, G., Kurtaran, A. et al. (2003) Imaging gastrointestinal tumours using vascular endothelial growth factor-165 (VEGF165) receptor scintigraphy. *Ann. Oncol.*, **14**, 1274–1277.
12. Li, S., Peck-Radosavljevic, M., Kienast, O., Preitfellner, J., Havlik, E., Schima, W. et al. (2004) Iodine-123-vascular endothelial growth factor-165 (^{123}I-VEGF165). Biodistribution, safety and radiation dosimetry in patients with pancreatic carcinoma. *Q. J. Nucl. Med. Mol. Imaging*, **48**, 198–206.
13. Li, S., Peck-Radosavljevic, M., Koller, E., Koller, F., Kaserer, K., Kreil, A. et al. (2001) Characterization of ^{123}I-vascular endothelial growth factor-binding sites expressed on human tumour cells: possible implication for tumour scintigraphy. *Int. J. Cancer*, **91**, 789–796.
14. Ferrara, N. (2004) Vascular endothelial growth factor: basic science and clinical progress. *Endocrinol. Rev.*, **25**, 581–611.
15. Cai, W., Chen, K., Mohamedali, K.A., Cao, Q., Gambhir, S.S., Rosenblum, M.G. et al. (2006) PET of vascular endothelial growth factor receptor expression. *J. Nucl. Med.*, **47**, 2048–2056.
16. Wang, H., Cai, W., Chen, K., Li, Z.B., Kashefi, A., He, L. et al. (2007) A new PET tracer specific for vascular endothelial growth factor receptor 2. *Eur. J. Nucl. Med. Mol. Imaging*, **34**, 2001–2010.
17. Eliceiri, B.P. and Cheresh, D.A. (2000) Role of alpha v integrins during angiogenesis. *Cancer J. Sci. Am.*, **6**, S245–S249.
18. Hynes, R.O., Bader, B.L., and Hodivala-Dilke, K. (1999) Integrins in vascular development. *Braz. J. Med. Biol. Res.*, **32**, 501–510.
19. Ruoslahti, E. and Pierschbacher, M.D. (1987) New perspectives in cell adhesion: RGD and integrins. *Science*, **238**, 491–497.
20. Aumailley, M., Gurrath, M., Muller, G., Calvete, J., Timpl, R., and Kessler, H. (1991) Arg–Gly–Asp constrained within cyclic pentapeptides. Strong and selective inhibitors of cell adhesion to vitronectin and laminin fragment P1. *FEBS Lett.*, **291**, 50–54.
21. Haubner, R.H., Wester, H.J., Weber, W.A., and Schwaiger, M. (2003) Radiotracer-based strategies to image angiogenesis. *Q. J. Nucl. Med.*, **47**, 189–199.
22. Haubner, R., Kuhnast, B., Mang, C., Weber, W.A., Kessler, H., Wester, H.J. et al. (2004) [^{18}F]Galacto-RGD: synthesis, radiolabeling, metabolic stability, and radiation dose estimates. *Bioconjug. Chem.*, **15**, 61–69.
23. Poethko, T., Schottelius, M., Thumshirn, G., Herz, M., Haubner, R., Henriksen, G. et al. (2004) Chemoselective pre-conjugate radiohalogenation of unprotected mono- and multimeric peptides via oxime formation. *Radiochim. Acta*, **92**, 317–327.
24. Poethko, T., Schottelius, M., Thumshirn, G., Hersel, U., Herz, M., Henriksen, G. et al. (2004) Two-step methodology for high-yield routine radiohalogenation of peptides: ^{18}F-labeled RGD and octreotide analogs. *J. Nucl. Med.*, **45**, 892–902.
25. Shields, A.F., Grierson, J.R., Dohmen, B.M., Machulla, H.J., Stayanoff, J.C.,

Lawhorn-Crews, J.M. et al. (1998) Imaging proliferation in vivo with [F-18]FLT and positron emission tomography. Nat. Med., 4, 1334–1336.

26. Lee, Y.S., Jeong, J.M., Kim, H.W., Chang, Y.S., Kim, Y.J., Hong, M.K. et al. (2006) An improved method of ^{18}F peptide labeling: hydrazone formation with HYNIC-conjugated c(RGDyK). Nucl. Med. Biol., 33, 677–683.

27. Prante, O., Einsiedel, J., Haubner, R., Gmeiner, P., Wester, H.J., Kuwert, T. et al. (2007) 3,4,6-Tri-O-acetyl-2-deoxy-2-[^{18}F]fluoro-glucopyranosyl phenylthiosulfonate: a thiol-reactive agent for the chemoselective ^{18}F-glycosylation of peptides. Bioconjug. Chem., 18, 254–262.

28. Cai, W., Zhang, X., Wu, Y., and Chen, X. (2006) A thiol-reactive ^{18}F-labeling agent, N-[2-(4-^{18}F-fluorobenzamido)ethyl] maleimide, and synthesis of RGD peptide-based tracer for PET imaging of alpha v beta 3 integrin expression. J. Nucl. Med., 47, 1172–1180.

29. Glaser, M., Solbakken, M., Turton, D.R., Pettitt, R., Barnett, J., Arukwe, J. et al. (2009) Methods for ^{18}F-labeling of RGD peptides: comparison of aminooxy [^{18}F]fluorobenzaldehyde condensation with "click labeling" using 2-[^{18}F]fluoroethylazide, and S-alkylation with [^{18}F]fluoropropanethiol. Amino Acids, 37, 717–724.

30. Kolb, H., Walsh, J., Liang, Q., Zhao, T., Gao, D., Secrest, J. et al. (2009) ^{18}F-RGD-K5: a cyclic triazole-bearing RGD peptide for imaging integrin $\alpha_v\beta_3$ expression in vivo. J. Nucl. Med., 50 (Suppl. 2), 329.

31. Morrison, M.S., Ricketts, S.A., Barnett, J., Cuthbertson, A., Tessier, J., and Wedge, S.R. (2009) Use of a novel Arg–Gly–Asp radioligand, ^{18}F-AH111585, to determine changes in tumor vascularity after antitumor therapy. J. Nucl. Med., 50, 116–122.

32. Haubner, R., Weber, W.A., Beer, A.J., Vabuliene, E., Reim, D., Sarbia, M. et al. (2005) Noninvasive visualization of the activated alphavbeta3 integrin in cancer patients by positron emission tomography and [^{18}F]galacto-RGD. PLoS Med., 2, e70.

33. Beer, A.J., Haubner, R., Wolf, I., Goebel, M., Luderschmidt, S., Niemeyer, M. et al. (2006) PET-based human dosimetry of ^{18}F-galacto-RGD, a new radiotracer for imaging alpha v beta3 expression. J. Nucl. Med., 47, 763–769.

34. Beer, A.J., Grosu, A.L., Carlsen, J., Kolk, A., Sarbia, M., Stangier, I. et al. (2007) [^{18}F]galacto-RGD positron emission tomography for imaging of $\alpha_v\beta_3$ expression on the neovasculature in patients with squamous cell carcinoma of the head and neck. Clin. Cancer Res., 13, 6610–6616.

35. Schnell, O., Krebs, B., Carlsen, J., Miederer, I., Goetz, C., Goldbrunner, R.H. et al. (2009) Imaging of integrin $\alpha_v\beta_3$ expression in patients with malignant glioma by [^{18}F]galacto-RGD positron emission tomography. Neuro Oncol., 11, 861–870.

36. Bach-Gansmo, T., Bogsrud, T.V., and Skretting, A. (2008) Integrin scintimammography using a dedicated breast imaging, solid-state gamma-camera and ^{99m}Tc-labelled NC100692. Clin. Physiol. Funct. Imaging, 28, 235–239.

37. McParland, B.J., Miller, M.P., Spinks, T.J., Kenny, L.M., Osman, S., Khela, M.K. et al. (2008) The biodistribution and radiation dosimetry of the Arg–Gly–Asp peptide ^{18}F-AH111585 in healthy volunteers. J. Nucl. Med., 49, 1664–1667.

38. Kenny, L.M., Coombes, R.C., Oulie, I., Contractor, K.B., Miller, M., Spinks, T.J. et al. (2008) Phase I trial of the positron-emitting Arg–Gly–Asp (RGD) peptide radioligand ^{18}F-AH111585 in breast cancer patients. J. Nucl. Med., 49, 879–886.

39. Hanahan, D. and Weinberg, R.A. (2000) The hallmarks of cancer. Cell, 100, 57–70.

40. Kubota, R., Kubota, K., Yamada, S., Tada, M., Ido, T., and Tamahashi, N. (1994) Microautoradiographic study for the differentiation of intratumoral macrophages, granulation tissues and cancer cells by the dynamics of

fluorine-18-fluorodeoxyglucose uptake. *J. Nucl. Med.*, **35**, 104–112.

41. Shreve, P.D., Anzai, Y., and Wahl, R.L. (1999) Pitfalls in oncologic diagnosis with FDG PET imaging: physiologic and benign variants. *Radiographics*, **19**, 61–77; quiz 150–151.

42. Rasey, J.S., Grierson, J.R., Wiens, L.W., Kolb, P.D., and Schwartz, J.L. (2002) Validation of FLT uptake as a measure of thymidine kinase-1 activity in A549 carcinoma cells. *J. Nucl. Med.*, **43**, 1210–1217.

43. Buck, A.K., Herrmann, K., Shen, C., Dechow, T., Schwaiger, M., and Wester, H.J. (2009) Molecular imaging of proliferation *in vivo*: positron emission tomography with [^{18}F]fluorothymidine. *Methods*, **48**, 205–215.

44. Machulla, H.J., Blocher, A., Kuntzsch, M., Piert, M., Wei, R., and Grierson, J. (2000) Simplified labeling approach for synthesizing 3′-deoxy-3′-[^{18}F]fluorothymidine ([^{18}F]FLT). *J. Radioanal. Nucl. Chem.*, **243**, 4.

45. Weber W.A. (2010) Monitoring tumor response to therapy with ^{18}F-FLT PET. *J. Nucl. Med.* **51**, 841–844.

46. de Langen, A.J., Klabbers, B., Lubberink, M., Boellaard, R., Spreeuwenberg, M.D., Slotman, B.J. et al. (2009) Reproducibility of quantitative ^{18}F-3′-deoxy-3′-fluorothymidine measurements using positron emission tomography. *Eur. J. Nucl. Med. Mol. Imaging*, **36**, 389–395.

47. Shields, A.F., Lawhorn-Crews, J.M., Briston, D.A., Zalzala, S., Gadgeel, S., Douglas, K.A. et al. (2008) Analysis and reproducibility of 3′-deoxy-3′-[^{18}F]fluorothymidine positron emission tomography imaging in patients with non-small cell lung cancer. *Clin. Cancer Res.*, **14**, 4463–4468.

48. Chen, W., Delaloye, S., Silverman, D.H., Geist, C., Czernin, J., Sayre, J. et al. (2007) Predicting treatment response of malignant gliomas to bevacizumab and irinotecan by imaging proliferation with [^{18}F]fluorothymidine positron emission tomography: a pilot study. *J. Clin. Oncol.*, **25**, 4714–4721.

49. Kenny, L., Coombes, R.C., Vigushin, D.M., Al-Nahhas, A., Shousha, S., and Aboagye, E.O. (2007) Imaging early changes in proliferation at 1 week post chemotherapy: a pilot study in breast cancer patients with 3′-deoxy-3′-[^{18}F]fluorothymidine positron emission tomography. *Eur. J. Nucl. Med. Mol. Imaging*, **34**, 1339–1347.

50. Pio, B.S., Park, C.K., Pietras, R., Hsueh, W.A., Satyamurthy, N., Pegram, M.D. et al. (2006) Usefulness of 3′-[F-18]fluoro-3′-deoxythymidine with positron emission tomography in predicting breast cancer response to therapy. *Mol. Imaging Biol.*, **8**, 36–42.

51. Sohn, H.J., Yang, Y.J., Ryu, J.S., Oh, S.J., Im, K.C., Moon, D.H. et al. (2008) [^{18}F]Fluorothymidine positron emission tomography before and 7 days after gefitinib treatment predicts response in patients with advanced adenocarcinoma of the lung. *Clin. Cancer Res.*, **14**, 7423–7429.

52. Herrmann, K., Wieder, H.A., Buck, A.K., Schoffel, M., Krause, B.J., Fend, F. et al. (2007) Early response assessment using 3′-deoxy-3′-[^{18}F]fluorothymidine-positron emission tomography in high-grade non-Hodgkin's lymphoma. *Clin. Cancer Res.*, **13**, 3552–3558.

53. Pfannenberg, C., Aschoff, P., Dittmann, H., Mayer, F., Reischl, G., von Weyhern, C. et al. (2010) PET/CT with ^{18}F-FLT: does it improve the therapeutic management of metastatic germ cell tumors? *J. Nucl. Med.*, **51**, 845–853.

54. Everitt, S., Hicks, R.J., Ball, D., Kron, T., Schneider-Kolsky, M., Walter, T. et al. (2009) Imaging cellular proliferation during chemo-radiotherapy: a pilot study of serial ^{18}F-FLT positron emission tomography/computed tomography imaging for non-small-cell lung cancer. *Int. J. Radiat. Oncol. Biol. Phys.*, **75**, 1098–1104.

55. Martin, G.V., Cerqueira, M.D., Caldwell, J.H., Rasey, J.S., Embree,

L., and Krohn, K.A. (1990) Fluoromisonidazole. A metabolic marker of myocyte hypoxia. *Circ. Res.*, **67**, 240–244.

56. Chang, J., Wen, B., Kazanzides, P., Zanzonico, P., Finn, R.D., Fichtinger, G. et al. (2009) A robotic system for ^{18}F-FMISO PET-guided intratumoral pO2 measurements. *Med. Phys.*, **36**, 5301–5309.
57. Gaertner, F.C., Souvatzoglou, M., Brix, G., and Beer, A.J. (2010) Imaging of hypoxia using PET and MRI. *Curr. Pharma. Biotechnol.*, (accepted for publication).
58. Gronroos, T., Bentzen, L., Marjamaki, P., Murata, R., Horsman, M.R., Keiding, S. et al. (2004) Comparison of the biodistribution of two hypoxia markers [^{18}F]FETNIM and [^{18}F]FMISO in an experimental mammary carcinoma. *Eur. J. Nucl. Med. Mol. Imaging*, **31**, 513–520.
59. Piert, M., Machulla, H.J., Picchio, M., Reischl, G., Ziegler, S., Kumar, P. et al. (2005) Hypoxia-specific tumor imaging with ^{18}F-fluoroazomycin arabinoside. *J. Nucl. Med.*, **46**, 106–113.
60. Matsumoto, K., Szajek, L., Krishna, M.C., Cook, J.A., Seidel, J., Grimes, K. et al. (2007) The influence of tumor oxygenation on hypoxia imaging in murine squamous cell carcinoma using [^{64}Cu]Cu-ATSM or [^{18}F]fluoromisonidazole positron emission tomography. *Int. J. Oncol.*, **30**, 873–881.
61. Yuan, H., Schroeder, T., Bowsher, J.E., Hedlund, L.W., Wong, T., and Dewhirst, M.W. (2006) Intertumoral differences in hypoxia selectivity of the PET imaging agent ^{64}Cu(II)-diacetyl-bis (N^4-methylthiosemicarbazone). *J. Nucl. Med.*, **47**, 989–998.
62. Burgman, P., O'Donoghue, J.A., Lewis, J.S., Welch, M.J., Humm, J.L., and Ling, C.C. (2005) Cell line-dependent differences in uptake and retention of the hypoxia-selective nuclear imaging agent Cu-ATSM. *Nucl. Med. Biol.*, **32**, 623–630.
63. Krause, B.J., Beck, R., Souvatzoglou, M., and Piert, M. (2006) PET and PET/CT studies of tumor tissue oxygenation. *Q. J. Nucl. Med. Mol. Imaging*, **50**, 28–43.
64. Mankoff, D.A., Link, J.M., Linden, H.M., Sundararajan, L., and Krohn, K.A. (2008) Tumor receptor imaging. *J. Nucl. Med.*, **49** (Suppl. 2), 149S–163S.
65. Scheidhauer, K., Miederer, M., and Gaertner, F.C. (2009) PET-CT for neuroendocrine tumors and nuclear medicine therapy options. *Radiologe*, **49**, 217–223.
66. Harris, A.G. (1994) Somatostatin and somatostatin analogues: pharmacokinetics and pharmacodynamic effects. *Gut*, **35** (Suppl. 3), S1–S4.
67. Cimitan, M., Buonadonna, A., Cannizzaro, R., Canzonieri, V., Borsatti, E., Ruffo, R. et al. (2003) Somatostatin receptor scintigraphy versus chromogranin A assay in the management of patients with neuroendocrine tumors of different types: clinical role. *Ann. Oncol.*, **14**, 1135–1141.
68. Gabriel, M., Muehllechner, P., Decristoforo, C., von Guggenberg, E., Kendler, D., Prommegger, R. et al. (2005) ^{99m}Tc-EDDA/HYNIC-Tyr^3-octreotide for staging and follow-up of patients with neuroendocrine gastro-entero-pancreatic tumors. *Q. J. Nucl. Med. Mol. Imaging*, **49**, 237–244.
69. Antunes, P., Ginj, M., Zhang, H., Waser, B., Baum, R.P., Reubi, J.C. et al. (2007) Are radiogallium-labelled DOTA-conjugated somatostatin analogues superior to those labelled with other radiometals? *Eur. J. Nucl. Med. Mol. Imaging*, **34**, 982–993.
70. Miederer, M., Seidl, S., Buck, A., Scheidhauer, K., Wester, H.J., Schwaiger, M. et al. (2009) Correlation of immunohistopathological expression of somatostatin receptor 2 with standardised uptake values in ^{68}Ga-DOTATOC PET/CT. *Eur. J. Nucl. Med. Mol. Imaging*, **36**, 48–52.
71. Pool, S.E., Krenning, E.P., Koning, G.A., van Eijck, C.H., Teunissen, J.J., Kam, B. et al. (2010) Preclinical and clinical studies of peptide receptor radionuclide therapy. *Semin. Nucl. Med.*, **40**, 209–218.

72. Hellwig, D., Baum, R.P., and Kirsch, C. (2009) FDG-PET, PET/CT and conventional nuclear medicine procedures in the evaluation of lung cancer: a systematic review. *Nuklearmedizin*, **48**, 59–69; quiz N58–59.
73. Menda, Y. and Graham, M.M. (2005) Update on ^{18}F-fluorodeoxyglucose/positron emission tomography and positron emission tomography/computed tomography imaging of squamous head and neck cancers. *Semin. Nucl. Med.*, **35**, 214–219.
74. Czernin, J., Benz, M.R., Allen-Auerbach, M.S. (2010) PET/CT imaging: the incremental value of assessing the glucose metabolic phenotype and the structure of cancers in a single examination. *Eur. J. Radiol.*, **73**, 470–480.
75. Herrmann, K., Krause, B.J., Bundschuh, R.A., Dechow, T., and Schwaiger, M. (2009) Monitoring response to therapeutic interventions in patients with cancer. *Semin. Nucl. Med.*, **39**, 210–232.
76. Thorwarth, D., Geets, X., and Paiusco, M. (2010) Physical radiotherapy treatment planning based on functional PET/CT data. *Radiother. Oncol.*, **96**, 317–324.
77. Weber, W.A., Czernin, J., Phelps, M.E., and Herschman, H.R. (2008) Technology insight: novel imaging of molecular targets is an emerging area crucial to the development of targeted drugs. *Nat. Clin. Pract. Oncol.*, **5**, 44–54.
78. Even-Sapir, E., Lerman, H., Lievshitz, G., Khafif, A., Fliss, D.M., Schwartz, A. *et al.* (2003) Lymphoscintigraphy for sentinel node mapping using a hybrid SPECT/CT system. *J. Nucl. Med.*, **44**, 1413–1420.
79. Khafif, A., Schneebaum, S., Fliss, D.M., Lerman, H., Metser, U., Ben-Yosef, R. *et al.* (2006) Lymphoscintigraphy for sentinel node mapping using a hybrid single photon emission CT (SPECT)/CT system in oral cavity squamous cell carcinoma. *Head Neck*, **28**, 874–879.
80. Keski-Santti, H., Matzke, S., Kauppinen, T., Tornwall, J., and Atula, T. (2006) Sentinel lymph node mapping using SPECT-CT fusion imaging in patients with oral cavity squamous cell carcinoma. *Eur. Arch. Otorhinolaryngol.*, **263**, 1008–1012.
81. Wagner, A., Schicho, K., Glaser, C., Zettinig, G., Yerit, K., Lang, S. *et al.* (2004) SPECT-CT for topographic mapping of sentinel lymph nodes prior to gamma probe-guided biopsy in head and neck squamous cell carcinoma. *J. Craniomaxillofac. Surg.*, **32**, 343–349.
82. Husarik, D.B. and Steinert, H.C. (2007) Single-photon emission computed tomography/computed tomography for sentinel node mapping in breast cancer. *Semi. Nucl. Med.*, **37**, 29–33.
83. Lerman, H., Metser, U., Lievshitz, G., Sperber, F., Shneebaum, S., and Even-Sapir, E. (2006) Lymphoscintigraphic sentinel node identification in patients with breast cancer: the role of SPECT-CT. *Eur. J. Nucl. Med. Mol. Imaging*, **33**, 329–337.
84. Van der Ploeg, IM. *et al.* (2007) The additional value of SPECT/CT in lymphatic mapping in breast cancer and melanoma. *J Nucl Med*, **48**(11), 1756–1760.
85. Gallowitsch, H.J., Kraschl, P., Igerc, I., Hussein, T., Kresnik, E., Mikosch, P. *et al.* (2007) Sentinel node SPECT-CT in breast cancer. Can we expect any additional and clinically relevant information? *Nuklearmedizin*, **46**, 252–256.
86. Lerman, H., Lievshitz, G., Zak, O., Metser, U., Schneebaum, S., and Even-Sapir, E. (2007) Improved sentinel node identification by SPECT/CT in overweight patients with breast cancer. *J. Nucl. Med.*, **48**, 201–206.
87. Hamaoka, T., Madewell, J.E., Podoloff, D.A., Hortobagyi, G.N., and Ueno, N.T. (2004) Bone imaging in metastatic breast cancer. *J. Clin. Oncol.*, **22**, 2942–2953.
88. Minoves, M. (2003) Bone and joint sports injuries: the role of bone scintigraphy. *Nucl. Med. Commun.*, **24**, 3–10.
89. Even-Sapir, E. (2005) Imaging of malignant bone involvement by morphologic, scintigraphic, and hybrid modalities. *J. Nucl. Med.*, **46**, 1356–1367.

90. Romer, W., Nomayr, A., Uder, M., Bautz, W., and Kuwert, T. (2006) SPECT-guided CT for evaluating foci of increased bone metabolism classified as indeterminate on SPECT in cancer patients. *J. Nucl. Med.*, **47**, 1102–1106.
91. Seo, Y., Wong, K.H., Sun, M., Franc, B.L., Hawkins, R.A., and Hasegawa, B.H. (2005) Correction of photon attenuation and collimator response for a body-contouring SPECT/CT imaging system. *J. Nucl. Med.*, **46**, 868–877.
92. Romer, W., Reichel, N., Vija, H.A., Nickel, I., Hornegger, J., Bautz, W. et al. (2006) Isotropic reconstruction of SPECT data using OSEM3D: correlation with CT. *Acad. Radiol.*, **13**, 496–502.
93. Horger, M., Eschmann, S.M., Pfannenberg, C., Vonthein, R., Besenfelder, H., Claussen, C.D. et al. (2004) Evaluation of combined transmission and emission tomography for classification of skeletal lesions. *Am. J. Roentgenol.*, **183**, 655–661.
94. Utsunomiya, D., Shiraishi, S., Imuta, M., Tomiguchi, S., Kawanaka, K., Morishita, S. et al. (2006) Added value of SPECT/CT fusion in assessing suspected bone metastasis: comparison with scintigraphy alone and nonfused scintigraphy and CT. *Radiology*, **238**, 264–271.
95. Tharp, K., Israel, O., Hausmann, J., Bettman, L., Martin, W.H., Daitzchman, M. et al. (2004) Impact of ^{131}I-SPECT/CT images obtained with an integrated system in the follow-up of patients with thyroid carcinoma. *Eur. J. Nucl. Med. Mol. Imaging*, **31**, 1435–1442.
96. Yamamoto, Y., Nishiyama, Y., Monden, T., Matsumura, Y., Satoh, K., and Ohkawa, M. (2003) Clinical usefulness of fusion of ^{131}I SPECT and CT images in patients with differentiated thyroid carcinoma. *J. Nucl. Med.*, **44**, 1905–1910.
97. Ruf, J., Lehmkuhl, L., Bertram, H., Sandrock, D., Amthauer, H., Humplik, B. et al. (2004) Impact of SPECT and integrated low-dose CT after radioiodine therapy on the management of patients with thyroid carcinoma. *Nucl. Med. Commun.*, **25**, 1177–1182.
98. Avram, A.M., Fig, L.M., and Gross, M.D. (2006) Adrenal gland scintigraphy. *Semin. Nucl. Med.*, **36**, 212–227.
99. Gross, M.D., Avram, A., Fig, L.M., and Rubello, D. (2007) Contemporary adrenal scintigraphy. *Eur. J. Nucl. Med. Mol. Imaging*, **34**, 547–557.
100. Franzius, C., Hermann, K., Weckesser, M., Kopka, K., Juergens, K.U., Vormoor, J. et al. (2006) Whole-body PET/CT with ^{11}C-*meta*-hydroxyephedrine in tumors of the sympathetic nervous system: feasibility study and comparison with ^{123}I-MIBG SPECT/CT. *J. Nucl. Med.*, **47**, 1635–1642.
101. Even-Sapir, E., Keidar, Z., Sachs, J., Engel, A., Bettman, L., Gaitini, D. et al. (2001) The new technology of combined transmission and emission tomography in evaluation of endocrine neoplasms. *J. Nucl. Med.*, **42**, 998–1004.
102. Krausz, Y., Keidar, Z., Kogan, I., Even-Sapir, E., Bar-Shalom, R., Engel, A. et al. (2003) SPECT/CT hybrid imaging with ^{111}In-pentetreotide in assessment of neuroendocrine tumours. *Clin. Endocrinol.*, **59**, 565–573.
103. Hillel, P.G., van Beek, E.J., Taylor, C., Lorenz, E., Bax, N.D., Prakash, V. et al. (2006) The clinical impact of a combined gamma camera/CT imaging system on somatostatin receptor imaging of neuroendocrine tumours. *Clin. Radiol.*, **61**, 579–587.
104. Gabriel, M., Hausler, F., Bale, R., Moncayo, R., Decristoforo, C., Kovacs, P. et al. (2005) Image fusion analysis of ^{99m}Tc-HYNIC-Tyr^3-octreotide SPECT and diagnostic CT using an immobilisation device with external markers in patients with endocrine tumours. *Eur. J. Nucl. Med. Mol. Imaging*, **32**, 1440–1451.
105. Judenhofer, M.S., Wehrl, H.F., Newport, D.F., Catana, C., Siegel, S.B., Becker, M. et al. (2008) Simultaneous PET-MRI: a new approach for functional and morphological imaging. *Nat. Med.*, **14**, 459–465.